[illegible], MD.
Houston
May 26, 1986

1986

YEAR BOOK OF

VASCULAR SURGERY

The Year Book Series

Anesthesia: Drs. Miller, Kirby, Ostheimer, Saidman, and Stoelting

Cancer: Drs. Hickey, Clark, and Cumley

Cardiology: Drs. Harvey, Kirkendall, Laks, Resnekov, Rosenthal, and Sonnenblick

Critical Care Medicine: Drs. Rogers, Allo, Dean, Gioia, McPherson, Michael, Miller, and Traystman

Dentistry: Drs. Cohen, Hendler, Johnson, Jordan, Moyers, Robinson, and Silverman

Dermatology: Drs. Sober and Fitzpatrick

Diagnostic Radiology: Drs. Bragg, Keats, Kieffer, Kirkpatrick, Koehler, Miller, and Sorenson

Digestive Diseases: Drs. Greenberger and Moody

Drug Therapy: Drs. Hollister and Lasagna

Emergency Medicine: Dr. Wagner

Endocrinology: Drs. Schwartz and Ryan

Family Practice: Dr. Rakel

Hand Surgery: Drs. Dobyns and Chase

Hematology: Drs. Spivak, Bell, Ness, Quesenberry, and Wiernik

Infectious Diseases: Drs. Wolff, Gorbach, Keusch, Klempner, and Snydman

Medicine: Drs. Rogers, Des Prez, Cline, Braunwald, Greenberger, Wilson, Epstein, and Malawista

Neurology and Neurosurgery: Drs. DeJong, Currier, and Crowell

Nuclear Medicine: Drs. Hoffer, Gore, Gottschalk, Sostman, and Zaret

Obstetrics and Gynecology: Drs. Pitkin and Zlatnik

Ophthalmology: Dr. Ernest

Orthopedics: Dr. Coventry

Otolaryngology–Head and Neck Surgery: Drs. Paparella and Bailey

Pathology and Clinical Pathology: Dr. Brinkhous

Pediatrics: Drs. Oski and Stockman

Plastic and Reconstructive Surgery: Drs. McCoy, Brauer, Haynes, Hoehn, Miller, and Whitaker

Podiatric Medicine and Surgery: Dr. Jay

Psychiatry and Applied Mental Health: Drs. Freedman, Lourie, Meltzer, Nemiah, Talbott, and Weiner

Pulmonary Disease: Drs. Green, Ball, Menkes, Michael, Peters, Terry, Tockman, and Wise

Rehabilitation: Drs. Kaplan and Szumski

Sports Medicine: Drs. Krakauer, Shephard, and Torg, Col. Anderson, and Mr. George

Surgery: Drs. Schwartz, Jonasson, Peacock, Shires, Spencer, and Thompson

Urology: Drs. Gillenwater and Howards

Vascular Surgery: Drs. Bergan and Yao

1986 The Year Book of VASCULAR SURGERY

Editors

John J. Bergan, M.D.

Magerstadt Professor of Surgery and Chief, Division of Vascular Surgery, Department of Surgery, Northwestern University Medical School

James S.T. Yao, M.D., Ph.D.

Professor of Surgery, Department of Surgery, Northwestern University Medical School

Year Book Medical Publishers, Inc.
Chicago • London

Printed in U.S.A.

International Standard Serial Number: 0749–4041

International Standard Book Number: 0–8151–0675–0

The editor for this book was Debra Q. Severson and the production manager was H. E. Nielsen. The Managing Editor for the Year Book series is Nancy Gorham.

Table of Contents

The material covered in this volume represents literature reviewed up to July 1985.

Journals Represented

Acta Chirurgica Scandinavica
Acta Dermato-Venereologica
Acta Medica Scandinavica
Acta Pathologica et Microbiologica Scandinavica
Acta Radiologica (Diagnosis) (Oncology)
American Heart Journal
American Journal of Cardiology
American Journal of Gastroenterology
American Journal of Hematology
American Journal of the Medical Sciences
American Journal of Medicine
American Journal of Physiology
American Journal of Roentgenology
American Journal of Sports Medicine
American Journal of Surgery
American Surgeon
Annals of Emergency Medicine
Annals of Internal Medicine
Annals of Neurology
Annals of the Royal College of Surgeons of England
Annals of Surgery
Annals of Thoracic Surgery
Archives of Internal Medicine
Archives of Neurology
Archives of Pathology and Laboratory Medicine
Archives of Surgery
ASAIO Journal (American Society for Artificial Internal Organs)
Atherosclerosis
Arteriosclerosis
British Heart Journal
British Journal of Ophthalmology
British Journal of Surgery
Cancer
Cardiovascular Research
Chirurg
Circulation
Circulation Research
Clinical Orthopaedics & Related Research
Clinical Radiology
Cardiology
Contemporary Surgery
Cutis
Danish Medical Bulletin
European Journal of Clinical Investigation
European Neurology
Experimental and Molecular Pathology
Fortschritte auf dem Gebiete der Rontgenstrahlen und der Nuklearmedizin
International Surgery
Investigative Radiology
Israel Journal of Medical Sciences
Journal of the American College of Cardiology

Journal of the American Medical Association
Journal of Bone and Joint Surgery (American vol.)
Journal of Bone and Joint Surgery (British vol.)
Journal of the Canadian Association of Radiologists
Journal of Cardiovascular Surgery
Journal de Chirurgie
Journal of Clinical Investigation
Journal of Clinical Pathology
Journal of Clinical Ultrasound
Journal of Computer Assisted Tomography
Journal of Hand Surgery
Journal of Hypertension
Journal of Laboratory and Clinical Medicine
Journal of Neurosurgery
Journal of Pediatric Surgery
Journal of the Royal College of Surgeons of Edinburgh
Journal of Thoracic and Cardiovascular Surgery
Journal of Trauma
Journal of Urology
Journal of Sports Medicine
Klinische Wochenschrift
Laboratory Investigation
Lancet
Mayo Clinic Proceedings
Medicine
Metabolism
Neurology
Neurosurgery
New England Journal of Medicine
Pediatric Radiology
Plastic and Reconstructive Surgery
Presse Medicale
Proceedings of the National Academy of Sciences
Radiology
RoFo: Fortschritte auf dem Gebiete der Rontgenstrahlen und der Nuklearmedizin
Scandinavian Journal of Hematology
Scandinavian Journal of Thoracic and Cardiovascular Surgery
Schweizerische Medizinische Wochenschrift
Science
Southern Medical Journal
Stroke
Surgery
Surgery, Gynecology and Obstetrics
Thrombosis Research
Thorax
Thrombosis and Haemostasis
Virchosw Archiv A: Pathological Anatomy and Histology
Zentralblatt fur Neurochirurgie

Publisher's Preface

The 1986 YEAR BOOK OF VASCULAR SURGERY, a new title in the Year Book series, is devoted to a surgical subspecialty of increasing importance. During the last decade, the growth of new knowledge and techniques on peripheral vascular surgery has been impressive. Reflecting this growth, new fellowship programs have been and are being established at institutions around the country. In addition, the American Board of Surgery recently began issuing a certificate of special qualification in general vascular surgery, and the vascular societies are drawing increasing membership.

Vascular literature now makes up more than 30% of the general surgical literature and is spread throughout radiology, neurology, cardiology, and general medicine journals. The subject, discussed in the YEAR BOOK OF SURGERY since the first edition was published in 1901, merits treatment in a separate Year Book volume. The goal of the new YEAR BOOK OF VASCULAR SURGERY is to provide vascular surgeons, general surgeons, neurologists, cardiologists, and general internists with a thorough survey of the world's literature, commented upon by experts in the field.

We are pleased to welcome John Bergan and James Yao as Editors of the YEAR BOOK OF VASCULAR SURGERY. We hope the Year Book will be a valuable resource and a useful addition to your library.

Introduction

The first 40 years of life furnish the text, while the remaining 30 supply the commentary.—ARTHUR SCHOPENHAUER

The philosophy expressed above by the acerbic Schopenhauer is as applicable to the development of vascular surgery as it is to human existence. Therefore, as vascular surgery in the modern era approaches age 40, it is time that a YEAR BOOK be created for our subspecialty so that text and commentary are collected together for a series of yearly updated reviews.

A view of the circular nature of life aided Harvey as he investigated directions of the circulation. Such life circles continue to add a certain symmetry and pleasure to our existence. In the YEAR BOOK, we see a circle initiated by De Bakey, whose well-chosen articles and succinct, pointed commentary aided more than one generation of surgeons through their early practice and successful completion of the Board examination. That circle was completed by the development of this YEAR BOOK by its vascular surgery editors. A need for this volume and its promise of a continuation are evident simply from the sheer volume of the excellent literature within our chosen field. This enormous weight of publication could not be accommodated in the YEAR BOOK OF SURGERY no matter how prescient Seymour Schwartz and his editorial board became.

Our objective in planning this volume has been to select articles that will expand the knowledge of surgeons working in this difficult field. Many of our selections ordinarily would not be seen by working surgeons because the sources, based in physiology, radiology, circulation research, and even dermatology, are out of the mainstream of surgical experience. Many of the articles selected originated in other countries and were published there. They reflect varying levels of surgical sophistication and, in many instances, demonstrate a penetrating intelligence that gives us a sense of pride in our specialty.

Assembling this YEAR BOOK has given us the opportunity to scan more than 1,200 articles, to identify important but obscure facts reported in single cases, to detect trends and changes in practice, and, in at least one instance, to call attention to a truly classic paper. We have seen atrophie blanche linked to aortic origin atheroembolization, osteochondroma to genesis of popliteal aneurysm, and cystic adventitial disease to the knee joint.

This has been a grand experience, and we hope that vascular surgeons will enjoy browsing in this volume as much as we have enjoyed selecting and commenting on its contents.

We look forward with pleasure to next year.

John J. Bergan, M.D.
James S.T. Yao, M.D., Ph.D.

BASIC CONSIDERATIONS

1 Pathology of the Arterial Wall

Recent Advances in Molecular Pathology: The Effects of Hypertension on the Arterial Wall

Aram V. Chobanian, Margaret Forney Prescott, and Christian C. Haudenschild (Boston Univ.)

Exp. Mol. Pathol. 41:153–169, August 1984 1–1

Hypertension is a major risk factor for clinically important atherosclerotic disease, but the link between these states remains poorly understood. Recent studies indicate that major arterial intimal and medial abnormalities result from hypertension. They include functional changes in endothelial permeability and changes in the endothelial cells themselves, but endothelial cell loss leading to denudation of the intimal surface appears to be relatively infrequent. The frequency of attachment of blood cells to the aortic endothelium is markedly increased by deoxycorticosterone-salt treatment. Focal intimal thickening is a consistent concomitant of prolonged blood pressure elevation; it results from accumulation of both cellular and extracellular constituents. Whether the greater medial muscle mass in hypertension is a result of hypertrophic or hyperplastic changes is uncertain. Recently, interest has centered on the role of the endothelium in mediating the effects of vasodilators on arterial tissue. Studies with lathyritic agents suggest that increased vascular collagen contributes to elevated peripheral resistance in hypertension.

Correction of hypertension reverses some but not all of the intimal cellular abnormalities. Enhancement of atherogenesis by hypertension generally requires a critical concentration of circulating lipoproteins. Hypertension itself does not seem directly to influence arterial lipid metabolism. The most impressive cerebrovascular changes associated with hypertension typically occur in the smaller intracerebral vessels penetrating the brain parenchyma. More knowledge is needed about the effects of antihypertensive therapy on atherosclerosis and its clinical sequelae. Many of the arterial changes induced by hypertension are mimicked by those resulting from aging. Studies in rats have suggested that some of the arterial abnormalities attributed to aging may be prevented by lowering the blood pressure. Aging changes in arteries may be due in part to prolonged hemodynamic stresses on the vessel walls.

Accelerated Progression of Atherosclerosis in Coronary Vessels With Minimal Lesions That Are Bypassed

W. Linda Cashin, Miguel E. Sanmarco, Sharon A. Nessim, and David H. Blankenhorn (Univ. of Southern California)

N. Engl. J. Med. 311:824–828, Sept. 27, 1984 1–2

Accelerated progression of atherosclerosis after coronary bypass surgery is well documented in vessels in which the preoperative stenosis was greater than 50%. To assess the effect of coronary bypass on vessels with lesser degrees of stenosis, the authors studied 85 men, aged 40–59 years, who had undergone coronary bypass surgery. All subjects had repeat coronary angiography on entry into the trial. All patients were nonsmokers or ex-smokers with no diabetes, severe hypertension, or chronic arthritis. Seventy-nine percent had no cardiac symptoms. Average plasma cholesterol level was 246 mg/dl. A pairwise comparison of study-entry angiograms with preoperative angiograms using criteria of Bruschke et al. was made to determine the presence or absence of progression of atherosclerosis: vessels showing 0% to 24% and 25% to 50% stenosis on preoperative angiograms were said to have disease progression if they showed more than 50% and 75% stenosis on the study-entry angiogram, respectively.

Three (3%) of 93 coronary vessels with less than 50% stenosis that were not bypassed showed disease progression. Mean change of stenosis was 3.8% ± 1.3%. Fourteen (38%) of 37 vessels with less than 50% stenosis that had been bypassed showed disease progression. Mean change of stenosis was 27.9% ± 5.6%. Hence, comparison of disease progression on a per-vessel basis during an average follow-up period of 37 months showed that bypassed arteries progressed 10 times more frequently than those that were not bypassed. Significance testing on a per-patient basis revealed that disease progressed in only 1 (2%) of the 59 patients in whom no coronary artery was bypassed and whose arteries had less than 50% preoperative stenosis, compared to 12 (46%) of 26 patients in whom one or more bypass grafts were done to an artery with less than 50% stenosis ($P < .005$).

Even though coronary risk factors were not exceptionally high, an accelerated rate of atherosclerosis was seen in patients whose bypassed lesions had less than 50% stenosis. The pattern of acceleration in atherosclerosis observed is complex, involves multiple lesions, and is generally deleterious in the long run. Evidence have shown that venous bypass grafts tend to deteriorate after 7 to 12 years. The data show that the percentage of nonbypassed arteries with minimal atherosclerosis that had progression of disease after 36 months was less than the percentage of totally occluded venous grafts to vessels with equivalent atherosclerosis; this indicates that a nonbypassed vessel with less than 50% stenosis is more likely to deliver blood to the myocardium for at least 3 years than a venous bypass placed in a vessel with a similar degree of preoperative stenosis.

The authors conclude that minimally diseased coronary arteries should not be bypassed.

▶ The cause for the decrease in the rate of deaths from cardiovascular disease is unknown. Either better control of hypertension or decreased cigarette smoking may have an influence. What these articles point out is that hypertension produces changes in endothelial permeability and damage to endothelial cells. These may be reversible and, in fact, some of the changes otherwise attributable to aging can be reversed by control of hypertension. With that in mind, it is of some importance to note that bypassing minimal coronary artery lesions allows progression of those lesions. It is apparent that the decreased flow through the vessel enhances atherosclerotic development. There are many operations in vascular surgery in which increased flow through a vessel is produced. Whether or not this decreases the rate of atherosclerotic development is unknown and intriguing.

Dietary Omega-3 Fatty Acids Prevent Carbohydrate-Induced Hypertriglyceridemia

William S. Harris, William E. Connor, Stephen B. Inkeles, and D. Roger Illingworth (Oregon Health Sciences Univ., Portland)

Metabolism 33:1016–1019, November 1984 1–3

Dietary fish oils rich in ω-3 fatty acids can reduce levels of plasma triglycerides in both normal and hyperlipidemic subjects. The very low-density lipoprotein (VLDL) fraction is especially reduced by dietary fish oil. An attempt was made to determine whether dietary fish oil can prevent the usual marked increases in levels of plasma triglyceride and VLDL that occur after a high-carbohydrate intake.

Seven mildly hypertriglyceridemic but otherwise healthy subjects aged 22 to 54 years, were included in the study. None were obese. Mean fasting level of triglyceride was 187 mg/dl, and mean level of plasma cholesterol was 202 mg/dl. The two high-carbohydrate diets contained 75% of calories as carbohydrates; the baseline diet contained 45% as carbohydrates. Either peanut oil and cocoa butter or fish oil provided fat calories amounting to 15% of high-carbohydrate diets. A total of 50 gm of fish oil was taken daily in a 3,000-kcal diet and provided 8.5 gm of eicosapentenoic acid and 5.5 gm of docosahexaenoic acid. Cholesterol intake was about 70 mg per 1,000 kcal in all diets.

The dietary effects on levels of plasma triglyceride are compared in Figure 1–1. The rise in levels of triglyceride with the high-carbohydrate control diet was due almost entirely to an increase in the VLDL fraction, which was more than doubled. The level of plasma triglyceride was reduced 61% when fish oil was substituted, usually within 3 days. Total levels of cholesterol fell significantly with the fish oil diet, chiefly because of a decrease in level of VLDL cholesterol. The fish oil diet also reversed the increase in concentrations of apolipoprotein C-III caused by the high-carbohydrate control diet.

These findings support the hypothesis that ω-3 fatty acids reduce the levels of VLDL by inhibiting synthesis of VLDL. The effect is seen even

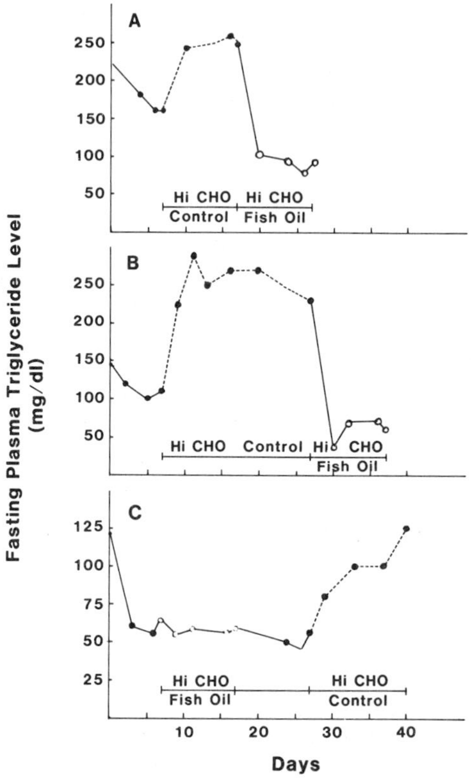

Fig 1–1.—Effects of baseline (●——●), control (●----●), and fish oil (○——○) diets on plasma triglyceride levels in 3 subjects. **A**, reversal of carbohydrate-induced hypertriglyceridemia by dietary fish oil; **B**, persistence of hypertriglyceridemia (more than 20 days) and subsequent reversal by fish oil; and **C**, prevention of carbohydrate-induced hypertriglyceridemia by fish oil. (Courtesy of Harris, W.S., et al.: Metabolism 33:1016–1019, November 1984.)

in the face of a high-carbohydrate intake. Further studies of the kinetics of VLDL are needed to determine how dietary ω-3 fatty acids influence synthesis of VLDL.

Atherosclerosis: Progression, Regression, and Resolution

M. Rene Malinow (Oregon Health Sciences Univ., Portland)

Am. Heart J. 108:1523–1537, December 1984 1–4

Despite clinical impressions that atherosclerosis is progressive, animal studies have shown that atherosclerotic plaques can decrease in size when atherogenic stimuli are removed, and sequential angiographic studies in human subjects also suggest that atherosclerotic stenoses can enlarge under certain circumstances. The concept of anatomical progression of atherosclerosis is based mainly on static microscopic studies and series of autopsies. Withdrawal of dietary cholesterol has been associated with shrinkage of induced atherosclerotic lesions in several animal species, including nonhuman primates. Most anatomical evidence for regression in human beings is circumstantial. Some studies have indicated that patients with malignant disease have less severe atherosclerosis than others. Reported rates or regression in human subjects vary widely. Up to 20% of patients in serial angiographic studies have been reported to show regression of lesions. Intensive treatment reducing the plasma cholesterol concentration has been found to lead to regression of femoral arterial disease.

Depletion of lipids and a reduction in both cell numbers and extracellular material account for angiographic regression of atherosclerosis in man. Other mechanisms could include lysis or retraction of superimposed thrombi; incorporation of thrombi into the arterial wall, followed by organization, contraction, or channel formation; release of spasm; arterial ectasia or dilatation; medial thinning with outward bulging of the plaque; and plaque ulceration. Various animal studies have suggested the importance of local mechanisms in regression. The hemodynamic consequences of regression remain to be determined, and studies are needed to find how to influence the course of regression. Prevention will remain easier until regression of atherosclerosis can be consistently induced.

A Study of Atherosclerosis Regression in *Macaca mulatta:* Changes in Abdominal Aorta and Carotid and Coronary Arteries From Animals With Atherosclerosis Induced for 38 Months and Then Regressed for 24 or 48 Months at Plasma Cholesterol Concentrations of 300 or 200 mg/dl

T. B. Clarkson, M. G. Bond, B. C. Bullock, K. J. McLaughlin, and J. K. Sawyer (Bowman Gray School of Medicine, Wake Forest Univ., Winston–Salem, N.C.)

Exp. Mol. Pathol. 41:96–118, August 1984 1–5

Regression of atherosclerosis at different sites was investigated in young adult male rhesus monkeys that were fed an atherogenic diet for 38 months, followed by diets with varying cholesterol contents to maintain plasma cholesterol concentrations of about 200 or 300 mg/dl over 2 or 4 years. Atherosclerosis was assessed in the coronary and carotid arteries and in the abdominal aorta.

Coronary atherosclerosis regressed in a majority of animals after 4 years, but not after 2 years, when the plasma cholesterol concentration was kept at 200 mg/dl. Among those with higher cholesterol concentrations, coronary involvement progressed in about half and regressed in the rest. Most monkeys with progressive involvement were genetic hyperresponders to dietary cholesterol, whereas those with regressive changes were chiefly hyporesponders, although the two groups had similar plasma lipid concentrations during the follow-up phase. Changes in atherosclerosis in the abdominal aorta were similar to those in the coronary arteries. In both instances, regression was not seen in animals that had a ratio of total serum cholesterol to high-density lipoprotein cholesterol exceeding 3.5. No regression of atherosclerosis was evident in the common carotid arteries or in the carotid bifurcation at 4 years.

The potential for regression of atherosclerosis induced over the long term in macaques appears to be comparable with that of lesions induced over the short term. A period of 4 years appears to be necessary to discern significant differences between monkeys maintained at total plasma cholesterol concentrations of 200 and 300 mg/dl.

Cod Liver Oil in the Prevention of Intimal Hyperplasia in Autogenous Vein Grafts Used for Arterial Bypass

R. W. Landymore, C. E. Kinley, J. H. Cooper, M. MacAulay, B. Sheridan, and C. Cameron (Dalhousie Univ., Halifax)

J. Thorac. Cardiovasc. Surg. 89:351–357, March 1985 1–6

Fibrous intimal hyperplasia is the most frequent cause of late graft failure after coronary bypass surgery. Intimal thickening appears to be platelet mediated. The unsaturated fatty acid eicosapentenoic acid, found in salt water fish and cod liver oil, decreases platelet aggregation and total platelet counts. The effects of cod liver oil on platelet-mediated intimal hyperplasia in autogenous vein grafts were examined in dogs having segments of external jugular vein interposed between divided femoral arteries. A 2% cholesterol diet was given, and study animals received cod liver oil capsules containing 1.8 gm of eicosapentenoic acid daily from 1 week before vein implantation to 6 weeks afterward.

Lipid supplementation led to a significant rise in the serum cholesterol value in both groups. No significant change in bleeding times or platelet counts occurred in either group. Marked intimal hyperplasia was observed in control animals, but much less hyperplasia was seen in those given eicosapentenoic acid. Mean intimal thickness increased from 4 μm to 86 μm in the control group and from 4 μ to 25 μm in the study animals.

Eicosapentenoic acid appears to inhibit platelet-mediated intimal hyperplasia in canine autogenous vein grafts used for arterial bypass. The findings suggest that cod liver oil might be useful in preventing intimal hyperplasia in vein grafts used for myocardial revascularization. Eicosapentenoic acid has been ingested by Eskimos for more than 100 years without apparent adverse effects. Substitution of this unsaturated fatty acid for arachidonic acid in platelet membranes results in decreased thromboxane A_2 activity and a reduction in platelet aggregation.

▶ These four articles supplement observations made by Kromhout et al. (*N. Engl. J. Med.* 312:1205–1209, 1985) on the inverse relationship between fish consumption and 20-year mortality from coronary artery disease as corroborated by Stamler and Paul (Shekelle, R. B., et al.: *N. Engl. J. Med.* 304:65–70, 1981) in the Western Electric Study. They can be considered valid observations.

The inverse relationship between fish consumption and coronary heart disease is most commonly explained by the effect of N-3 polyunsaturated fatty acids (e.g., eicosapentenoic acid) upon bleeding time and platelet aggregation. However, it may be that other constituents present in fish may influence mortality from coronary artery disease. Kromhout himself has suggested that one of these constituents might be selenium.

As more observations are accumulated, vascular surgeons may find ways in which to prevent progression of atherosclerosis in patients who require direct arterial reconstruction.

2 Biochemical Interactions of the Arterial Wall

Premature Development of Iliac Artery Stenosis in Asymptomatic Type II Hyperlipoproteinemia

Paolo Rubba, Alfredo Postiglione, Biagio De Simone, Fulvio Faccenda, Gabriele Riccardi, and Mario Mancini (Univ. of Naples)

Arteriosclerosis 4:625–629, Nov.–Dec. 1984 2–1

Although the plasma pattern of type II hyperlipoproteinemia (HLP) has consistently been associated with the premature development of coronary heart disease, the evidence relating increased plasma concentrations of low-density lipoproteins (LDL) to premature atherosclerosis of the lower limbs is conflicting. Using the echo-Doppler technique (Duplex Scanner III, ATL Mark V) with spectral analysis of the Doppler signals, possible common and external iliac artery stenosis was evaluated in 35 consecutive male patients, 40–60 years of age, with asymptomatic type II HLP (23 type IIA, 12 type IIB) and in 54 normocholesterolemic male controls, all 50 years of age.

Duplex scanning detected arterial wall abnormalities in 19 (27%) of the 70 limbs in patients with type II HLP, but in only 6 (5.5%) of the 108 control limbs ($P < .001$). Six of the 19 abnormal limbs had stenosis of 16% to 50% and 13 had stenosis of 1% to 15%. Only 2 of the 6 limbs with abnormal findings in the normocholesterolemic group had stenosis of 16% to 50%. No flow-reducing stenosis was detectable in either group. The severity of vascular involvement did not differ significantly between type IIA and type IIB patients.

Patients with type IIA and type IIB HLP have a higher incidence of wall abnormalities and stenoses of the iliac arteries than do normocholesterolemic controls of the same age and gender. This suggests that increased LDL concentration in type II HLP is associated with premature development of arteriosclerosis obliterans in the iliac arteries.

▶ Hopefully, echo-Doppler and Duplex Scanning will allow direct observation of atherosclerotic lesions. Treatment plans aimed at regression of arterial lesions can be evaluated more accurately by such monitoring.

Familial Apolipoprotein AI and Apolipoprotein CIII Deficiency: Subclass Distribution, Composition, and Morphology of Lipoproteins in Disorder Associated With Premature Atherosclerosis

Trudy M. Forte, Alex V. Nichols, Ronald M. Krauss, and Robert A. Norum

J. Clin. Invest. 74:1601–1613, November 1984 2–2

The risk of developing coronary heart disease varies inversely with plasma levels of high-density lipoprotein (HDL). The importance of this association was emphasized by finding in 2 sisters, 34 and 32 years of age, with extraordinarily low levels of HDL cholesterol, which is linked with premature atherosclerosis, xanthomas, and corneal clouding. Both sisters had a severe deficiency of plasma apolipoprotein AI (apo AI) and apolipoprotein CIII (apo CIII), as well as diminished levels of the apolipoproteins AII, E, CI, and CII. Characteristics of the lipoprotein classes isolated from the plasma of these 2 sisters were compared with those in healthy age-matched and sex-matched controls.

Plasma triglyceride levels in the patients were 31 mg/dl and 51 mg/dl, respectively, and the respective serum cholesterol levels were 130 mg/dl and 122 mg/dl. However, no plasma HDL cholesterol was detectable in either patient. The S_f° 0–20 lipoproteins had a single peak with S_f° rates of 7.4 and 7.6, respectively, which was similar to that in controls. The concentration of low-density lipoprotein (LDL) (S_f° 0–12) particles, though within the normal range, was 35% greater than that in controls. The levels of intermediate-density lipoproteins (IDL) and very low-density lipoproteins (VLDL) (S_f° 20–400) were extremely low. The calculated mass of HDL was 15.4 mg/dl and 11.8 mg/dl in the respective patients. Although HDL was not detectable by analytic ultracentrifugation, polyacrylamide gradient gel electrophoresis (gge) showed that the patients possessed 2 major HDL subclasses: $(HDL_{2b})_{gge}$ at 11.0 nm and $(HDL_{3b})_{gge}$ at 7.8 nm. The major peak in the controls was $(HDL_{3a})_{gge}$, which was not seen in the patients. Gradient gel analysis of LDL showed that the patients had 2 LDL peaks, a major one of 27 nm and a minor one at 26 nm. Electron microscopy showed that the structure of the patients' lipoprotein fractions was indistinguishable from that of the controls. In the patients, HDL particles were spherical and contained a cholesteryl ester core, suggesting that lecithin/cholesterol acyltransferase was functional in the absence of apo AI. The effects of postprandial lipemia (100-gm fat meal) were investigated in 1 patient. Major findings were the appearance of a 33-nm particle in the LDL density region of 1.036–1.041 gm/ml and the presence of discoid particles, accounting for 12% of the total particles, in the HDL region. The latter finding suggests that this patient has delayed transformation of discs to spheres.

The concurrent deficiency of apo AI and apo CIII suggests a dual defect in lipoprotein metabolism, one involving triglyceride-rich lipoproteins and the other involving HDL. The apo CIII deficiency may result in accelerated catabolism of triglyceride-rich particles and an increased rate of LDL formation. Also, the apo CIII deficiency would favor the rapid uptake of apo E-containing remnants by the liver and peripheral cells. Because HDL levels are very low, excess cellular cholestrol would not be removed by the reverse cholesterol transport mechanism and premature atherosclerosis would thus occur.

Accumulation of IgG and Complement Factor C3 in Human Arterial Endothelium and Atherosclerotic Lesions
Göran K. Hansson, Jan Holm, and John G. Kral (Univ. of Göteborg)
Acta Pathol. Microbiol. Immunol. Scand. (A) 92:429–435, 1984 2–3

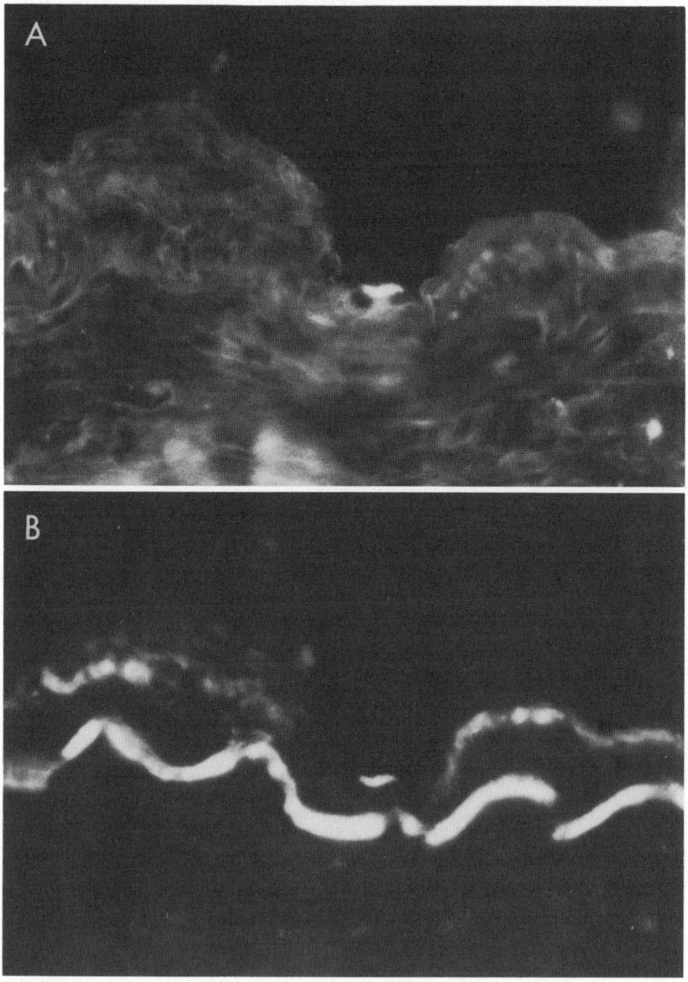

Fig 2–1.—Intima of cystic artery, incubated with tetramethyl-rhodamine isothiocyanate (TRITC)-conjugated anti-IgG and fluorescein isothiocyanate (FITC)-conjugated anti-C3; original magnifications ×400. **A,** photographed in red light, showing distribution of TRITC*-anti-IgG. Notice intense reaction in endothelial cell and reaction of limited intensity in subendothelial intima. **B,** photographed in green light, showing distribution of FITC-anti-C3. Notice intense reaction in same endothelial cell as showed IgG in **A.** (Courtesy of Hansson, G.K., et al.: Acta Pathol. Microbiol. Immunol. Scand. (A)92:429–435, 1984.)

Endothelial cell death leads to binding of IgG to cytoskeletal intermediate filaments in the dead cell, which may also bind complement factors. Accumulations of IgG and complement factors may promote the binding of granulocytes and monocytes to the vessel wall, and this could be an initiating factor in atheroslcerosis. The localization of IgG and complement factor C3 in normal and atherosclerotic human arteries was studied by a fluorescent antibody technique. Atherosclerotic arterial segments were obtained from the lower extremities of 8 patients aged 54 to 70 years who were operated on for intermittent claudication. Nonatherosclerotic cystic vessels were obtained during 8 cholecystectomies in patients aged 35 to 60 years. No subject with inflammatory symptoms was sampled.

Immunoglobulin G was demonstrated in the endothelial cell cytoplasm in cystic arteries (Fig 2–1), and such cells were more abundant in atherosclerotic lesions. Deposits of C3 were also present in the cytoplasm of many endothelial cells in cystic arteries; only IgG-positive cells contained C3. Factor C3 was especially prevalent in the subendothelial zone and the necrotic core of atherosclerotic plaques. The fibrous cap exhibited less intense C3 fluorescence.

Both IgG and C3 accumulate in human atherosclerotic lesions. Immunoglobulin G is found in endothelial cells, probably in relation to cell injury, and C3 is present in many IgG-containing cells. The findings suggest that immune components have a role in endothelial cell destruction and in adhesion of white blood cells. This could be important for both arterial tissue repair and atherogenesis.

▶ The search continues for the cause of premature atherosclerosis.

Lipid Angiogenic Factor From Omentum

Harry S. Goldsmith, Ann L. Griffith, Alan Kupferman, and Nicholas Catsimpoolas (Boston Univ.)

JAMA 252:2034–2036, Oct. 19, 1984 2–4

The investigations of Goldsmith and colleagues, which showed that vascular connections developed rapidly between transposed omental tissue and the brain and spinal cord in dogs and monkeys, led to an investigation of this phenomenon that occurs even in the absence of cerebral ischemia, which suggests that an angiogenic factor causes the response.

The omentum was removed from adult female cats along with subcutaneous fat to be used as a non-omental lipid control. Pieces of the omentum were placed in a blender containing phosphate-buffered saline (PBS). The homogenate was then centrifuged, and three fractions were produced: a pellet, a turbid homogenate, and a cream-colored lipid cake. An aqueous suspension was prepared by homogenizing 4-gm portions of the omental lipid cake with 4 ml of PBS; this was called the PBS homogenate of the omental lipid cake. To produce the lipid extract, portions of the cake were homogenized with 21 ml of choloroform-methanol solvent at room temperature. For the preparation of the PBS homogenate of subcutaneous fat, a 3-gm portion of the fatty tissue was homogenized in 4 ml of PBS. All these materials, plus PBS alone to serve as a control, were subjected to angiogenic testing by injecting 50-μl of the material intrastromally into the cornea of New Zealand white rabbits. The angiogenic response was graded 0 to 4+ (no angiogenesis to formation of dense blood vessels).

Excellent angiogenic activity was noted after a single injection of the chloroform-methanol extract made from the omental lipid cake. The angiogenic response developed rapidly and with intense activity. A panus with formation of interstitial blood vessels became evident 3 to 4 days after injection. By 7 to 10 days, blood vessels had formed a dense and richly structured network within the cornea. Histologic study showed multiple capillaries within the corneal stroma. Minimal angiogenic activity was noted with the PBS homogenates of the total omentum and of the lipid cake.

A lipid material obtained from the omentum contains a potent angiogenic factor extractable in a chloroform-methanol solvent mixture. This may have important therapeutic implications when an increased number of capillaries are clinically needed, i.e., wound healing, bone fracture repair, burns, and tissue and organ ischemia. Since the angiogenic activity of the omentum is activated minimally when the peritoneal cavity is violated, the possibility of an inhibitory angiogenic factor in the omentum is raised. Therefore, inhibition of angiogenic activity may have important clinical implications as in tumor angiogenesis. Studies are currently underway concerning the purification of the omental lipid factor in order to determine its structural characteristics.

3 Platelet and Endothelial Actions and Interactions

The Mesothelial Cell as a Nonthrombogenic Surface

L. J. Nicholson, J. M. F. Clarke, R. M. Pittilo, S. J. Machin, and N. Woolf (London)

Thromb. Haemost. 52:102–104, Oct. 31, 1984 3–1

Prosthetic vascular grafts fare less well than tissue grafts, partly because of the absence of a cellular lining having the properties of vascular endothelium. Endothelial cells are difficult to culture from adult veins; moreover, if adequate veins are available, they ordinarily would be used in place of prosthetic grafts. Mesothelium appears to be a promising nonthrombogenic material for use in lining prosthetic vascular implants.

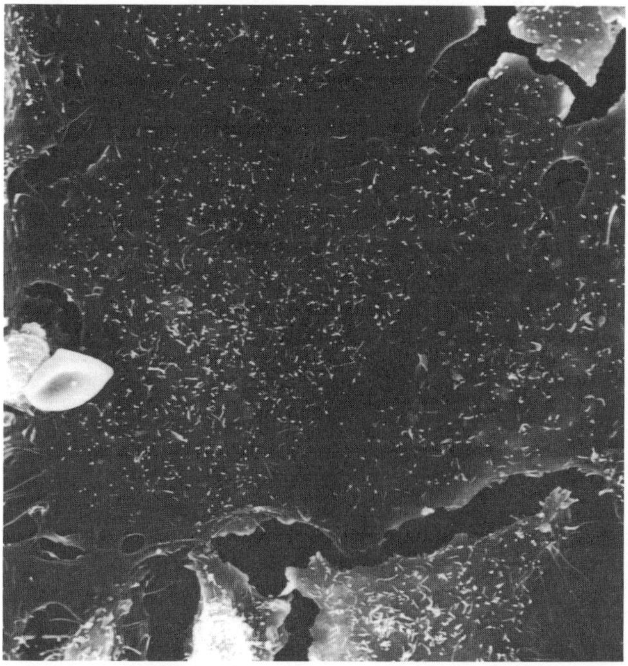

Fig 3–1.—Scanning electron microscopy of mesothelial cells after exposure to flowing blood. There is some loss of surface microvilli and some cell separation. A red blood cell can be seen, but there are no adhering platelets. Bar, 5 μm. (Courtesy of Nicholson, L.J., et al.: Thromb. Haemost. 52:102–104, Oct. 31, 1984.)

Mesothelial cells were harvested from the omentum of rats and from adult human omentum, and cultured in Ham F-12 nutrient mixture supplemented with hydrocortisone, insulin, antibiotics, and fetal calf serum. Cells cultured on plastic film were exposed to blood at a pulsatile flow rate of 160 ml/minute.

The morphologic features of cultured mesothelial cells were distinct from those of cultured fibroblasts. No fibroblasts remained on the plastic film after exposure of confluent monolayers of cells to blood; only adhering platelets were seen. There was some evidence of focal loss of surface microville. Some cells were shed from the film on exposure to flowing blood, but most remained adherent (Fig 3–1).

This technique may prove useful in preparing mesothelial cells for later use in vascular surgery. Rat mesothelial cells are nonthrombogenic and can support blood flow in vitro. Studies are in progress in which the canine infrarenal aorta is replaced with a vascular prosthesis seeded with mesothelial cells.

Luminal Release of Prostacyclin and Thromboxane A_2 by Arteries Distal to Small-Caliber Prosthetic Grafts

Harry L. Bush, Jr., Joseph A. Jakubowski, Suchen L. Hong, Melissa McCabe, Daniel Deykin, and Donald C. Nabseth (Boston)

Circulation 70(Suppl. 1):I-11–I-15, September 1984 3–2

Development of myointimal hyperplasia distal to prosthetic grafts may be related to a specific local imbalance of prostacyclin and thromboxane A_2 that results in exaggerated adherence of platelets. The authors evaluated the luminal release of the proaggregatory, vasoconstrictory metabolite thromboxane A_2 and the antiaggregatory, vasodilatory metabolite prostacyclin by arteries distal to prosthetic grafts in 12 dogs. Control segments were excised from both iliac arteries, and a 5-cm segment of polytetrafluoroethylene was grafted end to end. One iliac artery was circumferentially dissected from the distal anastomosis to the inguinal ligament; the contralateral iliac artery was not dissected. After excision each artery was evaluated for its ability to produce prostacyclin and thromboxane A_2.

Nineteen of the 24 grafts were patent at the time of excision. The amount of prostacyclin produced by the dissected iliac arteries distal to patent grafts was not significantly higher than that produced by the control ilial segments. The undissected arteries, however, produced a significantly greater amount of prostacyclin than either the dissected or control arteries. Both the dissected and undissected iliac arteries produced significantly more thromboxane A_2 distal to patent grafts than did the control iliac segments, but the difference between the dissected and undissected arteries was not significant.

The results demonstrate that only those arteries that are not surgically dissected maintain a normal balance of prostacyclin and thromboxane A_2. Thus, the dissected artery may be more susceptible to platelet interaction and myointimal hyperplasia.

▶ It is astounding to think that the mesothelial cell may substitute for the endothelial cell in seeding small-caliber prostheses. But it is disappointing to find that thromboxane-prostacyclin imbalance is produced by dissection of arteries and implantation of small-vessel prostheses and as such is unavoidable in today's vascular surgery.

The Role of Endothelial Injury and Platelet and Macrophage Interactions in Atherosclerosis

Russell Ross, Agostino Faggiotto, Daniel Bowen-Pope, and Elaine Raines (Univ. of Washington)

Circulation 70(Suppl. 3):III77–III82, November 1984 3–3

Investigators have long suggested that some form of endothelial change is an important antecedent to the arterial wall changes that culminate in atherosclerotic lesions. This concept forms the basis of the response to injury hypothesis of atherosclerosis. The definition of endothelial injury is imprecise. If endothelial injury is prolonged, as may occur at certain anatomical sites such as bifurcations and platelet and macrophage interactions, cell proliferation, new connective tissue deposit, and lipid accumulation could lead to development of the fibrous plaque (Fig 3–2). The hypothesis implies that lesions might regress if the source of injury were removed.

Relatively few longitudinal data are available on the events occurring at specific sites in the arterial wall, especially at the cellular level, under conditions of chronic hypercholesterolemia. Available data from monkeys suggest that the smooth muscle proliferative lesions of atherosclerosis are preceded by endothelial breaks, exposure of macrophages, and platelet interactions. The observations suggest that growth factors such as platelet-derived growth factor (PDGF), macrophage-derived growth factor (MDGF), and possibly endothelial cell-derived growth factor (EDGF) may have roles in the development of lesions.

A better understanding of the way in which endothelial cells may be altered in relation to the hypercholesterolemic environment and to the macrophages in fatty streaks might promote new means of prevention and treatment of atherosclerosis.

Epidemiologic Characteristics of Platelet Aggregability

T. W. Meade, M. V. Vickers, S. G. Thompson, Y. Stirling, A. P. Haines, and G. J. Miller (Harrow, England)

Br. Med. J. 290:428–432, Feb. 9, 1985 3–4

No measure of in vivo platelet function has been established as a marker of risk of thrombosis. Platelet aggregability was examined in 685 male and 273 female participants in a prospective study of the role of hemostasis in the pathogenesis of arterial disease. Dose-response aggregometry was performed using adenosine diphosphate (ADP) and adrenaline as aggre-

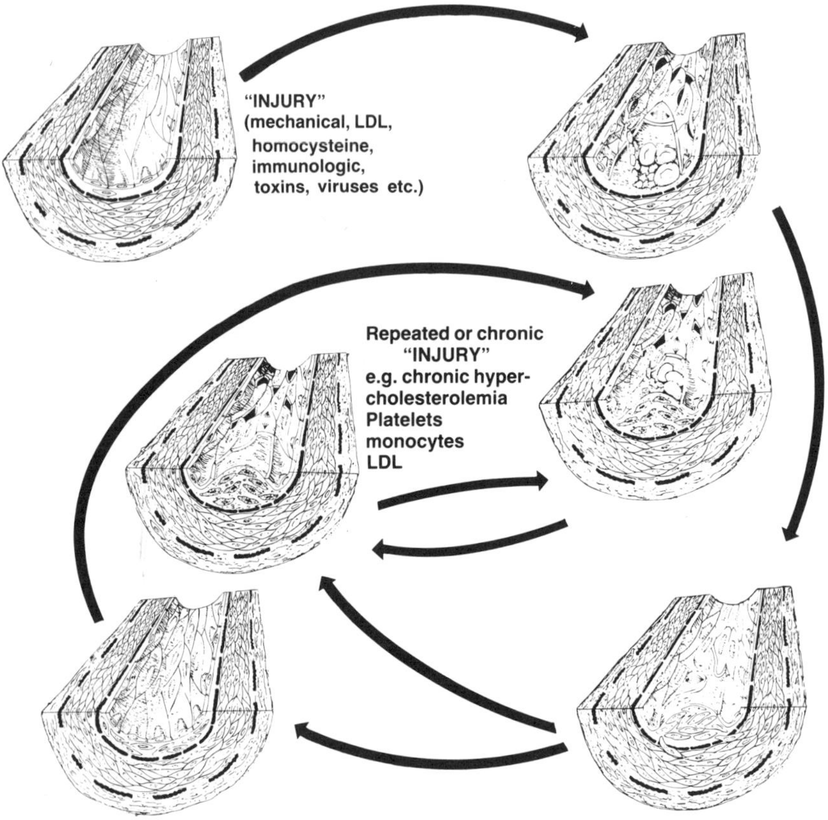

Fig 3–2.—Response to injury hypothesis of atherosclerosis. Series of events are postulated to occur in which endothelial injury results in range of responses from altered function with no morphological alteration to injury sufficient to cause exposure of subendothelium, with interactions among monocytes, macrophages, and platelets. Endothelial injury indicated in this diagram represents maximal response in which cell-cell detachment and cell-connective tissue detachment lead to subendothelial denudation. Platelet interactions with connective tissue or with macrophages lead to possible deposit of growth factors such as PDGF, which can then induce migration and proliferation of smooth muscle cells derived from media of artery into intima. If injury ceases and endothelium regenerates, it is postulated that lesion may be reversible, and resultant effect would be slightly thickened intima. However, if injury is continuous for prolonged period, there may be sequence of injury and repair, followed by reinjury and repair, leading to proliferative lesions that may compromise vascular supply. (Courtesy of Ross, R., et al.: Circulation 70:III77–III82, November 1984; by permission of the American Heart Association, Inc.)

gating agents. The main analyses were based on the level of ADP at which primary aggregation occurred at half-maximal velocity. Twenty-four of the 635 white men had had episodes of ischemic heart disease. Electrocardiographic evidence of possible ischemia was present in 54 subjects.

Platelet aggregability increased with advancing age in both men and women. It was greater in white persons than in black persons, especially among men, and it tended to decrease with a higher level of habitual alcohol consumption. Aggregability was less in smokers, especially among men. It increased with the plasma fibrinogen level but could not be related to obesity, oral contraceptive use, blood cholesterol or triglyceride levels, or recent aspirin consumption. Platelets were somewhat more aggregable in subjects with myocardial ischemia, but not to a significant degree.

Platelet aggregability was strongly associated with the plasma fibrinogen in this study. It may be an oversimplification to consider aggregability to be an intrinsic feature of platelets themselves. If platelet function depends on external influences such as the plasma fibrinogen or thrombin production to an appreciable degree, it may be helpful to modify these effects rather than rely solely on the use of platelet-active agents.

Flow Effects on Prostacyclin Production by Cultured Human Endothelial Cells

John A. Frangos, Suzanne G. Eskin, Larry V. McIntire, and C. L. Ives (Houston)

Science 227:1477–1479, Mar. 22, 1985 3–5

Various endothelial cell functions such as arachidonic acid metabolism may be influenced by blood flow-induced membrane stresses. Prostacyclin production appears to be affected by shear stress. The platelet aggregation-inhibiting effect of prostacyclin may contribute to the nonthrombogenicity of the endothelial lining of vessel walls. The vasodilating effect of prostacyclin could help regulate local blood flow.

Prostacyclin production by primary human endothelial cell cultures was examined in relation to pulsatile and steady flow shear stress in a flow chamber. The onset of flow led to a sudden rise in prostacyclin production, which decreased to a steady rate within several minutes. Steady-state production of prostacyclin was more than twice as great in cells exposed to pulsatile shear stress as in those exposed to steady shear stress and 16 times greater than in cells in stationary culture.

Production in prostacyclin by human vascular endothelium under physiologic flow conditions may be significantly greater than in cells cultured under stationary conditions. Lower concentrations of prostacyclin in veins than in arteries may be explained by the relative lack of pulsatile flow and the lower shear stress in veins. The findings support a controlling role for blood flow in endothelial cell function.

Platelet Function and Biosynthesis of Prostacyclin and Thromboxane A_2 in Whole Blood After Aspirin Administration in Human Subjects

Jawahar L. Mehta, Paulette Mehta, Larry Lopez, Nancy Ostrowski, and Ernie Aguila (Gainesville)

J. Am. Coll. Cardiol. 4:806–811, October 1984 3–6

Small doses of aspirin may inhibit platelet thromboxane A_2 while sparing vascular prostacyclin synthesis. However, leukocytes also synthesize thromboxane A_2 and prostacyclin. The effects of 40, 325, and 650 mg of aspirin given once orally on the production of thromboxane A_2 and prostacyclin by all blood components was examined in 15 normal subjects. Serum concentrations of thromboxane B_2, which reflect thromboxane A_2 production by platelets and leukocytes, and 6-keto-prostaglandin $F_{1\alpha}$ ($PGF_{1\alpha}$), which reflects prostacyclin synthesis by leukocytes, were determined.

Aspirin, 40 mg, inhibited platelet aggregation and adenosine triphosphate release for 24 hours. In contrast, platelet function was inhibited for 4–7 days in subjects given 325 or 650 mg. Significant inhibition of thromboxane B_2 synthesis occurred for at least 7 days with either the 325- or the 650-mg dose but only for 4 days with the 40-mg dose ($P < .05$). Recovery of thromboxane B_2 began 2 days after aspirin administration in all cases. Inhibition of 6-keto-$PGF_{1\alpha}$ production by 40%–60% lasted for 4 days with the 40-mg dose; in contrast, whole blood generation of prostacyclin was inhibited 90% by the larger doses for 7 days. Decreases in whole blood thromboxane A_2 and prostacyclin concentrations with any dose of aspirin were of similar magnitude.

Inhibition of platelet function and biosynthesis of thromboxane A_2 and prostacyclin in whole blood by aspirin in doses of 40–650 mg is dose-dependent. Since vessel wall synthesis of prostacyclin is suppressed in atherosclerosis, production by prostacyclin by leukocytes may be important. Further, with leukocytes being incorporated in the intra-arterial platelet thrombus, activated leukocytes may exert a regulatory role in thrombogenesis by producing prostacyclin via platelet-generated cyclic endoperoxidases.

▶ Genesis of atherosclerosis is inextricably linked with platelet, endothelial cell, and leukocyte or macrophage interaction. The preceding four articles comment upon the production of prostacyclin by endothelial cells, the epidemiologic characteristics of platelet aggregation, and the effects that heparin and aspirin have on both. With that in mind, the next study is of particular relevance.

Platelets, Carotids, and Coronaries: Critique on Antithrombotic Role of Antiplatelet Agents, and Exercise, and Certain Diets

Edward R. Eichner (Univ. of Oklahoma)

Am. J. Med. 77:513–523, September 1984 3–7

Interactions among platelets and vascular endothelial cells appear to be important in complications of atherosclerosis and possibly in the development of atherosclerosis itself. The interaction is modulated by platelet-produced thromboxane A_2 and the endothelial production of prostacyclin, which can be influenced by "antiplatelet" drugs. Platelet-endothelial interaction has been implicated in the formation and subsequent embolization of platelet thrombi in the carotid and coronary arteries.

Aspirin has variably been found to protect all patients or men only from stroke and coronary death. No good rationale is known for aspirin to benefit only men. Aspirin seems to offer secondary prevention against myocardial infarction and coronary death. Mixed effects have been obtained from aspirin and other antiplatelet agents in patients with angina, but a recent VA study strongly suggests benefit from aspirin in men with unstable angina. The exact dosage of aspirin used is probably unimportant. Sulfinpyrazone seems to have some antithrombotic effect, but this is no greater than that obtained with aspirin, and it may be reasonable to use aspirin alone or with a β-blocker in patients with myocardial infarction.

Exercise may tip the "thromboxane-prostacyclin balance" in the "antithrombotic" direction. Exercise promotes fibrinolysis and can increase prostacyclin release while it reduces platelet aggregability. The weight of epidemiologic evidence increasingly suggests that regular exercise protects against coronary heart disease in human beings. Some diets appear to be more "antithrombotic" than others. A fatty fish diet or fish oil supplements reduce platelet aggregability and increase the bleeding time. It is likely that diet and exercise, as well as drugs, can influence the interaction between platelets and their environment in clinically important ways.

Selective Thromboxane Inhibition: A New Approach to Antiplatelet Therapy

Marc Fisher, Bonnie Weiner, Ira S. Ockene, James S. Hoogasian, Anita M. Natale, John R. Arsenault, Mark H. Johnson, and Peter H. Levine
Stroke 15:813–816, Sept.–Oct. 1984 3–8

Antiplatelet drugs (e.g., aspirin) are often used to prevent stroke. Aspirin inhibits the formation of both thromboxane A_2, a potent platelet aggregator, and prostacyclin, a potent antiaggregator. Platelet aggregation might also be inhibited by selective suppression of thromboxane formation. A study was made of the effects of UK-38,485, an imidazole derivative that selectively inhibits thromboxane production while sparing prostacyclin production, on serum levels of thromboxane B_2 (TXB_2), the stable hydrolysis product of thromboxane A_2 (TXA_2), and on serum prostacyclin levels (PGI_2) in swine. The animals received either a single dose of UK-38,485 in the amount of 0.5 mg/kg intravenously or 10 mg/kg orally, or 10 mg/kg orally per day for 10 days.

A single 0.5 mg/kg intravenous dose of UK-38,485 produced maximal inhibition of TXB_2 production at 1 hour, but significant inhibition remained 6 hours after injection ($P < .05$). Serum PGI_2 levels were unaffected. A single 10 mg/kg dose of UK-38,485 given orally reduced mean serum TXB_2 levels to 14% of baseline values at 6 hours and to 28% of baseline at 24 hours. The effects at 6 hours, but not at 24 hours, were significant ($P < .05$). Again, serum PGI_2 levels were not significantly changed. Oral administration of UK-38,485 for 10 days resulted in prolonged inhibition of the serum TXB_2 level ($P < .01$). There was a trend toward a significantly higher level of TXB_2 by day 10, but the degree of suppression remained significant. Mean serum PGI_2 levels were significantly elevated on days 2, 8, and 10 ($P < .05$), but not on days 4 and 6. There were no observable hemorrhagic or other side effects in any of the study groups.

The results further support the proposal that drugs such as UK-38,485 should be considered as potential prophylactic agents in the prevention of stroke or other vascular disorders in which platelets play an important role.

▶ Many treatment methods reduce platelet aggregability. It is refreshing to learn that at least one of them, exercise, does not involve the administration of a drug.

Effect of Heparin on Platelet Aggregation

H. I. Saba, S. R. Saba, and G. A. Morelli (Tampa, Fla.)

Am. J. Hematol. 17:295–306, 1984 3–9

The effects of heparin on platelets remain uncertain. Paradoxical thrombosis has been described during the use of heparin, but reductions in

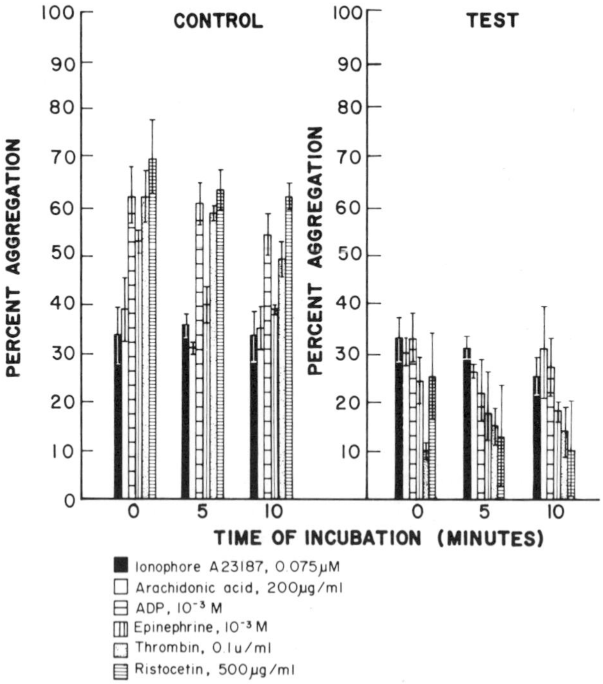

Fig 3–3.—Effect of heparin on washed platelets (WP); aggregation in presence of different agents. Aliquots (0.4 ml) of WP were incubated with 10 units of heparin. At 0.5 and 10 minutes these samples were aggregated with different agents. Results are expressed as mean percent of aggregation ± standard deviation. (Courtesy of Saba, H.I., et al.: Am. J. Hematol. 17:295–306, 1984.)

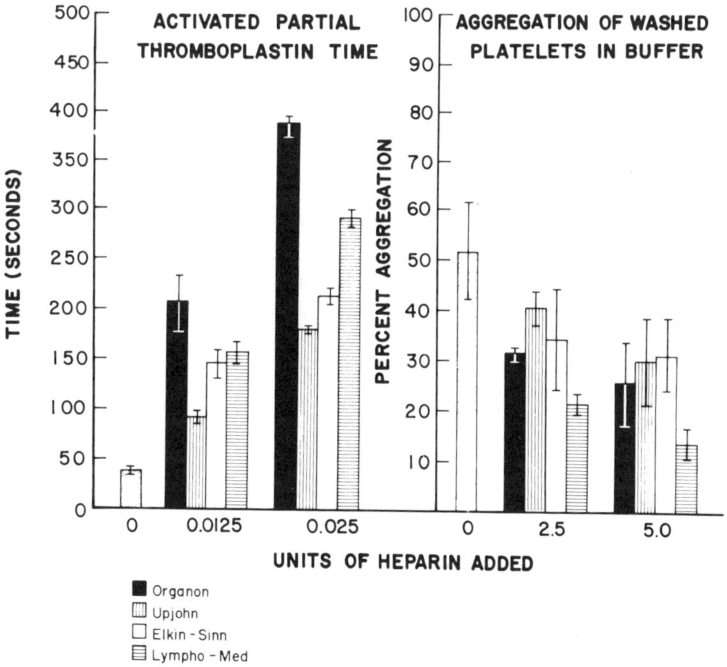

Fig 3–4.—Differences in anticoagulant and antiaggregatory activity of heparin. Heparin anticoagulant action in PTT system: 0.1-ml aliquots of platelet-poor plasma were combined with 0.1 ml of different heparin solutions (abscissa) and 0.1 ml of APTT reagents; 0.1 ml of 0.025 *M* of $CaCl_2$ was added and clotting time was measured. Results are expressed as mean clotting time ± standard deviation (ordinate). Heparin inhibitory activity on platelet aggregation: 0.4-ml samples of WP in buffer were incubated with different amounts of heparin solutions (abscissa) for 5 minutes at 37 C. Aggregations were performed by using 0.05 ml of 1×10^{-4} *M* adenosine diphosphate. Buffer replaced heparin for all controls. Results are shown as mean percent of aggregation ± standard deviation (ordinate). (Courtesy of Saba, H.I., et al.: Am. J. Hematol. 17:295–306, 1984.)

collagen- and epinephrine-induced platelet aggregation have also been noted. The present study examined the effects of heparin on isolated platelets resuspended in modified Tyrode's solution and on platelets in platelet-rich plasma. Gel-filtered, washed, and formaldehyde-fixed platelets were examined in the former system.

Heparin caused mild potentiation of platelet aggregation in the PRP system, but significant inhibitory activity was seen when it was added to isolated platelets (Fig 3–3). Inhibitory activity was especially evident in the presence of ristocetin. The activity appeared to be specific and not related to impurities in the heparin preparations; it was effectively neutralized by both heparinase and protamine. Differences in the anticoagulant and platelet antiaggregatory activity of heparin are shown in Figure 3–4. Heparin enhanced the generation of thromboxane in isolated platelets, but platelets pretreated with heparin failed to respond to preformed thromboxane.

In addition to potentiating the production of thromboxane in platelets, heparin also may alter the platelet membrane and interfere with the ability of platelets to respond to agonists of platelet aggregation. If the factors in plasma that block the antiaggregatory activity of heparin differ in different subjects or are altered in pathologic states, this could exlain the observation that not all heparin-treated patients show enhanced platelet aggregation or thrombocytopenia, or both.

Improved Graft Patency in Patients Treated With Platelet-Inhibiting Therapy After Coronary Bypass Surgery

B. Greg Brown, Ramon A. Cukingnan, Timothy DeRouen, Lacy V. Goede, Maylene Wong, Henry J. Fee, Jack A. Roth, and Joseph S. Carey

Circulation 72:138–146, July 1985 3–10

Vein graft patency declines over time after myocardial revascularization. Most occlusive episodes in the first 2 postoperative months are thrombotic. Measures to limit platelet adhesion and aggregation and counter the release of α-granules would be expected to improve graft patency. Platelet inhibitor therapy was evaluated in 147 consecutive male coronary bypass patients aged 34 to 70 years. Treatment began an average of 67 hours after operation. Patients received 325 mg of aspirin three times daily, alone or with 75 mg of dipyridamole three times daily. Treatment was given to 127 patients who received a total of 399 grafts.

No patient-specific variables could be related to graft occlusion in treated or placebo patients. The significant graft-specific variables included arterial diameter, severity of stenosis, graft flow, reactive hyperemia, collaterals, and graft type. Twenty-one percent of grafts in the placebo group were occluded. The relative risks of graft occlusion were 0.47 in patients given aspirin and 0.50 in those given aspirin and dipyridamole. Benefit was associated with fewer occlusions of grafts in which flow exceeded 40 ml per minute and those supplying arteries with a luminal diameter exceeding 1.5 mm. Grafts lacking reactive hyperemia had an occlusion rate of 32% in placebo patients; the relative risk of occlusion averaged 0.26 with platelet inhibition. Graft occlusion was associated with a poorer clinical outcome.

Substantial benefit was associated with platelet-inhibiting therapy in this series of coronary bypass patients. The use of 325 mg of aspirin three times daily, starting within 48 hours of operation, is recommended. Further study is needed to determine whether dipyridamole should also be used; no significant added benefit was found in this study.

Increased Platelet Sensitivity and Thromboxane B_2 Formation in Type II Hyperlipoproteinemic Patients

Elena Tremoli, Paola Maderna, Susanna Colli, Gabriele Morazzoni, Marina Sirtori, and Cesare R. Sirtori (Milan)

Eur. J. Clin. Invest. 14:329–333, October 1984 3–11

The correlation among hyperlipidemia, abnormalities of platelet function, and production of arachidonic acid metabolites is not well established. Platelet aggregation induced by collagen, adenosine diphosphate, and epinephrine was monitored in 150 type II hyperlipidemic patients and compared with that in 105 age-matched normocholesterolemic patients. Malondialdehyde and thromboxane B_2 formation in platelets of type IIA patients were also compared with those of age-matched controls to investigate the role of the prostaglandin metabolic pathway in platelets from patients at high risk of thrombotic complications. Determinations of total plasma cholesterol and triglyceride concentrations and lipoprotein fractionation were performed. Only 18 patients showed ECG alterations indicative of coronary heart disease, 4 had symptoms of cerebrovascular disease, and 3 had symptomatic peripheral vascular disease.

On the basis of the plasma lipid and lippoprotein profile, a diagnosis of type IIA hyperlipidemia was established in 115 patients, and type IIB was present in the other 35. Threshold aggregation concentrations (TAC) were significantly lower in type II patients than controls for all three aggregating agents; no significant difference was detected in TAC between type IIA and type IIB patients. A large portion of type II patients (44%) showed a normal aggregation response to each aggregating stimulus; only 56% of type II patients exceeded the 95th percentile of TAC in controls. No significant correlation was shown between age, sex, and plasma cholesterol concentration and platelet aggregatory response. Malondialdehyde formation in platelet-rich plasma stimulated with thrombin and collagen was greater in platelets from type IIA patients ($P < .001$). Production of thromboxane B_2 by platelets from type IIA patients was higher ($P < .001$) and exceeded the highest level found in controls. No correlation could be detected between thromboxane B_2 release and plasma cholesterol concentration.

Platelet hyperaggregability is a consistent phenomenon in type IIA patients. This response is not correlated with the plasma cholesterol concentration or the presence of atherosclerosis. The observed increase in arachidonic acid metabolism at the platelet level, with resulting increased thromboxane formation, suggests a specific alteration of platelets in type II patients. However, it may also reflect a more general metabolic derangement involving different sites at which prostaglandins and thromboxanes are generated. The use of diets and drugs affecting arachidonic acid oxidation should be considered in the prevention of thrombotic episodes in type II hyperlipidemic patients.

▶ Platelet thromboxane-heparin interactions are important to all of us in vascular surgery. The preceding three abstracts present some data which are at variance with observations. With regard to these interactions, the state of our science is simply one of data gathering. Hopefully, such data gathering will lead to a useful hypothesis in the future.

4 Coagulation Abnormalities

Evolution of Antithrombin III During the Postoperative Period
Jean-Jacques Rodzynek, Pierre Leautaud, Jacqueline Damien, Marie-Pierre Rosa, and Jean-Paul Govaerts (Free Univ. of Brussels)
Scand. J. Haematol. 33:207–211, August 1984 4–1

Antithrombin III (AT III), the chief inhibitor of thrombin, when deficient is associated with an increased risk of thromboembolic complications. The postoperative course of AT III was examined prospectively for 8 days in 57 consecutive patients undergoing major abdominal operations without prophylactic anticoagulant administration. Cases of appendectomy and herniorrhaphy were excluded. The 30 men and 27 women were aged 23 to 87 years. The most frequent procedures were colectomy, cholecystectomy, and gastrectomy.

Twenty-eight patients (49%) had deep venous thrombosis on phlebography 8 days after operation. Seventeen had distal and 11 had proximal venous thrombosis. The AT III concentration rose slightly after a transient fall immediately after operation. Mean values were significantly below baseline on the first 2 days. The courses of AT III values were similar in patients with and without deep venous thrombosis (Fig 4–1). A low pre-

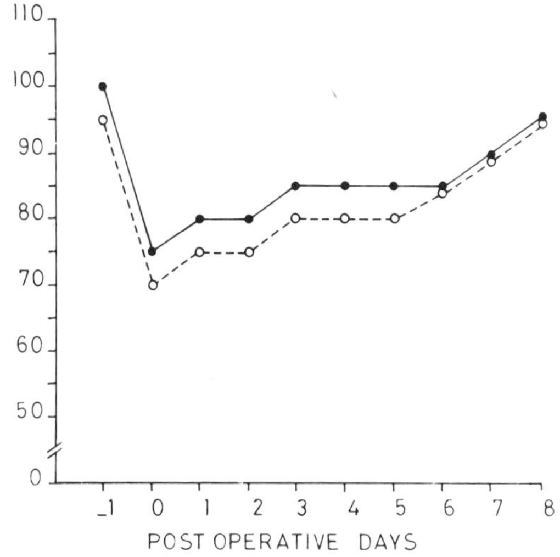

Fig 4–1.—Mean value of antithrombin III during the postoperative period in relation to the presence or absence of DVT. Closed circles show absence of DVT. Open circles show presence of DVT. (Courtesy of Rodzynek, J.-J., et al.: Scand. J. Haematol. 33:207–211, August 1984).

operative AT III value was not associated with an increased occurrence of postoperative deep venous thrombosis. Thrombosis was more frequent in patients with abnormal AT III concentrations at the end of intervention, but not significantly so.

The AT III concentration was not a reliable marker of the risk of postoperative deep venous thrombosis in this series of abdominal surgical patients. Low preoperative AT III values in patients with liver disease were not associated with an increased risk of thromboembolism. It is possible that a postoperative fall in AT III concentration is the result of hemodilution.

Fibrinogen, Factor VIII-Related Antigen, Antithrombin III and α_2-Antiplasmin in Peripheral Arterial Disease

M. Christe, A. Delley, G. A. Marbet, L. Biland, and F. Duckert (Basel)

Thromb. Haemost. 52:240–242, December 1984 4–2

Fibrinogen, factor VIII-related antigen (VIIIR:Ag), antithrombin III, and α_2-antiplasmin values were determined in 89 males seen in 1980 and 1981 with peripheral arterial disease and in 217 without arterial disease. The former had a blood pressure difference greater than 50 mm Hg between the arm and the dorsalis pedis artery.

Values for VIIIR:Ag and α_2-antiplasmin were significantly higher in the patients with peripheral artery disease. Antithrombin III values in this group were higher in patients with a normal exercise ECG than in those with abnormal tracings. Among the subjects without arterial disease, the ratio of α_2-antiplasmin to antithrombin III was significantly higher in those with abnormal exercise ECGs suggesting coronary disease. Fibrinogen and VIIIR:Ag values were higher in patients with a history of myocardial infarction, but age differences may have been responsible. Patients with cerebral circulatory disorder had higher VIIIR:Ag and α_2-antiplasmin values than those without this complication. Higher α_2-antiplasmin values tended to be associated with extension of arterial disease.

Patients with peripheral arterial disease have higher fibrinogen and VIIIR:Ag values than normal subjects. Elevations of these factors are seen in coronary heart disease, and fibrinolytic activity and antithrombin III values tend to be reduced. An imbalance between antithrombin III and α_2-antiplasmin may contribute to the development of arterial disease.

▶ Articles 4–1 and 4–2 link coagulant or lytic abnormalities to arterial disease and define the dynamics of antithrombin III in the postoperative period. The curious fact that antithrombin III deficiency in the postoperative period is not associated with deep venous thrombosis is linked to Ratnoff's comments in a following article in which he muses upon the lack of correlation between lifelong hemostatic changes and infrequent thrombotic episodes.

Two Different Mechanisms in Patients With Venous Thrombosis and Defective Fibrinolysis: Low Concentrations of Plasminogen Activator or Increased Concentration of Plasminogen Activator Inhibitor

Inga Marie Nilsson, Harald Ljungnér, and Lilian Tengborn (Univ. of Lund)
Br. Med. J. 290:1453–1456, May 18, 1985 4–3

The functional importance of the tissue plasminogen activator (TPA) inhibitor in patients with thrombosis is unclear. Fibrinolytic components and TPA inhibitor concentrations were studied in 100 patients with recurrent deep venous thrombosis or pulmonary embolism and no other known disease. The 60 men and 40 women had a mean age of 43 years. Fifty-seven healthy subjects with a mean age of 33 years served as controls. Plasminogen activators were estimated by the fibrin plate method, amidolytically, and by immunoradiometric assay.

All patients had normal platelet counts, clotting times, and concentrations of factors V and VIII. Sixty-seven patients had normal TPA values with all methods after the venous occlusion test. Inhibitor concentrations were also normal, except for a slight increase in 1 patient in this group. Twenty-two other patients had normal activator values by immunoradiometric assay alone and significantly increased concentrations of TPA inhibitor. Eleven patients had low activator values by all assays. All but 1 of them had normal inhibitor values.

Defective fibrinolysis in patients with venous thrombosis may be associated with defective synthesis and release of TPA and with an increased concentration of TPA inhibitor. The dose of activator used for thrombolysis will depend on the concentration of inhibitor. A means is needed for reducing the inhibitor in patients with high concentrations. The anabolic steroid stanozolol has been reported to reduce inhibitor in patients with normal concentrations.

New Approaches to Thrombolytic Therapy

Desire Collen and Henri R. Lijnen (Univ. of Leuven, Belgium)
Arteriosclerosis 4:579–585, Nov.–Dec. 1984 4–4

Tissue-type plasminogen activator (t-PA) is a serine protease distinct from urokinase that was purified from cultures of a stable human melanoma cell line. It has a molecular weight of about 70,000 and is composed of a single polypeptide chain, which is converted to a two-chain molecule by limited plasmic action. Activation is strikingly enhanced by the presence of fibrin, which increases the affinity of plasminogen for fibrin-bound t-PA. Plasmin formed on the fibrin surface may be protected from rapid inactivation by α_2-antiplasmin. The mechanisms regulating the removal of t-PA from the blood are poorly understood. Efficient thrombolysis in vivo appears to be regulated via adsorption of t-PA and plasminogen on the fibrin surface and the in loco generation of plasmin. Coronary thrombolysis has been consistently achieved with t-PA, without systemic activation of the fibrinolytic system. Limited experience suggests the potential of recombinant t-PA for coronary thrombolysis.

Prourokinase, the zymogen precursor of urokinase, also exhibits a degree of fibrin specificity. It is a true proenzyme, which, in a radiolabeled clot lysis assay, lysed clots in a manner similar to t-PA, with equivalent efficacy and fibrin specificity. Studies in rabbits with recombinant prourokinase have shown thrombolysis without associated activation of the fibrinolytic system. Higher concentrations were necessary, however, than when t-PA was used. It is likely that t-PA has greater specific thrombolytic activity in man as well.

▶ Safe lytic therapy awaits release and distribution of tissue-type plasminogen activator. From a practical point of view, deep venous thrombosis is seldom associated with defective fibrinolysis.

Thrombosis and the Hypercoagulable State

Oscar D. Ratnoff (Case Western Reserve Univ.)

Circulation (Suppl. 3) 70:III72–III76, November 1984 4–5

Clinical observations long have indicated that thrombosis may begin in areas of low blood flow or where blood viscosity is increased. Stasis presumably promotes the detachment of platelets from flowing blood and the local accumulation of activated clotting factors. The concept of the hypercoagulable state implies that thrombi can form when coagulation is enhanced or when protective mechanisms such as fibrinolysis are impaired. Clotting is the visible result of the conversion of plasma fibrinogen into an insoluble fibrin network after thrombin has cleaved the small fibrinopeptide fragments from the fibrinogen molecule. Clotting via the extrinsic pathway starts with exposure of plasma to injured tissue. Clotting can occur in the absence of tissue thromboplastin if blood comes into contact with certain "foreign" substances such as some forms of collagen or basement membranes.

Increased concentrations of plasma clotting factors have been implicated in the hypercoagulable state. Fibrinogen concentrations are often extremely high in clinical settings associated with a high risk of thrombosis. Women using oral contraception have high titers of Hageman factor. Hereditary deficiencies of protein clotting factors do not, however, prevent thromboembolic disorders. The titers of activated forms of clotting factors may sometimes reach critical values in the circulation, as in vascular damage or when clot-promoting substances are released from tumor tissue or from stimulated monocytes. Qualitative changes in clotting factors might predispose to thrombosis. Thrombosis has also been related to qualitative platelet abnormalities that enhance their aggregability. Impaired clot dissolution would be expected to increase the risk of significant thrombosis.

Future work on the role of cells in initiating and modifying intravascular clotting will be of interest. It remains to be determined why patients with lifelong hemostatic changes have few thrombotic episodes.

Thrombocytopenia in a Prospective, Randomized, Double-Blind Trial of Bovine and Porcine Heparin

David Green, Gary J. Martin, Sandor H. Shoichet, Noel DeBacker, John S. Bomalaski, and Richard N. Lind (Chicago)

Am. J. Med. Sci. 288:60–64, September 1984 4–6

Thrombocytopenia complicating heparin therapy reportedly occurs in fewer than 1% to 30% of treated patients. To ascertain the types of thrombocytopenic response to heparin, a prospective, double-blind clinical study was conducted in 141 patients randomized to receive either bovine or porcine heparin. Fifty-two patients received fewer than 6 days of heparin therapy and thus were not included in the final statistical analysis. Of the 89 patients who received heparin for 6 or more days, 45 received bovine heparin and 44 received porcine heparin.

Therapeutic partial thromboplastin times (PTTs) were achieved in all patients with mean daily doses ranging from 15,000 to 40,000 units. Severe thrombocytopenia developed in 2 patients (platelet count less than 20,000/μl). Both were randomized to receive bovine heparin, but 1 inadvertently received 2 doses of porcine heparin. Laboratory studies suggested that thrombocytopenia in these 2 patients was immunologically mediated, and platelet reactivity to both bovine and porcine heparin was demonstrated. A decrease in platelet count of more than 50,000/μl occurred in 20 of the 89 patients, but in 7 the platelet count increased subsequently even though they continued to receive heparin therapy. The decreased platelet count in the other 13 patients persisted until the end of therapy. Ten of the latter patients had received bovine heparin, with a mean decrease in platelet count of 88,000/μl, and 3 had received porcine heparin, with a mean decrease in platelet count of 68,000/μl. In none of these 20 patients did the platelet count fall below 150,000/μl. In the remaining 74 patients, including the 7 who had a decrease in platelet count followed by an increase in it, there was a statistically significant increase in the platelet count over pretherapy values ($P < .005$): 58,000 ± 81,000 for the bovine group and 79,000 ± 91,000 for the porcine group.

The results suggest that platelet counts often decline during periods of heparin treatment, but severe thrombocytopenia is relatively rare. It is recommended that platelet counts be obtained at regular intervals (every 3 days) during the course of heparin therapy. An increase in platelet count presumably reflects cessation of platelet consumption and may be considered an indicator of successful therapy.

▶ Both porcine and bovine heparin are implicated in immunologically mediated thrombocytopenia; but in fact, severe thrombocytopenia is rare during heparin administration.

An Endothelial Cell-Dependent Pathway of Coagulation

David Stern, Peter Nawroth, Dean Handley, and Walter Kisiel

Proc. Natl. Acad. Sci. USA 82:2523–2527, April 1985 4–7

The endothelial cell, though considered to be antithrombogenic, recently has been shown to participate in procoagulant reactions. Cultured endothelial cells now have been found to promote activation of the coagulation pathway when factor XI_a is added, leading to activation of factors IX, X, and prothrombin and finally the formation of fibrin strands that are closely associated with the cells. The final step is cleavage of fibrinopeptide A

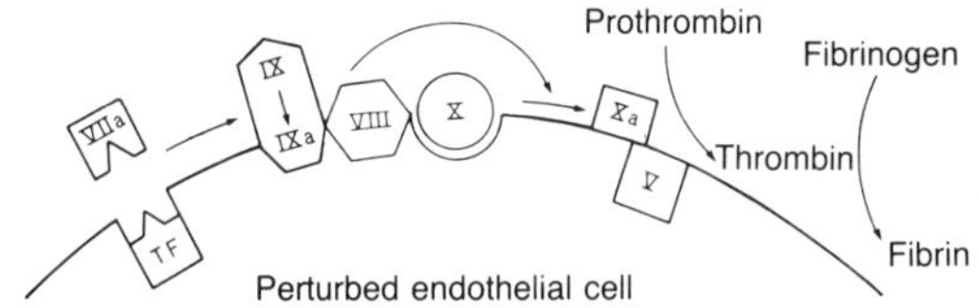

Fig 4–2.—Schematic of endothelial cell procoagulant pathway on surface of a perturbed endothelial cell. *TF,* tissue factor. (Courtesy of Proc. Natl. Acad. Sci. USA 82:2523–2527, April 1985.)

from fibrinogen and fibrin clot formation. In these studies endotoxin-treated endothelial cells from bovine aorta generated fibrinopeptide A in the presence of factors VII_a, IX, VIII, and X and prothrombin and fibrinogen factors. The addition of platelets augmented thrombin formation about 15-fold, as compared with endothelium alone. Anti-human factor V IgG reduced this effect.

It appears that endothelial cells can participate actively in procoagulant reactions when coagulation is initiated with factor XI_a. The reactions may well be involved in generating the baseline levels of thrombin and fibrinopeptide A that are found in vivo. Moreover, the endotoxin-perturbed endothelial cell provides a model of the thrombotic state that involves factor VII_a (Fig 4–2). After factor VII_a activates cell-bound factor IX, cell-associated factors IX_a and VIII can activate factor X and the factor X_a that is formed can interact with endothelial cell factor V, promoting thrombin formation. Thrombin then cleaves fibrinogen, resulting in a fibrin clot. These reactions provide a simple endothelial cell-dependent mechanism for initiation of coagulation at the site of an injured or diseased vessel wall.

5 Miscellaneous Topics

The Effect of Vascular Fellowships on General Surgical Residency Training

Bruce A. Perler and George D. Zuidema (Johns Hopkins Med. Inst.)

Ann. Surg. 200:247–254, September 1984 5–1

Evaluation and treatment of patients with vascular disease form an important part of general surgical training. A study was undertaken to learn whether establishment of vascular fellowships might detract from general surgical training. Questionnaires were sent to directors of 41 approved vascular fellowship programs, 41 residency directors in the same institutions, and 40 residency directors in university programs without approved fellowships.

The overall response rate was 74%; 93% were returned from fellowship directors, 63% from same-institution residency directors, and 65% from residency directors without vascular fellowships. Over the past 10 years, increased volume of case load per resident was more common in fellowship (61%) than in nonfellowship institutions (42%). In institutions with fellowships, general surgical residents performed an average of 71 major vascular operations and first-assisted in 44, whereas residents in nonfellowship institutions performed 65 major vascular operations and assisted in 47; the difference was insignificant. Despite this, 38% of general surgery directors and 34% of fellowship directors indicated that the fellowship reduced the vascular surgery case loads of residents. They observed that the residents participated in 103 major vascular operations as against 124 in institutions that showed no decline in resident case loads. In an overall qualitative assessment of the effect of fellowships, 79% of fellowship directors and 62% of same-institution general surgery directors indicated that the fellowship improved the quality of vascular surgery training. Only 15% of fellowship directors and 3% of same-institution residency directors believed that the fellowship had weakened the residency training. Seventy-one percent of fellowship directors, 85% of same-institution residency directors, and 89% of residency directors in nonfellowship institutions believed that the residents were receiving adequate training in vascular surgery. No fellowship director plans to abolish the program, although 8% plan to reduce the number of fellows to increase general surgery resident participation. Fifteen percent of nonfellowship institutions have begun vascular fellowship programs, and another 23% plan to begin such fellowships.

The data show a significant increase in vascular surgical volume in both fellowship and nonfellowship institutions. It also shows that compared with 1969, when 23% of residents performed major vascular operations, 76% and 79% of fellowship and nonfellowship residents perform an average of 40 major vascular operations during their training. The growth in vascular surgical volume has enhanced the operative experience of residents, though a portion of that benefit may have been lost to the fellows. The fellow's level of operative activity is greater in institutions that reported that the fellowship detracted from the residents' case loads, and this appears to be the reason for the decline in residents' case loads. Despite the opinion that the fellowship has withdrawn cases from the residents the residency directors believe that the fellowship has a positive effect on residents' training. The quality of training is not synonymous with nor determined only by quantity of operations.

Establishment of vascular fellowships has enhanced residency training among most institutions studied.

▶ This presentation at the American Surgical Association Meeting and the commentary made on it indicate that vascular surgery residencies strengthen the experience of general surgery residents in performing vascular surgery. Clearly, the vascular training programs studied did not subtract from the experience of general surgical residents.

The Uses and Abuses of Life-Table Methods in Vascular Surgery

C. J. Underwood, E. B. Faragher, and D. Charlesworth (Manchester, England)

Br. J. Surg. 71:495–498, July 1984 5–2

If graft patency curves are to be of real value, they must be estimated to an acceptable degree of precision. This requires that a study be conducted for a period longer than the time frame of interest to ensure that sufficiently large numbers of patients are followed for that period. However, at any given point along a patency curve, the observed patency rate is not an accurate estimate of the true probability of a graft remaining patent. Because the number of grafts at risk decreases with time through loss to follow-up examination, the efficacy of the patency curve also diminishes. Thus, it is necessary to know, for any curve, at what point even its general shape is no longer informative.

A life-table was calculated from graft patency data for use in vascular research, and the following recommendations were made: Graph patency curves should be presented as step graphs rather than as continuous graphs. Also, the number of patients remaining in a study should be indicated at intervals along the patency curve. The claimed length of follow-up observation should be defined by the point at which the patency curve ceases to be reliable rather than by the patient followed for the longest period of time. When possible, the frequency of patient review, especially in the early stage of a study, should be increased so as to increase the accuracy of the curve. Greater effort should be given to studying larger numbers of patients, even if this entails setting up large multicenter studies. Also, a set of definitive guidelines should be drawn up for presentation of graft patency data to editors of the major vascular journals.

▶ Life-table evaluation of patency is traditional in vascular surgery; but the real flaws in its use are indicated by this article.

Patterns of Atherosclerosis and Their Surgical Significance
Michael E. De Bakey, Gerald M. Lawrie, and Donald H. Glaeser (Baylor College of Medicine)
Ann. Surg. 201:115–131, February 1985 5–3

Previous reports have acknowledged the development of atherosclerosis in distinctive patterns and rates of progression. These characteristic atherosclerotic patterns may be classified according to predominant anatomical site or distribution as (I) the coronary arterial bed, (II) the major branches of the aortic arch, (III) the visceral branches of the abdominal aorta, (IV) the terminal part of the abdominal aorta and its major branches (Fig 5–1), and (V) a combination of two or more of these categories occurring simultaneously. The records of 13,827 patients admitted once or more for treatment of arterial atherosclerotic occlusive disease from 1948 to 1983 were retrospectively analyzed for age, sex, and incidence, time, and patterns of occurrence of a new category, or recurrence within the same category.

Category IV was the most common pattern (42.4%), followed by category I (32.1%); category III was the least common (2.6%). Atheroscle-

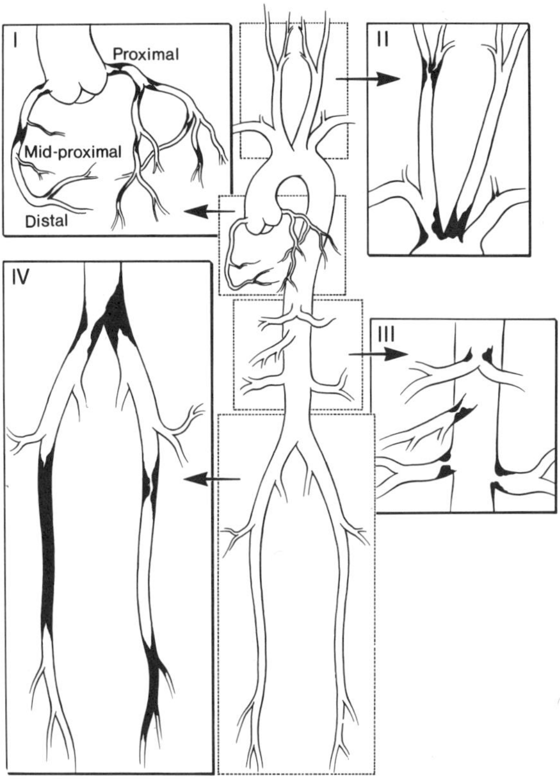

Fig 5–1.—Predominant anatomical sites *(black)* and distribution of atherosclerotic occlusive disease in four major arterial beds. (Courtesy of De Bakey, M.E., et al.: Ann. Surg. 201:115–131, February 1985.)

rotic lesions tended to be segmental, well localized, and usually in the proximal or midproximal portions of the arterial bed; these patterns were amenable to effective surgical treatment directed toward restoration of normal circulation. Less commonly, the arteriosclerotic process occurred predominantly in the distal portion of the arterial bed, making the lesions usually unamenable to effective surgical treatment. Patients in categories I and III were significantly younger than those in other categories. Although men predominated in all categories, significantly more women were in categories II and III. However, female patients behaved like male patients in all aspects of the study. The rates of progression of the disease were classified as rapid (0 to 36 months), moderate (37 to 120 months), and slow (longer than 120 months). The rapid and moderate rates occurred most frequently in categories II and IV and the slow rate in category I. The tendency to development of recurrence in the same category and in a new category was significantly greater in younger patients and was not affected by sex. Patients in category V had the highest probability of developing a new category, whereas those in category I had the lowest probability. Patients originally in category II had a greater tendency to subsequent development of category IV and patients originally in category IV to development of category II.

Patients with atherosclerotic occlusive arterial disease are at risk of development of new or recurrent critical lesions. They require careful and continuing follow-up.

▶ De Bakey has made many contributions to cardiovascular surgery, some of which were technical and others innovative. However, his contribution, with the most fundamental impact, has been the concept of the segmental nature of atherosclerosis. If this concept is accepted, surgeons can treat the several segmental manifestations of the disease as they appear rather than merely accepting the fact that it is as yet an incurable problem. What flows from De Bakey's concept is that each arterial segment produces its own syndrome of symptoms, and each syndrome of symptoms has its own natural history.

Skin Blood Flow Reduction Induced by Cigarette Smoking: Role of Vasopressin

Bernard Waeber, Marie-Denise Schaller, Jürg Nussberger, Jean-Paul Bussien, Karl G. Hofbauer, and Hans R. Brunner (Univ. of Lausanne, Switzerland)
Am. J. Physiol. 247:H895–H901, December 1984 5–4

Cigarette smoking appears to increase the risk of cardiovascular complications. Inhalation of nicotine-containing smoke triggers vasopressin secretion, and this potent vasoconstrictor may act on the coronary arteries. The effects of a vascular arginine vasopressin (AVP) antagonist [$d(CH_2)_5Tyr(Me)AVP$] and its vehicle on blood pressure (BP) and cutaneous blood flow responses to cigarette smoking were examined in 12 healthy men aged 18–46 years, all habitual smokers. The subjects smoked 2 nonfiltered cigarettes, each containing 1.8 mg of nicotine, within a 10-

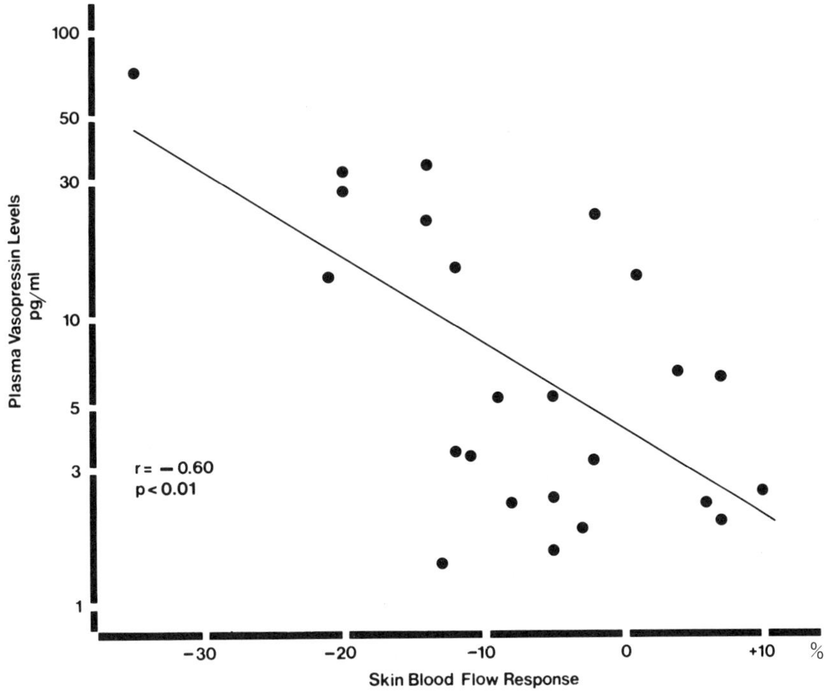

Fig 5–2.—Relationship between skin blood flow response to smoking and plasma vasopressin levels achieved afterward. (Courtesy of Waeber, B., et al.: Am. J. Physiol. 247:H895–H901, December 1984.)

minute period, and afterward received an intravenous injection of 5 μg/kg of the AVP antagonist or physiologic saline.

The plasma AVP level rose from 1.3 to 12.7 pg/ml after smoking, with no change in plasma osmolality. Epinephrine levels increased, but norepinephrine did not change consistently. Blood pressure and heart rate responses to smoking were unchanged by injection of the AVP antagonist, but the smoking-induced reduction in cutaneous blood flow was completely reversed by the anatagonist. The effect of smoking on cutaneous blood flow tended to be greater in subjects with the highest plasma AVP levels (Fig 5–2). Pallor after smoking usually was abolished by the AVP antagonist.

The reduction in cutaneous blood flow induced by smoking appears to be related to stimulation of vasopressin secretion. The effect was prevented by a specific vascular vasopressin antagonist in this study. It seems important to assess the effects of smoke-stimulated vasopressin release on other vascular beds, especially the coronary arteries.

The Magnitude and Nature of the Decrease in Coronary Heart Disease Mortality Rate

Manning Feinleib (Nat'l. Center for Health Statistics, Hyattsville, Md.)
Am. J. Cardiol. 54:2C–6C, Aug. 27, 1984 5–5

Since 1950, the age-adjusted cardiovascular mortality in the United States has fallen by 40%, with most of the decrease taking place in the most recent 16 years. Mortality from other causes has also decreased, but at a rate of 20%. Cardiovascular disease remains the leading cause of death in the United States, but the associated mortality has fallen below 50% and continues to decline. The effects of this decrease are evident in terms of life expectancy. Between 1970 and 1980, life expectancy increased by 2.7 years for white men, 2.5 years for white women, 3.7 years for black men, and 4.0 years for black women. If the mortality remained unchanged between 1968 and 1978, the number of deaths attributable to coronary heart disease (CHD) among persons aged 35–65 years would have been 300,000. In 1978, the rate of CHD deaths was 25% lower than would have been expected based on the 1968 rate. All states report a decrease in CHD deaths, but the extent of this decrease varies by region. Attempts to analyze the reduction in mortality must take into account the incidence, which reflects a change in primary prevention factors, and case fatality, which reflects improvement in the treatment of disease. Although data from various centers concerning the morbidity of cardiovascular disease are conflicting and difficult to interpret, there is some indication of improvement in all major risk factor behaviors in the United States. There also is some evidence that associates improved medical care with reduced CHD mortality. These improvements include advancements in medical and surgical services, the widespread establishment of coronary care units, improved diagnosis and follow-up capabilities, and more sophisticated drug treatments. Improved surgical techniques have probably affected the decrease in cardiovascular mortality. In 1982, some 37,000 heart valves were implanted, as were 171,000 pacemakers; also, 170,000 coronary bypass procedures were performed and almost 500,000 cardiac catheterizations carried out. Although it is clear that the dramatic decrease in cardiac deaths is not a statistical artifact and that this decrease continues, it is important that the actual nature of this decrease be determined and that factors influencing this trend be elucidated.

LESIONS OF THE ARTERIES

6 Aneurysms

Degenerative and Atherosclerotic Aneurysms of the Thoracic Aorta: Determinants of Early and Late Surgical Outcome
Carlos E. Moreno-Cabral, D. Craig Miller, R. Scott Mitchell, Edward B. Stinson, Philip E. Oyer, Stuart W. Jamieson, and Norman E. Shumway (Stanford Univ.)
J. Thorac. Cardiovasc. Surg. 88:1020–1032, December 1984 6–1

Prognostic factors on which to base clinical decisions in cases of thoracic aortic aneurysm are largely uncharacterized. Predictors of mortality were identified by multivariate discriminant analysis in 175 consecutive patients operated on for ascending and descending thoracic aortic aneurysms between 1962 and 1982. Only degenerative and atherosclerotic aneurysms were included in the series. Aortic dissections and traumatic, thoracoabdominal, arch, and false aneurysms were excluded. Ascending aortic aneurysms were present in 124 patients and descending aortic aneurysms in 51. Aortic valve replacement was necessary in 85% of the former. Mean follow-up was nearly 5 years.

Hospital mortality was 6.5% in the group with ascending aortic aneurysms and 18% in the descending group. Half the former deaths were due to myocardial failure and low cardiac output and one third of the latter to generalized sepsis. Cardiac arrhythmias were common in the early postoperative period. Two patients required reoperation for prosthetic valve endocarditis. Major cardiovascular procedures were necessary in 21 patients in all, including 17 in the ascending group. Actuarial survival rates at 5 and 10 years for discharged patients were 79% and 54%, respectively, in the ascending group and 70% and 49% in the descending group. Surgical priority was a determinant of hospital mortality in both groups. Advanced age was also a factor in the ascending group and congestive heart failure in the descending group. Late mortality in the ascending group correlated with advanced age. Both hypertension and preoperative congestive failure were determinants of late mortality in the descending group.

The adverse effects of various factors on late survival after operation for thoracic aortic aneurysm can be combated by earlier referral, an aggressive medical-surgical approach, and close follow-up.

Aneurysm of the Thoracic Aorta: Review of 260 Cases
Virginia Pressler and J. Judson McNamara (Univ of Hawaii)
J. Thorac. Cardiovasc. Surg. 89:50–54, January 1985 6–2

A review of data on 176 thoracic aortic aneurysms in 1980 indicated a 47% incidence of rupture in 135 patients managed without surgical procedure. Another 84 patients now have been added with a current emphasis on surgical treatment. A total of 126 patients have been treated operatively, 67 patients on an emergency basis and 59 patients electively. Half the patients in the series had dissecting aneurysms. Most lesions involved the descending aorta. Mean patient age was 64 years. Patients who had surgical procedure had a mean age of 61 years compared with 70 years for those managed without operation. Both atherosclerosis and hypertension were frequent in this patient population. All 7 patients with Marfan's disease were managed surgically; most had multiple operations.

The operative mortality was 21%, but it was only 8% in patients having elective aortic resection. In the past 5 years operative mortality was 5% in elective cases and 16% in emergency cases. The 5-year survival rate was 50% for electively operated patients, 30% for all surgical patients, and 21% for those who did not have an operation. Patients with dissecting aneurysms were more likely than others to be operated on and more likely to have emergency operation. Five of the 7 patients with Marfan's disease were alive at last follow-up. An abdominal aortic aneurysm was present in 29% of the patients. Only 2% of the patients died of ruptured abdominal aortic aneurysm.

Prompt surgical procedure has improved the outcome for patients with thoracic aortic aneurysm. Abdominal aortic aneurysms are frequent in these patients, and the entire aorta should be evaluated. Operative mortality can be minimized by resecting thoracic aortic aneurysms before they become symptomatic or cause acute problems.

Rigid Intraluminal Prosthesis for Replacement of Thoracic and Abdominal Aorta

Paschal M. Spagna, Gerald M. Lemole, Michael D. Strong, and N. Peter Karmilowicz

Ann. Thorac. Surg. 39:47–52, January 1985 6–3

The results of aortic substitution with a rigid intraluminal prosthesis in 80 patients operated on between 1976 and 1984 are reported. The Bard prosthesis was used in all but the first 5 patients. Indications for the procedure included 32 dissecting aneurysms (18 ascending and 14 descending), 16 atherosclerotic aneurysms of the ascending aorta, 13 atherosclerotic aneurysms of the descending aorta, 3 thoracoabdominal aneurysms, 2 arch aneurysms, and 14 abdominal aortic aneurysms. Mean follow-up was 25 months (range, 1 to 85).

Five deaths occurred in the immediate postoperative period, all among patients with aortic dissection. One of these deaths was the result of uncontrollable intraoperative hemorrhaging from the dissected aorta. Another 4 deaths occurred within 30 days of operation. One patient died of hemorrhage 40 hours after operation, despite two explorations for control. Six of these 9 early deaths occurred in patients older than age 65 years. Early postoperative complications occurred in 6 patients, 4 of whom required reoperation for bleeding. In 1 patient, a spool dislodged on the first postoperative day, requiring reoperation. There were 6 late deaths, 1 occurring 6 months after operation in a patient with empyema. No late complications of thrombosis, erosion, pseudoaneurysm formation, or hemorrhage were encountered. Postoperative angiograms of 20 patients showed normally functioning grafts with no hemodynamic gradients.

The results are extremely encouraging. The authors now use the Bard prosthesis whenever possible in all aortic substitutions. However, in about 40% of the patients it is necessary to remove one spool and suture either the proximal or the distal end of the graft because of the close proximity of the aneurysm to the coronary ostia or the origin of the subclavian artery. With some modifications, it is believed that this technique can soon have wider application.

▶ These reviews of clinical experience provide information about the results of surgical intervention in patients with thoracic aneurysm, but do not define the natural history of the unoperated lesion.

The intraluminal prosthesis is an interesting and increasingly useful device.

Commentary upon this paper, presented at the Twentieth Annual Meeting of the Society of Thoracic Surgeons, emphasized the continuing specter of paraplegia following resection of thoracic aneurysms as noted in the next two articles.

Prevention of Ischemic Spinal Cord Injury Following Aortic Cross-Clamping: Use of Corticosteroids

John C. Laschinger, Joseph N. Cunningham, Jr., Matthew M. Cooper, Karl Krieger, Ira M. Nathan, and Frank C. Spencer

Ann. Thorac. Surg. 38:500–507, November 1984 6–4

The incidence of neurologic injury after aortic cross-clamping for lesions of the thoracic and thoracoabdominal aorta has remained relatively constant at 1% to 14% regardless of the surgical technique or the method of protecting the spinal cord.

Dogs weighing 25 to 30 kg underwent aortic cross-clamping to determine whether ischemic tolerance of the spinal cord can be enhanced pharmacologically by corticosteroids to prevent postoperative paraplegia. Prior to proximal aortic cross-clamping, baseline measurements of spinal cord blood flow and function were obtained. Blood flow was evaluated with radioactive microspheres, and function was determined by assessment of somatosensory evoked potential (SEP).

Group 1 dogs (6) had aortic cross-clamping for 5 minues after complete loss of SEP was documented. Group 2 (9) underwent aortic cross-clamping for 10 minutes after loss of SEP. Group 3 (6) also had aortic cross-clamping for 10 minutes after SEP loss; however, this group was given methyprednisolone intravenously, 30 mg/kg, 10 minutes prior to cross-clamping and 4 hours after operation. After release of the cross-clamp, serial evaluations of spinal cord blood flow and neurologic status were carried out for 7 days.

Group 1 animals recovered uneventfully without neurologic injury. Six of 9 dogs in group 2 (67%) sustained severe postoperative neurologic injury. In contrast, the mcthyprednisolone-treated animals in group 3 demonstrated complete recovery without residual neurologic deficit. Measurements of blood flow in the spinal cord at the time of loss of SEP showed similar degrees of spinal cord ischemia in all groups. There were no significant differences among the three groups in the duration of aortic cross-clamping prior to loss of SEP.

This study indicates that short periods (5 minutes) of proximal aortic cross-clamping are well tolerated, whereas longer periods (10 minutes) are associated with a high incidence of paraplegia. Such injury can be prevented if an adequate dose of methyprednisolone is given before and after cross-clamping. Beneficial effects of steroids do not appear to be related to changes in blood flow of the spinal cord but may be related to the protective effects on cellular and subcellular components. Steroids may markedly reduce the increased intracranial pressure resulting from hypertension proximal to the cross-clamp which is one of the proposed causes of spinal cord ischemia. Clinical investigations with the use of high-dose steroids as an important adjunct in extending the safe period of proximal aortic cross-clamping during operations on the thoracoabdominal aorta appear to be indicated.

Surgical Experience in Descending Thoracic Aneurysmectomy With and Without Adjuncts to Avoid Ischemia

James J. Livesay, Denton A. Cooley, Rogelio A. Ventemiglia, Carlos G. Montero, R. Keith Warrian, David M. Brown, and J. Michael Duncan (Houston)

Ann. Thorac. Surg. 39:37–46, January 1985 6–5

The outcomes of surgical treatment of descending thoracic aneurysms in 360 patients operated on between 1971 and 1983 were reviewed.

Distal aortic perfusion was provided during resection by temporary bypass in 75 patients (group 1) or by shunt in 22 (group 2). Aortic cross-clamping without adjunctive perfusion was used in the other 263 patients during the latter part of the study. The overall survival rate was 88%. Age greater than 70 years, atherosclerotic disease, renal failure requiring dialysis, and the need for an emergency procedure significantly increased the risk of early mortality and morbidity. The use of adjunctive perfusion did not reduce the incidence of death (11.8%), paraplegia (6.5%), or renal failure (6%), and bleeding complications requiring reoperation were significantly increased in groups 1 and 2. The risks of paraplegia and of renal failure were only 3% and 4%, respectively, when the aneurysm was localized to the proximal half of the descending thoracic aorta. However, the incidence of each complication increased to 8% when the aneurysm was localized to the distal portion of the descending thoracic aorta and to 9% and 7%, respectively, when the aneurysm involved the entire descending thoracic aorta. The need for emergency operation and cross-clamping times exceeding 30 minutes also increased the risk of paraplegia. The risk of renal failure was significantly increased by advanced age and atherosclerotic disease. The principal causes of death were hemorrhage, cardiac events, and multiple-organ failure.

With an experienced surgical team, the primary risks of descending thoracic aneurysmectomy are unrelated to the method of adjunctive perfusion, but are related to the patient's age, general health, and nature and extent of the aneurysm.

▶ The final answer on how to prevent postoperative paraplegia has not been uncovered. It seems that the technique of somatosensory evoked potentials is too sensitive to become clinically useful.

Aortic Dissection in Noonan's Syndrome (46 XY Turner)

Neil Shachter, Joseph K. Perloff, and Donald G. Mulder (Univ. of California, Los Angeles)

Am. J. Cardiol. 54:464–465, Aug. 1, 1984 6–6

Dissection of the ascending aorta is an uncommon but established complication of the 45 XO Turner syndrome, but it has not previously been reported in Noonan's syndrome, the Turner phenotype with normal chromosomal constitution. Such a case is described below.

Man, previously healthy but mentally retarded, presented with 24 hours of constant anterior chest pain. He was 160 cm in height and weighed 52.3 kg. Blood pressure was 100/70 mm Hg in both arms, and heart rate was 110 beats per minute. Neck webbing, low posterior hairline, micrognathia, pectus carinatum, low-set ears, and dystrophic nails were noted, as well as cubitus valgus and distal triaxial radius. The testes were small, and a left inguinal herniorraphy scar was noted. Computed tomography and aortographic study showed a type II dissection of the ascending aorta without coarctation. Results of karyotyping were normal. The ascending aorta was replaced with a Dacron graft. Microscopic study showed typical cystic medial necrosis.

Cardiac anomalies in Turner's syndrome include coarctation of the aortic isthmus, bicuspid aortic valve, and ascending aortic dissection. In Noonan's syndrome there may be a dysplastic pulmonic valve, hypertrophic cardiomyopathy and, less often, pulmonary artery stenosis, atrial septal defect, or patent ductus arteriosus. Hemostatic defects were not found in the present patient. Aortic dissection apparently may occur in Noonan's syndrome as well as in Turner's syndrome.

▶ This is an interesting variation on the dissecting aneurysm theme.

MRI of Chronic Posttraumatic False Aneurysms of the Thoracic Aorta

Elizabeth H. Moore, W. Richard Webb, Edward D. Verrier, Courtney Broaddus, Gordon Gamsu, Eugenio Amparo, and Charles B. Higgins (Univ. of California, San Francisco)

AJR 143:1195–1196, December 1984 6–7

Rupture of the thoracic aorta is a fairly common cause of death in deceleration injuries. In a small percentage of cases, the rupture is contained, creating a false aneurysm that may not be detected until months or years later when it is manifest as a mediastinal mass. These chronic false aneurysms most often occur at the level of the ligamentum arteriosum. A case is reported in which magnetic resonance imaging (MRI) was used for diagnosis and postoperative follow-up of a patient with a posttraumatic aortic false aneurysm.

Man, 30, who was asymptomatic, exhibited a middle mediastinal mass on a routine chest film taken 5 years after a motor vehicle accident. Contrast-enhanced transaxial computed tomographic (CT) scans of the chest showed local dilatation of the proximal descending aorta with an apparent septation. Oblique sagittal reformations in the plane of the aortic arch and proximal descending aorta showed a 5-cm enhancing vascular sac resembling a false aneurysm arising from the anterior wall of the proximal descending aorta at the level of the ligamentum arteriosum. Sagittal MRI better defined the location of the false aneurysm, its relation to the left subclavian artery, and the size of its communication with the aorta than did CT reformations, transaxial CT, or transaxial MRI. The absence of a significant magnetic resonance signal from the lumen of the false aneurysm on echo images indicated rapid flow in the false aneurysm. At operation the aortic segment containing the false aneurysm was isolated, and an 18-mm tubular Dacron graft was positioned within the aortic lumen, acting as a stent through the level of the rupture. Part of the false aneurysm was removed and the rest was wrapped around the graft. Repeat sagittal MRI 3 days after operation showed normal flow in the aortic conduit and high signal intensity from clotted blood in the residual false aneurysm sac.

One major advantage of MRI over CT is its ability to produce sagittal and coronal images without degradation of spatial resolution, allowing mediastinal vessels to be imaged along their axes. As observed in a second patient with chronic false aneurysm, the appearance of a direct sagittal

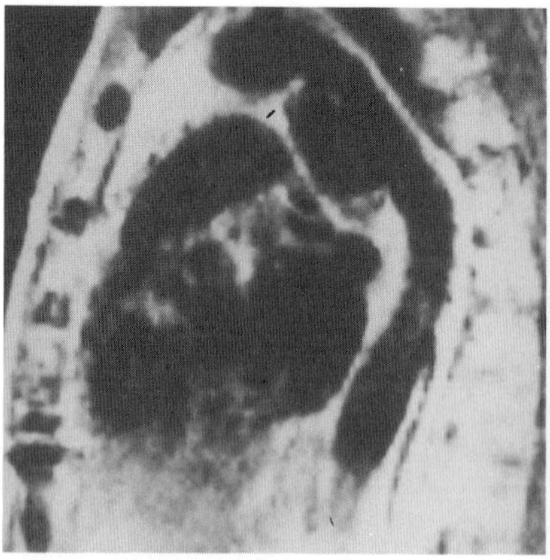
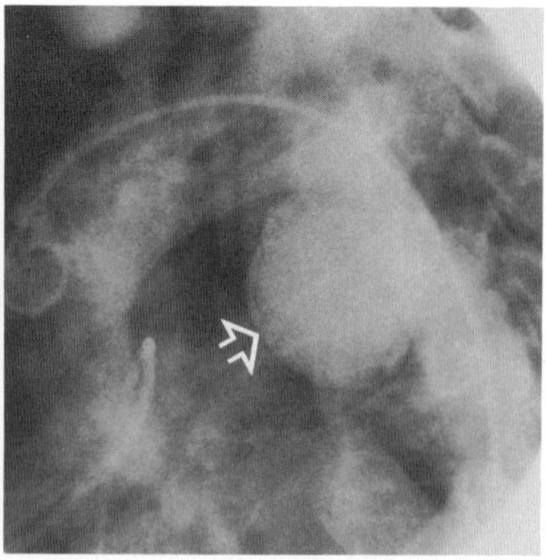

Fig 6–1 (left).—Direct sagittal MRI shows false aneurysm sac and its relation to left subclavian artery. Small area of high signal intensity within sac *(arrow)* may represent clot or wall thickening.

Fig 6–2 (right).—Cineaortogram in left anterior oblique projection in same patient shows rapid filling of false aneurysm sac with calcified rim *(arrow)*.

(Courtesy of Moore, E.H., et al.: AJR 143:1195–1196, December 1984.)

image was similar to that of an aortogram (Figs 6–1 and 6–2). Magnetic resonance imaging also allows, to some extent, evaluation of blood flow. The case described shows that MRI can be used successfully in the preoperative and postoperative evaluation of chronic posttraumatic aortic false aneurysms.

Significance of Symptoms and Signs in Patients With Traumatic Aortic Rupture

James T. Sturm, John F. Perry, Jr., Federick R. Olson, and James J. Cicero
(St. Paul, Minn.,-Ramsey Med. Center)
Ann. Emerg. Med. 13:876–878, October 1984 6–8

The records of 50 patients (40 males), aged 12–80 years, with traumatic aortic rupture (TAR) treated during 1968–1982 (group I) and 50 (39 males), aged 15–81, treated during 1977–1982 (group II) were reviewed. Symptoms and signs referable to chest and thoracic aorta were compared in these groups. In groups I and II, 86% and 84%, respectively, had sustained blunt chest trauma in motor vehicle accidents.

Each patient's chart was evaluated for chest pain, respiratory distress, thoracic back pain, hypotension, hypertension, and decreased femoral pulses. None of the symptoms or signs attained a statistically significant difference between group I and group II. The only significant difference between groups was in the injury severity score (ISS): the mean ISS for aortic rupture patients was 42.1, but was 19.9 for patients without aortic rupture.

The classic presenting symptoms and physical findings of TAR do not occur uniformly. Symptoms and signs of TAR are found with similar frequencies among patients with documented aortic rupture and patients with blunt chest trauma and normal aortograms. The history and physical findings classically associated with aortic rupture are both insensitive and nonspecific. Consequently, the presence or absence of TAR can not be accurately predicted on the basis of symptoms and signs. The only difference between patients with and without aortic rupture was that the former were more severely injured.

Symbas et al., in an analysis of the presenting symptoms and physical findings in 204 patients with ruptured thoracic aorta who survived to undergo operative repair, found that the most common presenting symptoms were chest pain, respiratory distress, and back pain. In contrast to the current study, that analysis revealed a 31% incidence of the acute onset of upper extremity hypertension. The authors, however, found that only 6% of aortic rupture patients had hypertension; arterial hypotension was much more common. The review by Symbas et al. showed a higher incidence of decreased femoral pulse amplitude and systolic cardiac murmers than did the present study. These differences might be explained in part by the fact that the authors' study included all hospitalized patients with aortic rupture, and the review of Symbas et al. was restricted to patients who survived to undergo operation. The infrequent occurrence of the characteristic symptoms and signs of aortic rupture in the present study has also been reported by Applebaum and Kirsh.

The chest x-ray film provides the first suspicion that TAR has occurred. The roentgenographic findings that suggest TAR include distortion of the aortic arch contour, wide mediastinum, opacification of the medial aspect of the left upper lung field, and tracheal shift to the right. These abnormalities also possess low sensitivity and specificity rates. The reported rates of normal aortograms among patients with blunt thoracic trauma vary between 68% and 89%. Besides aortic rupture, other causes of mediastinal widening must be considered when the chest roentgenograms of patients who have sustained blunt thoracic trauma are evaluated.

▶ It is useful to know that the chest x-ray film provides the first suspicion that thoracic aorta rupture has occurred.

The new technique of MRI would not be useful in the acute case, but it may be valuable to see the axial display of mediastinal vascular structures as obtained by a noninvasive technique.

Surgical Treatment of Infected Pseudoaneurysms After Replacement of the Ascending Aorta

Patricia Bakker-de Wekker, Ottavio Alfieri, Freddy Vermeulen, Paul Knaepen, Raf De Geest, and Joseph Defauw (Utrecht, Netherlands)

J. Thorac. Cardiovasc. Surg. 88:447–451, 1984 6–9

A radical approach to infected pseudoaneurysms after replacement of the ascending aorta involves considerable risk and is difficult technically, especially if the coronary arteries have been implanted in the graft. At St. Antonius Hospital a less radical approach combined with local antiseptic irrigation was evaluated in 3 patients with pseudoaneurysms that resulted from infection after replacement of the aortic valve and ascending aorta. The prosthetic material was not entirely removed in any case. Extensive, accurate debridement of the mediastinum was carried out, and the mediastinum was continuously irrigated with 1% povidone-iodine solution for 6 days after operation. Appropriate antibiotic therapy was continued for at least 6 weeks. The entire graft was replaced in 1 case and a part of the graft in the others.

All patients were deteriorating progressively and required urgent operation. All survived surgery and all were in excellent clinical condition 9 to 49 months after operation. The postoperative course of 1 patient was complicated by bronchopneumonia and renal failure. Studies done 8 to 36 months after operation by conventional angiocardiography or digital video-subtraction angiography showed an intact repair in all cases. One patient with Marfan's syndrome had a new dissection of the aortic arch.

Prompt surgery is necessary for infection of a thoracic aortic prosthesis, but expeditious restoration of the circulation and removal of only what seems necessary are preferable to systemic removal and replacement of the entire graft and the prosthetic valve. The prosthetic valve was not replaced in any of the present patients. Extensive debridement of the mediastinum and local antiseptic irrigation are essential. It may prove helpful to use an omental pedicle or a pectoralis major muscle flap around the ascending aortic prosthesis.

Surgery of Thoracoabdominal Aortic Aneurysms

Risto Pokela, Pentti Kärkölä, Matti Tarkka, Matti I. Kairaluoma, and Teuvo K. I. Larmi (Oulu Univ., Oulu, Finland)

Scand. J. Thorac. Cardiovasc. Surg. 18:179–189, 1984 6–10

Eight patients were successfully operated on between 1978 and 1982 for arteriosclerotic aneurysms of the thoracoabdominal aorta. The 6 men and 2 women had a mean age of 59 years. All patients but 1 had associated disease, most often hypertension and compensated congestive heart failure. All but one of the aneurysms produced symptoms; pain in the chest, abdomen, and back and claudication predominated. Two aneurysms ruptured before surgical treatment. One other patient had semielective surgery. A thoracoabdominal incision that split the left side of the diaphragm was made through the eighth intercostal space, using a retroperitoneal route. A temporary aortofemoral shunt was employed. Reattachment was performed in a stepped manner into ready made side-limbs in the woven Dacron graft. One patient in whom a shunt could not be used underwent perfusion cooling of the abdominal organs. Another was saved by autotransfusion.

There were no operative deaths, and no patient was paraplegic after the operation. Reoperation was necessary in 2 cases. Renal function was normal in 6 patients (table); 1 of the exceptions became abnormal preoperatively. Good graft function was the rule. Only 1 patient was symptomatic from thrombosis of a revascularized artery. All patients except 1 who died of lung cancer were doing well 20–60 months after surgery.

Renal Function After Repair of Thoracoabdominal Aortic Aneurysm*

Procedure	Case no.	Shunt time (min) RRA	Shunt time (min) LRA	Renal ischemic time (min) RRA	Renal ischemic time (min) LRA	Highest postoperative s-creatinine (μmol/l)	S-creatinine one month after operation (μmol/l)
Shunt and renal revascularization	1	129	†	30	–	505	Normal
	3	165	90	30	11	189	Normal
	8	55‡	35	55	20	176	117
Cooling and renal revascularization	6§	–	–	35	58	325	134
Shunt without renal revascularization	2	110		–	–	162	Normal
	4	90		–	–	139	Normal
	5	72		–	–	121	Normal
	7	65		–	–	87	Normal

*RRA, right renal artery; and LRA, left renal artery.
†Left renal aplasia.
‡Right renal artery occluded at control angiography.
§Preoperative serum creatinine level, 158 μmol/L (normal range, 50–115 μmol/L).
(Courtesy of Pokela, R., et al.: Scand. J. Thorac. Cardiovasc. Surg. 18:179–189, 1984.)

Thoracoabdominal aortic aneurysms can be treated surgically with acceptable morbidity and mortality figures. A woven Dacron graft with side-limbs for attaching the visceral and renal arteries is used, along with a temporary shunt. Elective surgery is preferred. An unpredictable risk of permanent paraplegia does exist.

Recurrent Aneurysms and Late Vascular Complications Following Repair of Abdominal Aortic Aneurysms

Gunnar Plate, Larry A. Hollier, Peter O'Brien, Peter C. Pairolero, Kenneth J. Cherry, and Francis J. Kazmier (Mayo Clinic)

Arch. Surg. 120:590–594, May 1985 6–11

Recurrences and late complications were analyzed in 1,087 patients who were followed for 6–12 years after repair of abdominal aortic aneurysm between 1970 and 1976. These patients, with a median age of 68 years, represented 98% of all patients having aneurysm repair during this period. About half of the patients had evidence of heart disease, and 40% were hypertensive.

Overall survival was 67.5% at 5 years and 41% at 10 years. Forty-eight late deaths were related to peripheral vascular morbidity. A total of 68 new arterial aneurysms were diagnosed in 59 patients, a median of 5 years after repair of the initial aneurysm. Five dissecting thoracic aneurysms were also diagnosed. Twenty deaths were due to thoracic aortic aneurysm rupture or dissection. Three of 5 patients who underwent thoracoabdominal aneurysms had fatal ruptures. Six of 11 more proximal abdominal aortic aneurysms ruptured fatally. There was 1 fatal rupture of an iliac artery aneurysm. Most femoral artery lesions were pseudoaneurysms occurring at a graft anastomosis. Ten aortoenteric fistulas were diagnosed; only 1 patient survived this complication. Recurrent aneurysm was associated with preoperative hypertension, even when patients with concurrent heart disease were excluded.

Recurrent aneurysm formation and graft complications are significant causes of late morbidity and mortality after abdominal aortic aneurysm repair. Close follow-up of these patients and control of hypertension may lead to better late survival. Elective repair of recurrent aneurysms should be carried out, if feasible, to reduce the risk of rupture and sudden death.

▶ It is refreshing to see the article from Finland on thoracoabdominal aneurysm repair, but one would hope that the side-arm technique reported has now changed to the much easier graft inlay method since this 1978–1982 study.

It has become increasingly obvious that patients surviving abdominal aortic aneurysm resection are at grave risk for formation of other aneurysms. This is consistent with the hypothesis that aortic aneurysms are associated with an as yet unexplained weakening of the arterial wall rather than mere atherosclerosis. The weakening then leads to arteriomegaly, elongation, and tortuosity of affected vessels as is often seen in aneurysm disease.

A Technique for Renal Preservation During Suprarenal Abdominal Aortic Operations

John L. Ochsner, Noel L. Mills, and Philip A. Gardner (Ochsner Clinic and Med. Found., New Orleans)

Surg. Gynecol. Obstet. 159:388–390, October 1984 6–12

Preservation of the renal parenchyma presents a problem unless the kidneys can be reperfused within 20 minutes of warm ischemic time in suprarenal abdominal aortic operations. A simple method of perfusing the kidneys with hypothermic solution to allow safe exclusion of renal blood flow has been used in 29 patients who required suprarenal aortic occlusions in 1975 through 1981.

The perfused solution consisting of 500 ml of lactated Ringer's solution to which 2,500 units of heparin and 100 ml of mannitol have been added is placed in an ice bath and chilled to approximately 4 C. Immediately prior to aortic clamping, a sterile intravenous tube set-up is passed onto the operative field, a 14-gauge Jelco needle is inserted into the aorta in the isolated occluded segment which is to be perfused with 500 ml of the chilled electrolyte solution at a pressure of 150 to 200 mm Hg for a period of approximately 2 minutes. Should the intra-aortic operation take more than 25 minutes, each kidney is reperfused by inserting a no. 5 or no. 8 infant feeding tube into the orifice of the renal artery.

Aortic occlusion of the 29 patients lasted from 10 to 52 minutes. The 1 death resulted from persistent bleeding from the prosthetic graft and hypotension. After operation the levels of blood urea nitrogen (BUN) and creatinine remained at or improved from the preoperative levels in 24 patients. Two patients had elevated levels of BUN due to postoperative prerenal azotemia secondary to congestive heart failure. Two patients had slightly increased levels of creatinine that became normal within a few days.

Hypothermic perfusion of the kidney is based on the principle of decreased renal metabolism with hypothermia. The 7% decrease in metabolism for each degree of decrease (centigrade) in temperature resulted in a highly protective effect in these cases because temperature of the kidneys decreased to less than 20 degrees. Because of the collateral circulation to the kidney, reperfusion of the organ is needed if prolonged periods of renal ischemia are necessary. The authors recommend this technique for preservation of renal function during reconstruction of a renal artery and aneurysmectomy and less frequently for operations involving thoracoabdominal aneurysms that extend down into the renal artery and for operations for visceral ischemia.

Abdominal Aortic Aneurysm in High-Risk Patients: Outcome of Selective Management Based on Size and Expansion Rate

Eugene F. Bernstein and Edmond L. Chan

Ann. Surg. 200:255–263, September 1984 6–13

Low mortality and improved 5-year survival after elective operations on abdominal aortic aneurysms justify an aggressive approach in most patients. However, in patients with associated severe debilitating disease or advanced age, the decision to operate remains a delicate balance of risks and benefits. The authors report the outcome of selective management of high-risk patients with small aneurysms and no symptoms. Ninety-nine high-risk patients with asymptomatic abdominal aortic aneurysms initially measuring 3 to 6 cm in largest transverse diameter were followed for 1 to 9 years (mean, 2.4) with repeat ultrasound studies every 3 months. Relative contraindications to aneurysmectomy included recent myocardial infarction, intractable congestive heart failure, severe pulmonary insufficiency, chronic renal failure, debilitation from cerebral vascular accidents, metastatic malignancy, and advanced age with aneurysm size of less than 5 cm. Elective operations were performed for aneurysmal enlargement greater than 6 cm or the development of symptoms. Operation included intraluminal graft placement and use of technical adjuncts as described by Whittemore et al. Another 11 patients whose aneurysms were initially larger than 6 cm and whose initial evaluation did not result in elective operation were also followed.

Serial echographic measurements showed a mean expansion rate of 0.4 cm per year for aneurysms smaller than 6 cm. Forty-one high-risk patients underwent elective resection, with 2 deaths. Thirty-four patients died of causes unrelated to aneurysms that were not operated on, and 21 patients are without symptoms. Three patients had aneurysm rupture and emergency operations, with 2 deaths. Overall, there were 4 deaths from elective aneurysm operations or rupture in the 99 high-risk patients with small aneurysms. Of the 11 patients with aneurysms larger than 6 cm, 5 underwent elective operations, with 1 death, and 3 had aneurysm rupture and died. The cumulative 5-year survival for these high-risk patients with small aneurysms was 63.7%.

The average expansion rate of 0.4 cm per year should be used only as a general guideline, since the course of individual aneurysms is unpredictable, with intervals of stability and slow and rapid expansion. Serial measurements are necessary to follow patients in whom elective operation is not initially indicated. Both ultrasound and computerized tomographic (CT) scanning offer equal, and essentially perfect, diagnostic capability; however, CT has been the method of choice in this study for it provides superior images in obese patients and is not hindered by intra-abdominal gas or distention. Also, anatomical resolution to 1 mm is frequently possible, and with limited abdominal CT, radiation exposure, time, and expense are minimized. Other pertinent data like the presence of an infected aneurysm are available and often helpful.

A protocol of serial echographic examinations at 3-month intervals permits elective aneurysm operations on high-risk patients with significant or rapid expansion or development of symptoms. It has limited rupture to only 3% and mortality due to rupture or operation to 4%. Further, improved criteria may emerge from recent advances in high-resolution CT.

▶ Bernstein has devised a protocol for managing high-risk patients with abdominal aortic aneurysm and has substantiated his suggestions with his own direct observation. His information is useful, and although the study was carried out with echography, in fact the same observations apply to the use of CT scanning or even lateral films of the abdomen when the aorta can be visualized by this technique. This is an important paper, as is the discussion that complements it.

Abdominal Aortic Aneurysm: The Case for Elective Resection

Allan R. Pasch, John J. Ricotta, Allyn G. May, Richard M. Green, and James E. DeWeese (Univ. of Rochester, N.Y.)

Circulation 70 (Suppl. 1):I-1–I-4, September 1984 6–14

The incidence of ruptured abdominal aortic aneurysms remains high. A review was made of the results of resection of 413 aneurysms in patients operated on during the 8-year period between 1974 and 1982, with special attention to associated costs.

Mortality during the last 2 years of the study period was 3.6%. This compares favorably with a mortality after elective resection of 5.6% in the past 9 years, 8.4% in 1966–1973, and 13% in 1955–1965. The incidence of ruptured abdominal aortic aneurysms also decreased, the rate being 22% in 1955–1965 and 13% in the past 9 years. However, mortality after resection of ruptured aneurysms is unchanged, remaining high at 70%. During 1980 and 1981, 129 aneurysms were resected, of which 20 were ruptured and 109 were resected electively. The total hospital costs were $364,000 for resection of ruptured aneurysms and $1,102,000 for elective resection, with a mean hospital cost of $18,223 and $10,114, respectively, per patient. Ancillary costs averaged $11,282 per patient after rupture, accounting for 62% of the total costs, compared with an average of $5,408 per patient treated electively, which accounted for only 52% of the total hospital costs. Patients operated on for ruptured aneurysm also had a significantly higher average cost per hospital day ($1,139 compared with $632) despite a similar duration of hospitalization. Mortality in 1981 after rupture was 57%, compared with 5% after elective procedures. For patients who survived for at least 24 hours, the mean hospital cost was $27,144 per patient after rupture and $10,114 for one treated electively, the ultimate cost per survivor being $34,369 after rupture and $10,866 after elective resection.

Using 1979 discharge data from hospitals in the United States, and assuming mortality of 5% after elective resection and 50% after aneurysmal rupture, it is estimated that $50 million and more than 2,000 lives could have been saved in 1979 if patients with abdominal aortic aneurysms had been identified and subjected to elective resection. All patients with demonstrated abdominal aortic aneurysms should undergo elective resection unless surgery is contraindicated. Screening of high-risk patients for asymptomatic aneurysms may prove cost effective.

▶ There is much valuable information in this article. Elective resection of aortic aneurysms decreases the number of ruptured aneurysms cared for. Also, the cost per case decreases. The increased rate of survival after surgery is the real bottom line.

Computed Tomography Vs. Aortography for Preoperative Evaluation of Abdominal Aortic Aneurysm

E.-M. Larsson, U. Albrechtsson, and J. T. Christenson (Univ. of Lund, Sweden)

Acta Radiol. (Diagn.) (Stockh.) 25:95–100, 1984 6–15

An attempt was made to learn whether computed tomography (CT) could replace aortography before surgery for patients with abdominal aortic aneurysm. A review was made of the findings in 28 patients having both studies in 1981–1983 before elective aneurysmectomy and aortic reconstruction. The 21 men and 7 women had a mean age of 68 years. The mean interval between the two studies was 3 weeks, and surgery was done an average of 38 days after the last of the examinations. Contrast enhancement was obtained with Isopaque, injected intravenously before each scan.

The upper limit of the aneurysm was correctly evaluated by CT in 25 of the 28 cases, and by aortography in 27. Computed tomography more accurately showed the distance from the upper limit of the aneurysm to the renal arteries. Renal artery stenosis was identified by aortography in 7 cases, and accessory renal arteries were demonstrated in 6 cases. Computed tomography did not show these findings. Both studies accurately showed the lower limit of the aneurysm. In showing the maximum transverse diameter of the aneurysm, CT was more accurate, and it more reliably demonstrated calcifications of the aneurysmal wall. Bleeding into the wall was shown by CT in 2 cases. Digital subtraction angiography provided the same information as aortography.

Computed tomography is recommended in place of aortography for the preoperative evaluation of patients having elective abdominal aortic aneurysm surgery. Aortography is indicated if the CT study shows a very tortuous aorta or if there are signs and symptoms of severe ischemic disease of the lower extremities, or hypertension with evidence of renovascular disease. Digital subtraction angiography may complement CT in the future.

Magnetic Resonance Imaging of Abdominal Aortic Aneurysms

Joseph K. T. Lee, David Ling, Jay P. Heiken, Harvey S. Glazer, Gregorio A. Sicard, William G. Totty, Robert G. Levitt, and William A. Murphy (Washington Univ.)

AJR 143:1197–1202, December 1984 6–16

Magnetic resonance imaging (MRI) was performed in 20 patients seen in 1983 and 1984 with proved abdominal aortic aneurysms. The study was done within 4 weeks of sonography in 15 and within 2½ weeks of computed tomography (CT) in 8. Seven patients had abdominal arteriography. Eight patients had repair of the aortic aneurysm within 6 days of MRI and another was operated on later. A spin-echo (SE) technique was used in all instances. Coronal scans were used in early cases but were then abandoned because the entire abdominal aorta usually could not be imaged on a single slice.

The MRI study correctly predicted the presence and origin of the aortic aneurysm in all patients who were operated on (Figs 6–3 and 6–4). It also accurately showed the status of the iliac arteries. Sonography was equivocal about the status of the iliac arteries in 2 instances. Computed tomography was of limited use in 2 patients who could not receive intravenous contrast medium. Measurements of the aneurysms by MRI and by CT-sonography differed by less than 5 mm in all cases. The MRI study detected aneurysms as small as 2.8 cm in diameter in patients who were not operated on. In only 1 of 9 cases did the MRI and sonographic measurements differ by more than 5 mm. Both arteriographic studies agreed with the MRI findings with regard to the extent of the aneurysm.

Transverse and sagittal MRI is a useful noninvasive means of evaluating abdominal aortic aneurysms. The examination takes less than 30 minutes. The study is more costly than sonography, and patients with aneurysm clips or a pacemaker cannot be examined. Claustrophobic patients may have difficulty with MRI. Sonography is the preferred screening study for patients suspected of having an aortic aneurysm, with MRI reserved for those in whom sonography is unsuccessful or the findings are equivocal.

▶ Much has been learned since the 1981–1983 experience reported here with CT evaluation of aortic aneurysms. Newer scanners give even better images, and information obtained in toto is greater than the information gained from routine aortograms. This has led us to use CT scanning in uncomplicated aortic aneurysm evaluation to the exclusion of aortography. On the other hand,

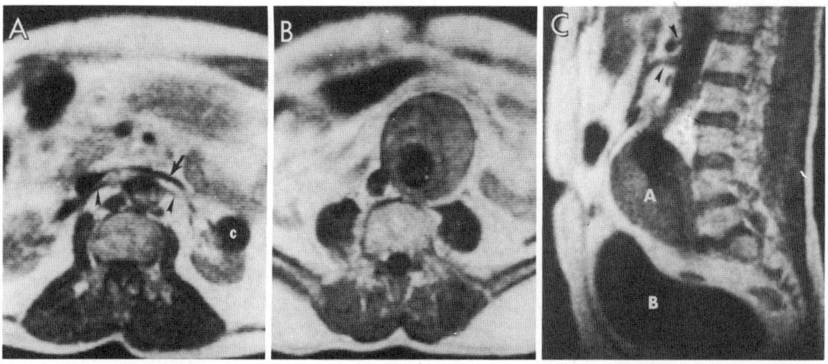

Fig 6–3.—Infrarenal aortic aneurysm. **A,** axial SE 900/30 scan. At level of renal arteries *(arrowheads),* aorta is normal in size. Left renal vein *(arrow)* and left renal cyst *(c)* are shown. Increased signal intensity in posterior aspect of aortic lumen is thought to be secondary to turbulent flow. **B,** axial SE 900/30 scan showing distal aortic aneurysm. **C,** sagittal SE 500/30 scan. Relation of aortic aneurysm *(A)* to origins of celiac and superior mesenteric arteries *(arrowheads)* is seen. *B,* bladder. (Courtesy of Lee, J.K.T., et al.: AJR 143:1197–1202, December 1984.)

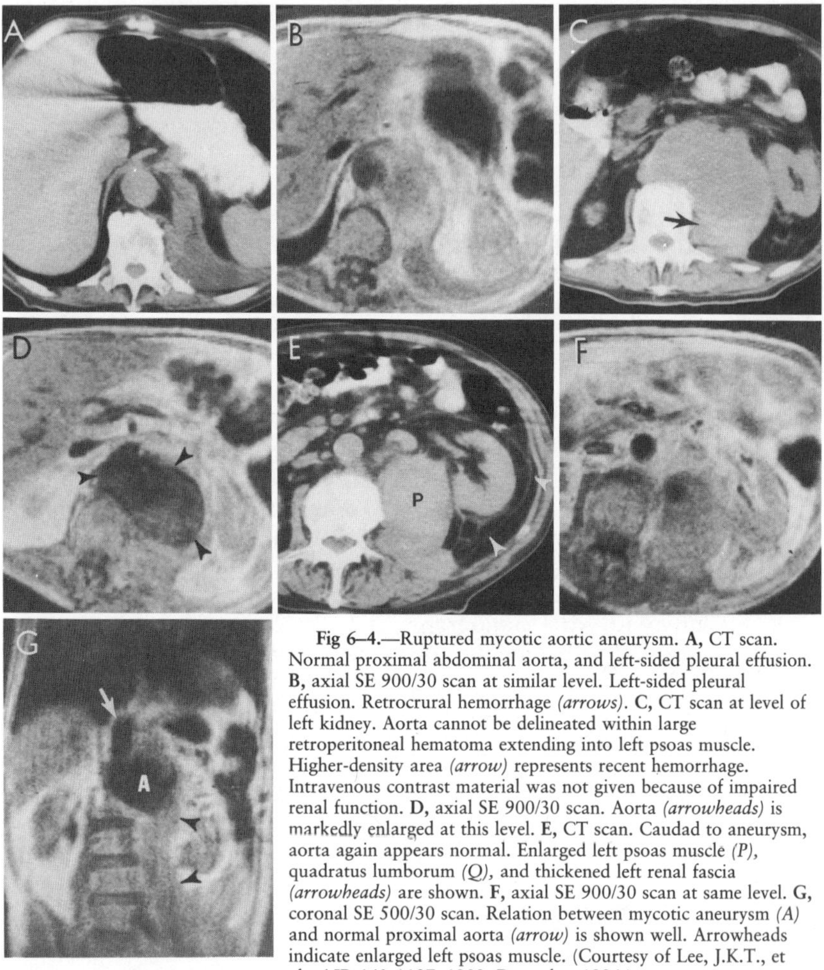

Fig 6–4.—Ruptured mycotic aortic aneurysm. **A,** CT scan. Normal proximal abdominal aorta, and left-sided pleural effusion. **B,** axial SE 900/30 scan at similar level. Left-sided pleural effusion. Retrocrural hemorrhage *(arrows)*. **C,** CT scan at level of left kidney. Aorta cannot be delineated within large retroperitoneal hematoma extending into left psoas muscle. Higher-density area *(arrow)* represents recent hemorrhage. Intravenous contrast material was not given because of impaired renal function. **D,** axial SE 900/30 scan. Aorta *(arrowheads)* is markedly enlarged at this level. **E,** CT scan. Caudad to aneurysm, aorta again appears normal. Enlarged left psoas muscle *(P)*, quadratus lumborum *(Q)*, and thickened left renal fascia *(arrowheads)* are shown. **F,** axial SE 900/30 scan at same level. **G,** coronal SE 500/30 scan. Relation between mycotic aneurysm *(A)* and normal proximal aorta *(arrow)* is shown well. Arrowheads indicate enlarged left psoas muscle. (Courtesy of Lee, J.K.T., et al.: AJR 143:1197–1202, December 1984.)

whenever the situation is complex or if occlusive disease or uncontrolled hypertension is present, an aortogram is mandatory.

Magnetic resonance imaging, on the other hand, is disappointing and can be looked upon as being in the same category today as the earliest CT body scans were some years ago. There may be hope for it in the future if the images improve.

Inflammatory Aneurysms of the Aorta

John L. Crawford, Cary L. Stowe, Hazim J. Safi, Charles H. Hallman, and E. Stanley Crawford (Houston)

J. Vasc. Surg. 2:113–124, January 1985 6–17

Cases of acute "inflammatory aneurysm" of the aorta were encountered in 1957–1984 in 28 men and 2 women, most of whom were older than age 60 years. All smoked heavily. About half were hypertensive and one third had coronary artery disease. All patients had large atherosclerotic aortic aneurysms that were readily palpable in the abdomen.

Aneurysmal disease involved the iliac arteries in 5 cases. Two patients had occlusive renal artery disease. Aortic aneurysmal disease appeared to be the focus of the inflammatory process in all cases (Fig 6–5). In some cases endarteritis involved the vasa vasorum and other vessels running through the aortic adventitia. A coagulum of fibrous and fatty tissue extended for varying distances in the retroperitoneal space. All patients but 2 were symptomatic. Twenty-six had surgery for a leaking aneurysm or impending rupture.

Computed tomography showed anterior and lateral aortic thickening outside a ring of medial or subintimal calcification. Ultrasonography showed a sonolucent halo surrounding the aneurysm.

Surgery consisted of inserting a graft from within the aneurysm. The aorta was clamped below the renal arteries in 13 patients, at the diaphragm in 11, and in the chest in 6. Mean clamp times were 43 minutes or less. One patient died after operation from myocardial infarction. Two patients with initially impaired renal function required hemodialysis, one of them permanently. Twenty of 29 who survived operation were alive at follow-up for a mean of 3 years. Signs of ureteral obstruction and hydronephrosis resolved without treatment in 3 cases. No patient had recurrent ureteral obstruction or other signs of retroperitoneal fibrosis during follow-up.

The cause of inflammatory aneurysmal disease is not known, but the aneurysm appears to be the initiating factor in the inflammatory process.

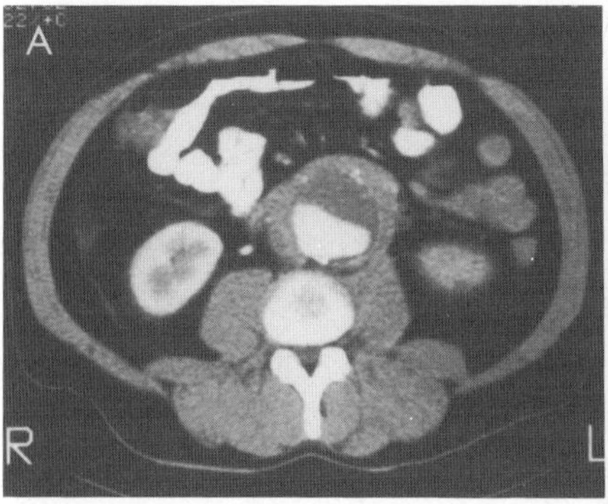

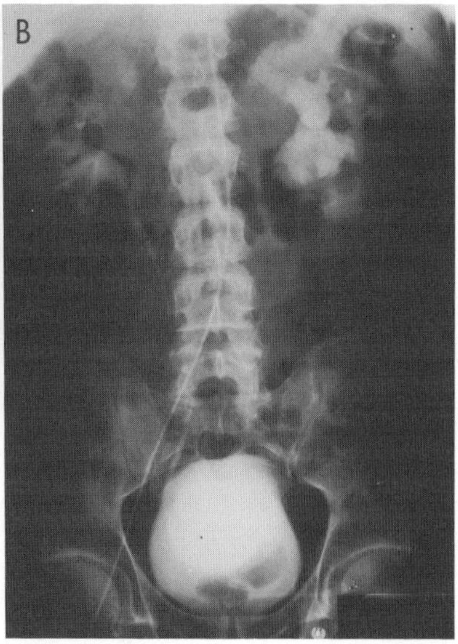

Fig 6–5.—Patient with inflammatory infrarenal abdominal aortic aneurysm. **A,** computed tomography scan shows typical appearance of inflammatory aneurysm with thickened anterior and lateral walls exterior to line of calcification in media and ureteral entrapment but thin or absent posterior wall. **B,** excretory urogram shows mild ureteral obstruction and hydronephrosis. (Courtesy of Crawford, J.L., et al.: J. Vasc. Surg. 2:113–124, January 1985.)

Both CT and ultrasonography aid in the precise diagnosis of this disorder. Early graft insertion is the preferred method of treatment. Steroid therapy may be used temporarily to relieve systemic symptoms and facilitate the treatment of severe bilateral ureteral obstruction and uremia. Steroid therapy alone should be restricted to patients with advanced associated disease that makes surgery too hazardous.

So-called Inflammatory Aneurysm of the Abdominal Aorta
Von E. Gmelin, E. Burmester, A. Valesky, and H.-D. Weiss
ROFO 141:56–60, July 1984 6–18

The authors described computer tomographic (CT) appearances of 4 patients with inflammatory aneurysm of the abdominal aorta accompanied by a retroperitoneal fibrosis. In 1972 some authors found excessive thickening of the aneurysmic wall.

Computer tomography shows, in addition to the typical changes due to an aortic aneurysm, horseshoe shaped, circular, homogeneous perianeurysmic masses (Fig 6–6), which enhance after intravenous contrast. On the basis of different etiologic explanations, several terms of retroperitoneal fibrosis were suggested: inflammatory aneurysm of the abdominal aorta, secondary retroperitoneal fibrosis of the aneurysm of the abdominal aorta, periaortic fibrosis, perianeurysmic retroperitoneal fibrosis, and inflammatory variant of the abdominal aortic aneurysm. It is thought that inflammatory infiltrates in the adventitia and differently marked fibroformations could be found in all abdominal aortic aneurysms. Therefore, this is not an independent disease but a special form of an arteriosclerotically contingent aneurysm with a special tendency to fibroformation. This belief is supported by the fact that no traceable fibrinogen is found in these fibrous structures. The frequency of inflammatory conditions among all

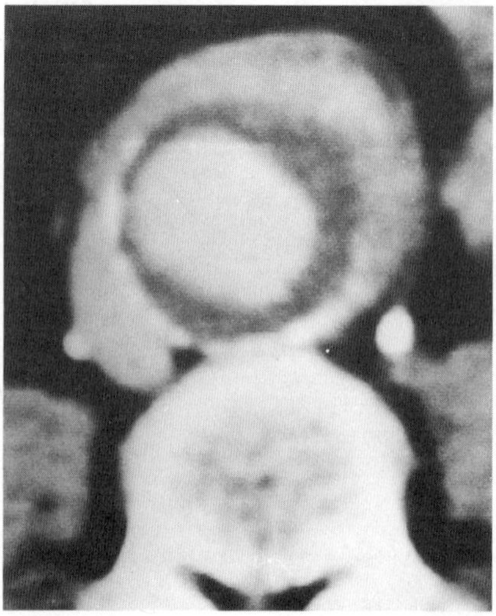

Fig 6–6.—Preoperative CT of inflammatory aneurysm of the abdominal aorta with cocardiform picture at the circular periaortic fibrosis. (Courtesy of Gmelin, V.E., et al.: ROFO 141:56–60, July 1984.)

aneurysms of the abdominal aorta fluctuates between 5% and 15%. The authors found 4 in 80 (5%) CT scans. The extent of the fibrosis and involvement of bordering organs corresponds with the primary retroperitoneal fibrosis. Ureter stenoses with medial deviation of ureters as well as stenoses of the inferior vena are described most frequently. The clinical symptoms varied with simultaneous phenomena; however, all patients complained of back pain for weeks or months. Bolus injection of contrast is necessary in order to differentiate the periaortic soft tissue formation from a dissection or retroperitoneal lymphoma. Distinction between these conditions is possible as a result of the various types of enhancement that occur in the aortic lumen, fibrosis, and lymphoma.

Treatment of choice consists of implanting a vascular prosthesis under fibrotic masses. Computer tomographic controls several months postoperatively document that fibrotic tissue disappears after successful operation.

▶ The search continues for the cause of the dense fibrofatty tissue infiltrate that surrounds some aortic aneurysms. The condition is inseparable from retroperitoneal fibrosis, formerly described by Urban as a cause of ureteral obstruction. It may also be linked to fibrinous mediastinitis, which has an identical appearance.

Computed tomography scanning of aortic aneurysms reveals the dense inflammatory process and alerts the surgeon to difficulties to be encountered in surgery, making yet another argument for use of CT prior to aneurysm resection.

It is interesting that patients become asymptomatic after surgery and that in Crawford's experience, ureterolysis was not required. Not all would agree, but it is fascinating that these two papers, from such different parts of the world, both conclude that the aneurysm appears to be the initiating factor in the inflammatory process. The lack of aneurysm formation in the many cases presenting to urologists would be contrary evidence to this hypothesis.

Renal Complications to Left Renal Vein Ligation in Abdominal Aortic Surgery

Jonas Rastad, Bo. Almgren, Staffan Bowald, Ingvar Eriksson, and Bengt Lundquist (Univ. of Uppsala)

J. Cardiovasc. Surg. 25:432–436, Sept.–Oct. 1984 6–19

Renal complications may be more frequent than previously recognized after left renal vein ligation to gain access to the proximal part of the abdominal aorta. The left renal vein was ligated in 31 of 579 patients undergoing operations for aneurysm or occlusive disease of the abdominal aorta between 1975 and 1982. Eighteen patients had a nonruptured aneurysm, 11 had a ruptured aneurysm, and 2 had occlusive disease. Mean age was 67 years. The vein was reconstructed by direct anastomosis in 3 patients. The left spermatic or adrenal veins were also ligated in 2 patients. Five of 17 patients in whom the renal arteries or suprarenal part of the aorta were clamped had in situ perfusion with cold Perfadex; mean time of warm renal ischemia in the other 12 was 19 minutes. Ten patients were in hypovolemic shock just before, during, or shortly after operation.

No death was directly attributed to division of the left renal vein. The serum creatinine concentration consistently increased, but this was transient in all but 6 cases. The increase was especially marked in patients in hypovolemic shock, but not in those with renal ischemia from clamping. Ten patients (32%) had permanent renal damage. Three of these patients had had clamping of the suprarenal part of the aorta, and 1 of them developed hypovolemic shock. Two patients required left nephrectomy because of massive bleeding from the renal capsule and parenchyma. Seven patients had transient macroscopic hematuria. Patients in whom the left renal vein was resutured did not develop permanent renal damage. Renal complications were infrequent in the 25 control patients who did not undergo division of the left renal vein.

Ligation of the left renal vein during abdominal aortic operations increases the risk of postoperative renal complications, and its use should be restricted. The procedure may be contraindicated in patients with no right kidney or with reduced renal function, and it should be considered with great caution in patients with ruptured aneurysm. Reanastomosis should be considered after intentional or inadvertent division of the vessel.

▶ Although there are flaws in this paper as a study, the observations are of value to all surgeons who operate on the aorta. A decision to divide the renal vein should not be taken lightly whether or not the aorta is to be clamped above the renal arteries. One would wish that the authors had divided the cases into those in which the renal vein was compressed by a large aneurysm and those not compressed at all. But perhaps this will be material for another study.

Significance of Positive Bacterial Cultures From Aortic Aneurysm Contents

J. A. C. Buckels, J. W. L. Fielding, J. Black, F. Ashton, and G. Slaney (Birmingham, England)

Br. J. Surg. 72:440–442, June 1985 6–20

Identification of sources of contamination and infection of vascular prostheses is important in avoiding the serious consequences of aortic graft sepsis. Aneurysm contents were cultured in 275 patients, who were among 546 undergoing infrarenal aortic aneurysm repair between 1961 and 1981. Either part of the intramural thrombus or a swab of the aneurysm wall was cultured immediately after the aneurysmal sac was opened. Aortic reconstruction was done by an inlay method, initially with Teflon and later with Dacron prostheses. Extra-anatomical bypass was done in 2 patients with primary aortoduodenal fistulas and 1 with operative findings suggesting an infected aneurysm.

Bacteria were cultured in 22 cases (8%). The incidences were 4% in

BACTERIA CULTURED RELATED TO TYPE OF ANEURYSM

Bacteria cultured	Elective	Acute	Ruptured	Total
Micrococus	5	–	2	7
S. aureus	–	2	3	5
E. coli	–	2	1	3
Alpha haemolytic streptococci	1	–	2	3
Proteus	1	–	1	2
Pneumococcus	–	–	1	1
Bacillus anitratum (Acinetobacter)	–	–	1	1
Salmonella indiana	–	–	1	1
Totals	7	4	12*	23*

*One culture grew 2 organisms.

(Courtesy of Buckels, J.A.C., et al.: Br. J. Surg. 72:440–442, June 1985. By permission of the publishers, Butterworth & Co., Ltd.)

elective cases, 9% in acute cases, and 17% in cases of rupture. The organisms isolated are shown in the table. Gram-positive organisms, especially *Micrococcus,* predominated. Organisms were sensitive in vitro to the antibiotics given prophylactically in 11 of 14 evaluable cases. Thirteen patients had graft sepsis. Seven of these patients had positive cultures of aneurysm contents. One infection developed 6 years after operation; the mean interval in the other cases was 37 days. Culture-negative infections occurred a mean of 13 months after operation. Only 1 patient with an infected graft survived.

Routine culture of the contents of aortic aneurysms is suggested to identify patients at high risk of graft sepsis. Those with positive cultures can be given prolonged organism-specific antibiotic therapy. Preoperative antibiotic therapy may eliminate organisms from aneurysms and reduce the risk of graft sepsis.

Acute Gastrointestinal Complications of Infrarenal Aortic Aneurysm Repair

M. Crowson, J. W. L. Fielding, J. Black, F. Ashton, and G. Slaney (Queen Elizabeth Hosp., Birmingham, England)
Br. J. Surg. 71:825–828, November 1984 6–21

Resection of an infrarenal aortic aneurysm may compromise the blood supply of the gastrointestinal tract. Early gastrointestinal complications associated with 472 aortic aneurysmectomies are reviewed.

Acute gastrointestinal complications developed in 31 (6.6%) patients after aortic aneurysmectomy. Such complications occurred in 19 of 174 patients with ruptured aneurysms (10.9%), 9 of 222 patients who underwent elective aneurysmectomy (4.1%), and in 2 of 72 patients with acute aneurysmectomies (2.7%). Complications included ischemic intestine in 9 patients, mechanical or paralytic ileus in 8, peptic ulceration in 7, undiagnosed gastrointestinal bleeding in 5, and paraprosthetic fistula in 2. All

7 patients with peptic ulcer complications had ruptured aneurysms. The risk of developing complications with a peptic ulcer was not significantly increased in patients with a previous history of peptic ulcer disease.

Five of 418 patients with no previous history of peptic ulceration (1.2%) developed postoperative complications, which were associated with a high mortality (80%). All 9 patients who developed ischemic bowel died. Gangrene developed in the distribution of the superior mesenteric artery in 2 patients, the inferior mesenteric artery in 6, and in both arteries in 1. The risk of developing an ischemic intestine was increased if the distal limb of a prosthesis was anastomosed directly to the external iliac artery. Overall, 21 patients died (67.7%) of acute gastrointestinal complications and accounted for 19.4% of total mortality. Thirty-three percent of mortality associated with gastrointestinal complications occurred with elective resection of an aneurysm, 18.9% occurred with ruptured aneurysm, and 7.1% followed acute aneurysmectomies.

The incidence of acute gastrointestinal complications after repair of an infrarenal aortic aneurysm was much higher in the group with ruptured aneurysms; however, these complications also accounted for 33.3% of mortality in patients who underwent elective aneurysmectomy.

All complications of peptic ulcer disease occurred in patients who had repair of ruptured aortic aneurysms, demonstrating the need for immediate and aggressive therapy. In patients noted to have active ulceration at the time of aneurysm resection, it would seem appropriate to undertake a definitive operation such as a vagotomy and pyloroplasty or, if time allows, a highly selective vagotomy to reduce the risk of contamination of the prosthesis. Endoscopy should establish the diagnosis in patients who bleed after operation and who should be treated aggressively by either operation or endoscopic coagulation.

Ischemic colitis can be due to an atherosclerotic coeliac axis and superior mesenteric artery which are further compromised by dividing the inferior mesenteric artery. This can be avoided by preoperative angiographic study to note the adequacy of the intestinal vessels or, if not appropriate, the patency of the major gut vessels should be insured at the time of resection. If bifurcated grafts inlaid with the distal limb are placed end to end onto the external iliac artery after ligation of the internal iliac artery, the inferior mesenteric artery or one or both of the internal iliac arteries should be included in the circuit. If the common iliac arteries are unsuitable for anastomosis, then (after closure of the distal ends) the graft limb can be anastomosed to the femoral arteries, thus providing retrograde flow through the internal iliac arteries.

▶ The Birmingham Study quite convincingly links positive cultures from aortic aneurysm contents to subsequent graft sepsis. It does so with a larger number of positive cultures than have been reported in other similar studies. The manuscript also reports a higher incidence of graft sepsis than is usual in reports from North America and reports sepsis in all 4 cases of primary aortoduodenal fistulas, two of which developed graft infection and died. Perhaps Sir Geoffrey is right: Contents of all aortic aneurysms should be cultured, and those with a positive culture should be given prolonged organism-specific antibiotic therapy.

Also from the Queen Elizabeth Hospital is this detailed study of gastrointestinal complications after aortic surgery that emphasizes, once again, that internal iliac artery revascularization is important in reconstructing the arterial stream after aortic aneurysm exclusion.

Primary Aortoduodenal Fistula: Manifestation, Diagnosis, and Treatment

Michael S. Sweeney and Thomas R. Gadacz (Baltimore)

Surgery 98:492–497, September 1984 6–22

Primary aortoduodenal fistulas can be particularly lethal, primarily because of their subtle manifestations, which lead to delays in diagnosis. Data are presented on a case of primary aortoenteric fistula that was successfully repaired. There is also a review of data on 118 cases of primary aortoduodenal fistula that have been reported in the world literature.

Man, 66, presented with a 10-hour history of weakness and melena. An episode of hematemesis in the emergency room prompted admission, at which time he was noted to have orthostatic hypotension and a hematocrit value of 33%. Both en-

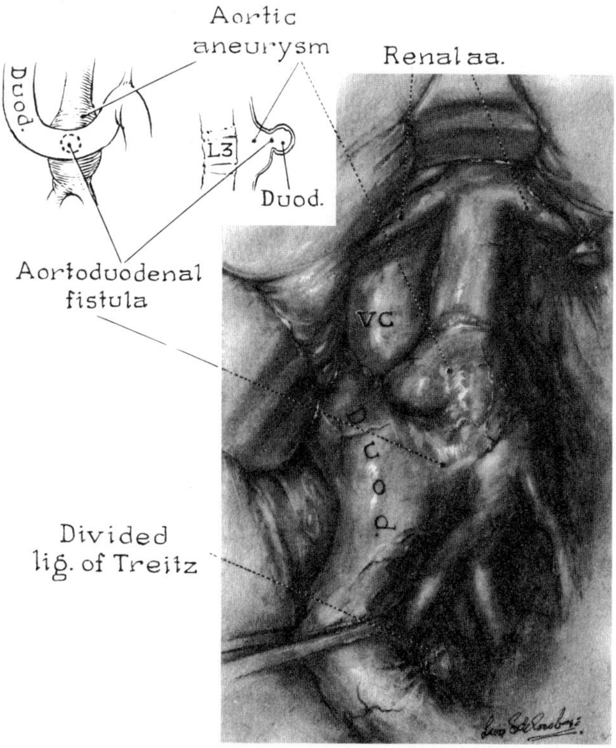

Fig 6–7.—Schematic drawing of operative findings in patient aged 66 years. (Courtesy of Sweeney, M.S., and Gadacz, T.R.: Surgery 98:492–497, September 1984.)

doscopy and flexible sigmoidoscopy failed to confirm a source of the bleeding. About 18 hours after restoration of normal hemodynamic status, he had another episode of massive hematemesis. Again, endoscopy failed to identify a source of bleeding. At laparotomy a pyloromyotomy showed the area of bleeding to be below the proximal duodenum. Closer examination revealed a fistula between the third portion of the duodenum and a 4 cm aorta aneurysm (Fig 6–7). After proximal control of the aorta was established, the fistula was dissected and the duodenal defect was closed with 2 layers of polypropylene suture. The aneurysm was then resected and a knitted Dacron tube graft was inserted. Cultures of the aneurysm wall were negative. The patient is doing well 2½ years after operation.

Symptoms that have been associated with primary aortoduodenal fistulas include flank pain, abdominal pain, hematemesis, melena, and abdominal mass. However, the triad of pain, hemorrhage, and a pulsatile mass is rarely encountered. Review of the 118 cases indicated that 32% of patients had some form of pain and fewer than 25% had a palpable abdominal mass before diagnosis or death. Hematemesis, with or without melena, as an initial symptom was present in only 64% of patients. Although it was an initial symptom in less than 5% of cases, "herald bleeding" followed by hypovolemic shock is an important finding. Routine abdominal films, barium studies, and endoscopy have not been effective diagnostic aids.

Only 33 of the 118 patients were operated on and only 21 of the 33 have survived operation. In 3 unique cases aneurysmorrhaphy was possible; in the other 18 operative success involved primary repair of the duodenal rent and replacement of the diseased aorta with an in situ Dacron graft. Because most patients undergo operation on an emergency basis, the latter operative approach is recommended as the standard treatment for primary aortoduodenal fistulas.

▶ It is important to differentiate between primary and secondary aortoduodenal fistulas when discussing these entities. The more favorable nature of the primary fistula has been referred to by Ernst (Daugherty, M., et al.: *J. Surg.* 86:399, 1979) and is emphasized in this abstract as well. However, the negative culture from the contents of the aneurysm in the present case differs from the findings of Slaney's group reported earlier. Undoubtedly, CT study of the abdomen would have revealed the aneurysm in this case and probably would have made the diagnosis of communication of the aneurysm and duodenum.

Aortic Aneurysm Secondary to Umbilical Artery Catheterization

P. W. Brill, P. Winchester, A. R. Levin, A. Y. Griffith, E. Kazam, and K. Zirinsky (New York Hosp.–Cornell Med. Center)

Pediatr. Radiol. 15:199–201, March 1985 6–23

Thirteen cases of aortic aneurysm complicating umbilical artery catheterization have been reported in the English language literature since 1970.

Previous staphylococcal sepsis is a consistent feature. A catheter-related thoracoabdominal aortic aneurysm was diagnosed by dynamic computed tomography (CT) and ultrasonography and successfully resected.

Girl, aged 14 months, was found to have a retrocardiac mass on chest roentgenography for respiratory infection. She had been born prematurely and had been in neonatal intensive care for 4 months with hyaline membrane disease, patent ductus, and bronchopulmonary dysplasia. Tracheal stenosis had resulted from prolonged intubation. An umbilical artery catheter had been in place for the first 2½ weeks of life, with its tip in the thoracic aorta at the T9–T10 level. Sepsis due to *Staphylococcus aureus* developed at 2½ weeks. The catheter was removed and intravenous methicillin given. Hypertension developed at age 5 weeks, and infarction of the right kidney secondary to catheter-related thrombosis was diagnosed. A vascular mass in the lower thoracic aorta was found on radionuclide scanning but recognized only in retrospect. Hypertension responded to hydralazine. Lung densities were attributed to bronchopulmonary dysplasia. Contrast CT demonstrated an aneurysm of the lower thoracic and upper abdominal aorta. Real-time ultrasonography and aortography confirmed the presence of a large saccular aneurysm, which was resected. The histologic findings were consistent with a healed mycotic aneurysm. No thrombus was present.

Aortic aneurysm formation secondary to umbilical artery catheterization is probably related to both localized trauma and infection. The absence of pulsations on real-time ultrasonography does not exclude a vascular mass. Radionuclide angiography with early static blood-pool imaging is a useful screening measure for infants at risk.

▶ Did you know that this condition occurred? We did not. The fact that an aneurysm can develop in an area of aortic wall infection with healing is important in understanding genesis of aneurysm. It fits with the hypothesis expressed by Zarins and Glagov. (Zarins, C. K., and Glagov, S.: *Aneurysms and Obstructive Plaques.* In Bergan, J., and Yao, J. *Aneurysms.* Grune and Stratton, New York, 1982).

Abdominal Aortic Aneurysms in Western Australia: Descriptive Epidemiology and Patterns of Rupture

W. M. Castleden, J. C. Mercer, and the Members of the West Australian Vascular Service (Nedlands, Australia)

Br. J. Surg. 72:109–112, February 1985 6–24

An 11-year review of abdominal aortic aneurysms was carried out in the geographically isolated population of Western Australia. All aneurysms presenting to hospitals and coroners between 1971 and 1981 were reviewed. Age and sex standardization of the 1,237 cases indicated that the prevalence increased during this period from 75 to 117 cases per 100,000 for men older than age 55 years, a rise of 57%, and from 17.5 to 34/100,000 for women of this age, a rise of 94%. A total of 123 autopsy cases were seen after sudden death from ruptured, undiagnosed aneurysm.

Elective resection was done in 225 cases, with a mortality of 4%, and emergency surgery in 253, with a mortality of 31%. The number of coroner cases of rupture declined during the review period. Both coroner cases and emergency admissions were more prevalent in the winter.

The hospital diagnosis of abdominal aortic aneurysm has increased rapidly from 1971 to 1981. Operation rates have increased faster than rates of diagnosis, but it is not clear that the increase in elective operations has consistently reduced the number of patients seen as emergencies for aneurysm operations. Only 53% of diagnosed males and 35% of females had surgical repair of their aneurysms in the last 2 years of the study. Temperature-related changes in blood pressure may partly explain the increase in aneurysm ruptures seen in the winter. It is uncertain whether abdominal aortic aneurysm is becoming more frequent, or whether it is being diagnosed better than in the past.

▶ Evidence is accumulating that abdominal aortic aneurysms are being seen with increased frequency, and this fact is not due simply to better methods of diagnosis. If this observation is accepted as a fact, then environmental factors may be important as suggested in this article. Perhaps the explanation is simple inhalation of cigarette smoke. Another observation is that, with increasing degrees of medical sophistication, ruptured aortic aneurysms are seen less frequently because elective operations are more often done. This had not occurred in Western Australia, where more than one half of aortic aneurysms encountered were those that ruptured.

Influence of the Rupture Site of Abdominal Aortic Aneurysms With Regard to Postoperative Survival Rate

S. Miani, P. Mingazzini, R. Piglionica, G. M. Biasi, and U. Ruberti (Univ. of Milan)

J. Cardiovasc. Surg. 25:414–419, Sept.–Oct. 1984 6–25

Mortality from ruptured abdominal aortic aneurysm still carries a mortality of about 50% despite substantial surgical experience. The influence of the site of rupture on postoperative survival was examined in a series of 226 patients with rupture of an abdominal aortic aneurysm who were operated on between 1965 and 1982. Males consistuted 89% of the series. Mortality was 53% in 193 cases of retroperitoneal rupture; 75% in 16 cases of intraperitoneal rupture, 38% in 13 cases of rupture into the vena cava, and 50% in 4 cases of enteric rupture. Overall mortality was 53.5%. Mortalities were 68% when renal insufficiency was present at operation and 56% when renal shutdown followed operation. Mortality increased with both advancing age and the need for blood.

Retroperitoneal rupture of abdominal aortic aneurysms carries a high mortality, chiefly because of postoperative renal shutdown. Renal function may be compromised by atheromatous embolization, sudden pressure changes, and hemoglobinuria in these cases. The even higher mortality associated with rupture into the peritoneal cavity is related to a sudden fall in pressure leading to irreversible shock. A significant number of aneurysms rupture into the inferior vena cava, producing a high-flow arteriovenous fistula. Reduced renal function resulting from the shunt, heart failure, and increased renal venous pressure constitute a secondary cause of death in these cases. The risk of a secondary aortoenteric fistula persists even after successful reconstructive operation.

Postoperative survival of patients with ruptured abdominal aortic aneurysms is related to the site of rupture.

Perianal Hematoma: An Unusual Feature of a Leaking Aortic Aneurysm

R. M. Antrum (Gen'l. Infirm., Leeds, England)

Br. J. Surg. 71:649, August 1984 6–26

The diagnosis of a ruptured aortic aneurysm can be difficult. A case is described in which a perianal hematoma was a physical manifestation of a leaking aortic aneurysm.

Man, 73, presented with acute abdominal pain that radiated through to the back. He was in shock, had impalpable femoral pulses, and had a tender aortic aneurysm. His perineum exhibited a tense, bulging, dark blue perianal hematoma with peau d'orange, which was discovered 2½ hours after the onset of symptoms. Laparotomy revealed an infra-renal aneurysm, 8 cm in diameter, that extended into both the internal and external iliac arteries. An extensive retroperitoneal hematoma, prominent on the left side, was observed, with obvious extension under the sigmoid mesentery into the pelvis. There was a small amount of free intraperitoneal blood. The aneurysm was observed to have ruptured posteriorly, just above the sigmoid mesentery. The aorta was controlled proximally and the aneurysmal involvement of the iliac arteries was managed by oversewing and ligating both common femoral arteries. A Dacron mesh graft was then inserted from below

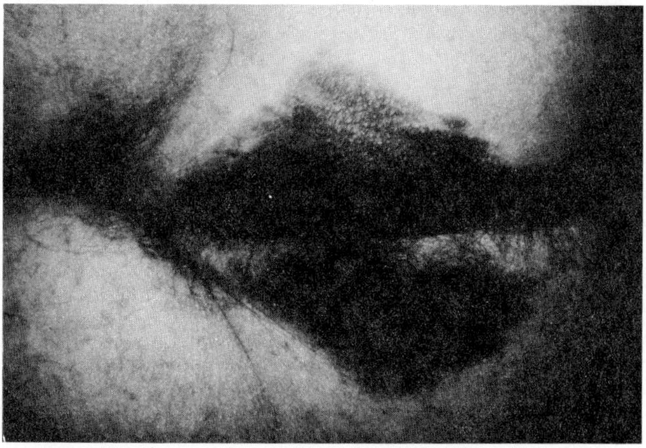

Fig 6–8.—Diamond-shaped perianal hematoma, 6 × 7 cm, day after admission to hospital. (Courtesy of Antrum, R.M.: Br. J. Surg. 71:649, August 1984. By permission of the publishers, Butterworth & Co., Ltd.)

the renal arteries to both common femoral arteries with end-to-end anastomoses. The hematoma had developed into a diamond-shaped lesion by the following day (Fig 6–8) and gradually disappeared over the next 30 days. The patient made a good recovery and has not been affected by the loss of both internal iliac arteries.

Accessory physical signs may be helpful in the diagnosis of a ruptured aortic aneurysm. Superficial bruising is seen occasionally in acute cases, but it is more likely to be present in patients who make an apparently satisfactory recovery after an acute extraperitoneal leak. Perianal hematoma as a physical manifestation of acute rupture of an aneurysm is rare and is caused by extraperitoneal rupture of the aneurysmal sac into the sigmoid mesocolon. The resulting hematoma then extends into Waldeyer's fascia, traverses the levator ani sling, and eventually appears as a bulging diamond-shaped perianal ecchymosis. This diamond-like appearance suggests that the hematoma initially takes the shape of the ischiorectal fossae, seeps through the perianal fascia into the shallow subcutaneous perianal space, and then dissipates into the skin overlying the urogenital triangle.

Determinants of Failure in the Treatment of Ruptured Abdominal Aortic Aneurysm

Jo Carol Gordon Hiatt, Wiley F. Barker, Herbert I. Machleder, J. Dennis Baker, Ronald W. Busuttil, and Wesley S. Moore (Univ. of California, Los Angeles)

Arch. Surg. 119:1264–1268, November 1984 6–27

Aggressive elective resection of abdominal aortic aneurysms has reduced the occurrence of rupture, but patients with rupture as the initial manifestation continue to be seen. A majority of free intraperitoneal ruptures are fatal, and survival after operation for contained rupture is poor. Factors related to death after treatment were examined in a series of 29 patients with ruptured abdominal aortic aneurysms who died after hospital admission at two centers between 1971 and 1981. All cases of free intraperitoneal rupture or contained retroperitoneal rupture were included. The 26 men and 3 women had an average age of 70 years.

Twelve patients were known to have an aneurysm before rupture but were not operated on electively. Another patient had had an aneurysm identified on a roentgenogram 8 months before rupture, but this was overlooked by the physician. Five patients in this group had a free intraperitoneal rupture. In 9 cases an error in diagnosis of aortic rupture led to delay in arrival in the operating room. Intraoperative technical errors resulting in venous injury were identified in 8 patients. In 4 instances there was undue delay in inducing anesthesia. Fifteen patients in all had a free intraperitoneal rupture; the other 14 had a contained retroperitoneal rupture. In 18 patients it was possible to resect the aneurysm and insert a prosthesis. The 16 perioperative deaths were related to myocardial injury from hemorrhage and hypotension. The patients who lived more than 24 hours had renal insufficiency besides cardiac injury. Coagulopathy was a factor in 6 cases.

Failure to operate electively was the chief correctable error associated with death in this series. Failure to make the correct diagnosis was the next most frequent fatal error. Most technical operative errors involved venous injury, especially of the left renal vein. Monitoring techniques as with the Swan-Ganz catheter improved intraoperative and postoperative surveillance.

▶ In these days of diminished teaching of anatomy, an article such as that which describes perianal hematoma presents a strong argument for a thorough understanding of anatomy. This finding is carefully explained here. The physical sign may be valuable to know.

In analyzing the influence of the rupture site upon survival after aortic aneurysm resection, the Milanese authors furnish us with the frequency of the various sites of rupture, emphasize the lethal nature of intraperitoneal rupture, and suggest that intracaval rupture is more frequent than one would have thought. This group of aortocaval fistulas had the lowest mortality, 38.4%, thus indicating that intracaval rupture can be considered a favorable event by comparison with intraperitoneal or retroperitoneal rupture. "Determinants of failure in treatment of aortic aneurysm" is an analysis of death following attempted repair of ruptured aortic aneurysm. Its conclusion is important. That is, that the chief determinant of failure was the failure to electively resect the aneurysm. It is unfortunate that placing this paper in a surgical journal is simply preaching to the confirmed.

True Aneurysms of the Hand Resulting From Athletic Injury: Report of Two Cases

Paul K. Ho, A. Lee Dellon, and E. F. Shaw Wilgis (Baltimore)
Am. J. Sports Med. 13:136–138, Mar.–Apr. 1985 6–28

Blunt athletic trauma has been shown to be a cause of vascular injury in the upper extremity but not of aneurysms of the hand. Two cases of hand aneurysm secondary to blunt athletic injury were encountered.

Man, 31, developed swelling and ecchymosis over the left hypothenar area with paresthesias in ulnar digits after being struck by a ball in the left palm. A 1.5-cm pulsatile mass was noted. X-ray film examination was negative, but a radio-nuclide study showed increased perfusion persisting as focally increased activity on the blood pool image. An aneurysm of the ulnar artery (Fig 6–9) was resected, and the defect was reconstructed with a reversed vein graft from the forearm using microvascular technique. Histopathologic study showed a true aneurysm. Symptoms remained absent on follow-up at 9 months, and the patient returned to sports activity. An Allen test confirmed a patent ulnar artery.

Woman, 35, presented with a mass in a web space 2 months after bruising the palm. An aneurysm of the ulnar digital artery of the long finger was resected, and reanastomosis of the vessel gave a good clinical result at 4 months.

The ulnar artery is susceptible to injury from the distal border of the continuation of the transverse carpal ligament to the palmar fascia. Diagnosis of the present cases was aided by three-phase nuclide scanning;

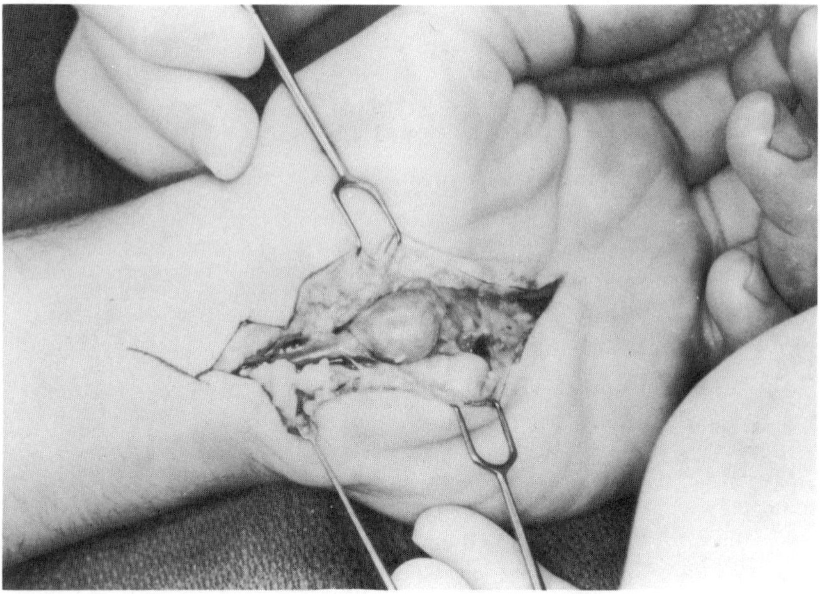

Fig 6–9.—Aneurysm of ulna artery just distal to Guyan's canal. (Courtesy of Ho, P.K., et al.: Am. J. Sports Med. 13:136–138, Mar.–Apr. 1985.)

increased uptake in the angiogram phase suggests arterial aneurysm. Aneurysm should be included in the differential diagnosis of upper extremity masses, especially if there is a history of trauma. Evaluation of the distal circulation will help in deciding on restitution of flow versus vascular ligation.

Granulomatous Radial Arteritis With Bilateral, Nontraumatic, True Arterial Aneurysms Within the Anatomical Snuffbox

David W. Leitner, Jeffrey S. Ross, and J. Ryder Neary

J. Hand Surg. 10A:131–135, January 1985 6–29

Only 4 cases of true aneurysm of the anatomical snuffbox were found in the English language literature. Two such aneurysms occurred in the same patient within a 1-month period.

Woman, 69, right-handed, reported vomiting, diarrhea, and extremity pain present for 8 days. The left knee, left wrist, and both ankles were most markedly affected. The joint swelling had begun shortly after the patient struck her left hand on an object and abraded the dorsum of the metacarpophalangeal joints of 3 fingers. A pansystolic murmur was noted as well as swelling of the left wrist and left axillary adenopathy. Fever of 101 F developed with a white blood cell count of 14,000. X-ray films of the left hand showed chronic osteoarthritic changes but no apparent osteomyelitis. A 2-cm pulsatile mass subsequently was noted in the left anatomical snuffbox, and brachial arteriography showed a radial aneurysm just proximal to the junction with the palmar arch. The aneurysm was excised, but similar symptoms developed in the right wrist 1 month later. An aneurysm also was found on this side and was excised. Both specimens exhibited marked thickening of the arterial wall and a mural thrombus. Many histiocytes were present in the arterial media, but multinucleated giant cells were not observed.

True aneurysms of the wrist and hand are relatively rare. Most reported true hand aneurysms are traumatic in origin and are found at the hypothenar eminence or in the area of the thenar eminence. Aneurysms of the anatomical snuffbox have not been ascribed to trauma. The present patient's symptoms were consistent with polymyalgia rheumatica, a clinical manifestation of granulomatous arteritis.

▶ Whereas these two articles call attention to aneurysms of the hand, the important finding in both is that damage to the media of the artery leads to arterial aneurysm. This is because destruction of the elastic and muscle fibers of the tunica media allows the vessel to dilate and then follow the well-known dicta of the Law of LaPlace.

Atherosclerotic Extracranial Carotid Artery Aneurysms

Robert M. Zwolak, Walter M. Whitehouse, Jr., James E. Knake, Barry D. Bernfeld, Gerald B. Zelenock, Jack L. Cronenwett, Errol E. Erlandson, Andris Kazmers, Linda M. Graham, S. Martin Lindenauer, and James C. Stanley (Univ. of Michigan)

J. Vasc. Surg. 1:415–422, May 1984 6–30

Most of the literature on aneurysms of the extracranial carotid artery are case reports that fail to define its natural history and a uniform approach to treatment. The authors report their experience with operative and nonoperative management of 24 atherosclerotic extracranial carotid artery aneurysms in 21 patients treated over a 25-year period. Included were 15 men, with a mean age of 58.7 years, and 6 women, with a mean age of 66.2 years. Atherosclerotic risk factors included arterial hypertension, cigarette smoking, insulin-dependent diabetes mellitus, and hyperlipidemia. Manifestations of extracarotid arterial atherosclerosis included coronary artery disease (19%), peripheral vascular occlusive disease involving the lower extremity (14%), and abdominal aortic aneurysms (14%). Neurologic symptoms, including amaurosis fugax, transient ischemic attacks, and stroke, were found in 50% of patients. An asymptomatic pulsatile neck mass was present in 33%. Aneurysms were mostly fusiform, were commonly found at the bifurcation of the common carotid artery, and ranged from 0.8 to 5.5 cm in diameter. Operations were performed on 18 aneurysms, including aneurysmectomy for 14 and aneurysmorrhaphy in 4. Six patients were followed conservatively.

There were no operative deaths. Transient perioperative neurologic deficits affected 3 patients (17%), whereas 1 patient (5%) had a permanent deficit. Transient cranial nerve injuries occurred in 3 patients and a permanent deficit in 1 patient. During a 7.6-year mean follow-up, no late strokes occurred among patients operated on. Three ipsilateral strokes occurred among patients not operated on, an incidence of 50%, during a mean follow-up of 6.3 years.

The atherosclerotic extracranial carotid artery aneurysms reported in this series represent 46% of 52 extracranial carotid artery aneurysms of all types diagnosed at the University of Michigan during the 25-year period. The pathogenesis is still poorly understood. The existence of a generalized arterial abnormality cannot account for this aneurysm, since it is infrequently associated with other peripheral aneurysms. Hypertension may be a contributing factor; however, it is not a universal finding. Clinical signs and symptoms are varied. Cerebral arteriography is a necessary preoperative study.

Operation with precise surgical technique is recommended for all patients with atherosclerotic extracranial carotid artery aneurysms. Despite perioperative neurologic deficits, prevention of late strokes as shown by an incidence of 50% with conservative treatment justifies operation. Treatment is directed toward aneurysm resection with restoration of arterial continuity; the choice of procedure is best determined by aneurysm size, configuration, and location. The authors recommend selective intraluminal shunting in the absence of adequate collateral blood flow, especially in patients who have had a stroke.

Medial Agenesis Associated With Multiple Extracranial Peripheral and Visceral Arterial Aneurysms

Patrick J. O'Hara, Norman B. Ratliff, Robert A. Graor, Andrew Novick, and Edwin G. Beven (Cleveland Clinic Found.)
J. Vasc. Surg. 2:298–306, March 1985 6–31

Two patients were encountered who had multiple peripheral and visceral aneurysms associated with the histologic features of intracranial saccular berry aneurysms. The presumed cause is medial agenesis of the arterial wall. The patients had no clinical or angiographic evidence of cerebrovascular aneurysm formation and no evidence of associated collagen-vascular disease. They were a boy, aged 9 years, with an abdominal aortic aneurysm and aneurysms of the humeral, brachial, hypogastric, profunda femoris, popliteal, tibial, renal, and other arteries; and a man, aged 52, with similarly extensive aneurysms. The patients successfully underwent segmental resection and grafting of symptomatic, expanding, or large aneurysms. Complete focal absence of the arterial media was observed in areas of aneurysm formation.

Multiple congenital, peripheral, and visceral aneurysms in the absence of clinical collagen-vascular disease are uncommon. The present patients had histologic evidence of complete focal absence of the arterial media similar to, but much more extensive than, that seen in intracranial berry aneurysm. No evidence of inflammation or vasculitis was seen. These patients probably had agenesis of the arterial media, with multiple peripheral and visceral aneurysms resulting. The defect may be a result of embryologic ischemia. When medial agenesis is a possibility, aneurysms should be carefully sought by peripheral, visceral, cerebral, and coronary angiography. Individual aneurysms should be repaired on the basis of conventional criteria.

Aneurysm of the Superior Mesenteric Artery: Its Diagnosis and Clinical Significance

Von A. Gebauer (Univ. of Munich)

ROFO 141:529–533, November 1984 6–32

This is a report about 4 patients with aneurysms of the superior mesenteric artery of arteriosclerotic, mycotic, and probably congenital etiology together with a review of the literature as to etiology, diagnostic possibilities, and therapy. One of the case histories is described.

Man, 62, suffered from chronic bronchitis, hypertension, diabetes mellitus, and absolute arrhythmia. He was admitted because of severe abdominal pain and suspicion of mesenteric artery embolism. Selective angiography of the superior mesenteric artery showed an embolus with high-grade stenosis of the main stem about 8 cm from its aortic origin. At 2 cm further out a complete occlusion was seen. Besides this, an aneurysm in the terminal branches was found. Six days after embolectomy a new mesenteric embolism developed and a laparotomy had to be performed. A partial resection of the jejunum and a resection of the ileum and ascending colon up to the hepatic flexure with jejunum-transversostomy were necessary. This included a resection of the jejunal arteric aneurysm.

Arteriography is definitive even though a diagnosis may be possible by sonography or computed tomography. The small size of the aneurysm and the variable location in the abdomen as well as artifacts caused by intestinal air make a sonographic diagnosis difficult. Even though an aneurysm of the superior mesenteric artery is rare, it has to be considered in the differential diagnosis of persistent abdominal problems of unknown origin. This is especially true for patients with a predisposing history such as endocarditis, sepsis, arteriosclerosis, and hypertension. Superior mesenteric artery(SMA) aneurysms are also found in connection with periteritis nodosa, as a complication of pancreatitis or in neoplasms with vascular erosion.

Because of the possibility of rupture followed by life-threatening bleeding, an adequate diagnostic test such as arteriography has to be considered early. The therapy of choice is the surgical removal of the aneurysm with reconstruction of the arterial arborisation, if necessary.

Inferior Mesenteric Artery Aneurysms

Linda M. Graham, Michael R. Hay, Kyung J. Cho, and James C. Stanley (Univ. of Michigan)

Surgery 97:158–163, February 1985 6–33

Aneurysms of the splanchnic arteries can present as organ- or life-threatening emergencies. The least frequent are inferior mesenteric artery (IMA) aneurysms; only 11 cases have previously been reported. Two patients were treated for asymptomatic IMA aneurysms during reconstructive operations for infrarenal aortic disease. The lesions were found incidentally during angiography in 1 and at operation in the other.

CASE I.—Man, 62, had a history of hypertension and several myocardial infarctions. An 8-cm pulsatile abdominal mass was present, representing a fusiform, clot-filled abdominal aortic aneurysm. Aneurysmal dilatations of the iliac, femoral, and right popliteal arteries were also present. There was a 1.5-cm fusiform aneurysm of the IMA just proximal to its primary branching. The IMA was suture-ligated proximally and the obliterated aneurysm left in place. The patient did well during 80 months of follow-up.

CASE II.—Man, 54, who was normotensive, had a 1-cm, clot-filled proximal IMA aneurysm, which was resected with a narrow segment of aorta. Examination of the aneurysm showed a dissecting mural thrombus, fragmentation of the internal elastic lamina, and decreases in the elastic and muscular components of the media.

Incidental IMA aneurysms will be found more often as aortic operations and angiography become more frequent. Aneurysms of the IMA have been arteriosclerotic, mycotic, and iatrogenic, as well as due to medial dissection. The natural history of IMA aneurysms is unclear, since few patients have been followed-up in deatil. Aneurysmectomy with IMA ligation is feasible if the splanchnic and pelvic circulation is otherwise normal. The distal ligature should be placed so as to preserve communications between the IMA branches. When the IMA is not reconstructed after aneurysmectomy, intraoperative assessment of the adequacy of blood flow to the distal part of the colon is important. The IMA should not be interrupted if it provides important collateral circulation to the pelvis or lower extremities in the presence of severe aortoiliac occlusive disease. Colon resection may be necessary in unusual circumstances. All 7 patients operated on for IMA aneurysms have had satisfactory results, despite reconstruction of the vessel in only 3.

▶ Although mesenteric artery aneurysms are rare, these abstracts are of value. The Graham et al. article, for example, is scholarly and complete with a reference list going back to 1861.

O'Hara's documentation of focal absence of the arterial media provides yet another hint as to the cause of unusual aneurysms, which may eventually throw light upon the cause of more central aortic dilations.

Ruptured Mycotic Aneurysm of the Superior Mesenteric Artery Secondary to Bacterial Endocarditis in a 6-Year-Old Girl

C. Christophe, W. Burniat, M. Spehl, C. Cogaert, N. Amalou, F. Delaet, D. Biarent, and N. Perlmutter (Alger, Algeria)

Pediatr. Radiol. 15:202–204, March 1985 6–34

A patient with mitral valve disease and probable bacterial endocarditis was found to have a false mycotic aneurysm on a branch of the superior mesenteric artery. It ruptured suddenly, but was successfully treated.

Girl, 6, referred for surgical treatment of postrheumatic mitral valve disease, had valve vegetations noted on ultrasonography. Several blood cultures were negative. Hepatosplenomegaly was present, as well as a retroumbilical mass that had grown slowly for 2 months and currently was grapefruit-sized and relatively hard, but mobile. Ultrasound study showed a sonolucent zone in the epigastrium below the normal pancreas, surrounded superficially by a more echogenic, heterogenous structure. The mass was 6 cm at largest diameter. Computed tomographic findings are shown in Figures 6–10 and 6–11. Shock ensued, and the abdominal mass no longer was palpable. Massive peritoneal bleeding was seen at laparotomy. A 4-mm bleeding fissure was seen in a branch of the superior mesenteric artery, with surrounding organized intramesenteric hematoma but rupture into the peritoneal cavity. The hematoma was removed, and the arterial branch was sutured. The mitral valve was replaced 2 days later.

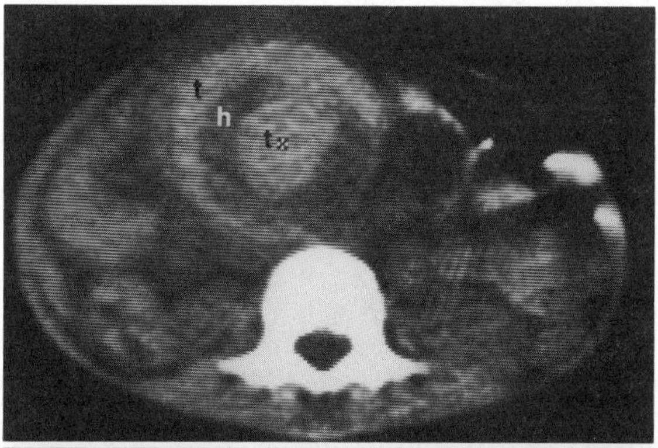

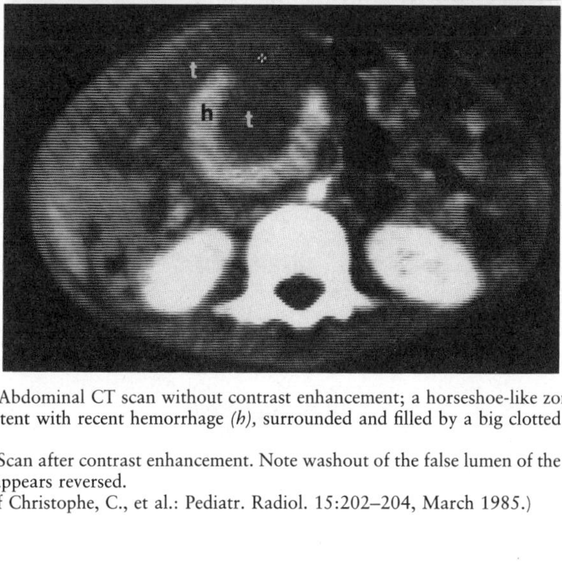

Fig 6–10.—Abdominal CT scan without contrast enhancement; a horseshoe-like zone can be seen of a density consistent with recent hemorrhage *(h)*, surrounded and filled by a big clotted hematoma *(t)* of higher density.

Fig 6–11.—Scan after contrast enhancement. Note washout of the false lumen of the pseudoaneurysm *(h)*: the image appears reversed.

(Courtesy of Christophe, C., et al.: Pediatr. Radiol. 15:202–204, March 1985.)

This patient appears to have had a secondary aneurysm associated with bacterial endocarditis and rheumatic heart disease. Superior mesenteric artery aneurysms usually are infective in origin, and most infective aneurysms are secondary to bacterial endocarditis. Small infected emboli presumably lodge in the vasa vasorum of the arterial wall, which is weakened by inflammation, resulting in formation of a false aneurysm after leakage into adjacent tissues that enclose the hemorrhage. Contrast computed tomography is a useful diagnostic procedure, and angiography can help localize the aneurysm. Expeditious management is necessary to prevent catastrophic bleeding.

Bacteriologic and Surgical Determinants of Survival in Patients With Mycotic Aneurysms

Spencer L. Brown, Ronald W. Busuttil, J. Dennis Baker, Herbert I. Machleder, Wesley S. Moore, and Wiley F. Barker (Univ. of California, Los Angeles)
J. Vasc. Surg. 1:541–547, July 1984 6–35

Mycotic aneurysms are a fulminant infectious process frequently resulting in rupture and death if the patient is not properly treated. The authors conducted a collective review of current literature on the bacteriology, etiology, and treatment of mycotic aneurysms to determine any significant relation between these factors and outcome. A review of the University of California medical records identified 10 patients with extrathoracic, extracranial mycotic aneurysms. Further, a search of the English language literature revealed 178 patients with 243 mycotic aneurysm.

The femoral artery was the most common location (38%), followed by the abdominal aorta (31%). Arterial injury (iatrogenic, traumatic, or self-induced by intravascular drug abusers) was the primary cause of 42% of mycotic aneurysms; in 25% of patients, no clear source of infection was identified. *Staphylococcus aureus* was cultured from 28% of mycotic aneurysms and *Salmonella* from 15%. Increasing involvement of gram-negative aerobes and anerobes was found. Optimal surgical treatment remained unresolved. Aortic aneurysms were repaired with in situ Dacron in 61% of patients, resulting in a 32% mortality rate and a 16% reinfection rate. Simple ligation of femoral artery mycotic aneurysms resulted in a 34% incidence of ischemia necessitating amputation. Ligation of 16 mycotic aneurysms of the mesenteric arteries, 14 of the superior mesenteric artery, and 2 hepatic mycotic aneurysms resulted in 33% of patients developing bowel ischemia necessitating resection. Seven carotid artery mycotic aneurysms were repaired by ligation, saphenous vein homograft, Dacron, or primary aneurysmorrhaphy with a vein patch, resulting in 1 rupture. Iliac artery mycotic aneurysms were treated by ligation or in situ Dacron graft. Mortality was 33%. Ligation of mycotic aneurysm of the brachial, radial, or ulnar artery was successful.

Though mycotic aneurysms are commonly in the femoral artery, the increasing incidence of intravascular drug abusers and of the use of catheters for hemodynamic monitoring has led to an increased incidence of peripheral mycotic aneurysms of the extremities. Coincident with the change in mycotic aneurysm cause from endocarditis to arterial trauma, *S. aureus* has become the most common pathogen. With use of broad-spectrum antibiotics, gram-negative aerobes and anerobes have become increasingly prevalent. Therefore, neither negative blood cultures nor intraoperative Gram stains should exclude the diagnosis. Persistent fever without a known source in the presence of a newly discovered aneurysm should alert the physician to the possibility of a mycotic lesion.

The operation of choice for each patient must be individualized. However, the following recommendations are made. Patients with mycotic aneurysms of the abdominal aorta, with a negative Gram stain and without purulence, should be treated with in situ Dacron and maintained for 6 to 8 weeks on oral antibiotic therapy. A positive Gram stain or purulence in an infrarenal aortic aneurysm necessitates an extra-anatomical bypass and prolonged oral antibiotic treatment. Patients with aneurysms at the level of the renal arteries must be treated with in situ Dacron and given lifelong antibiotic therapy. Aneurysms of the superior mesenteric artery must be excised and a saphenous vein bypass placed. Those of the femoral artery must be repaired with extra-anatomical bypass. Those of the upper extremities may be simply ligated if they occur between the thyrocervical trunk and the subscapular artery or distal to the profunda brachi.

▶ There's something old and something new in these two abstracts. What is old is the superior mesenteric artery aneurysm from bacterial endocarditis, which is well reported in older literature. What is new is the CT diagnosis of the site of rupture, which calls attention to the value of this modality of diagnosis. What is old in the UCLA abstract is, again, the large number of mycotic mesenteric arterial aneurysms; and, what is new is the unfortunate self-induced mycotic aneurysm of the intravascular drug abuser, a sad medical commentary on our society, in general, and the southern California atmosphere in particular.

Familial Aortic Aneurysms: Serum Concentrations of Triglyceride, Cholesterol, HDL-Cholesterol and (VLDL + LDL)-Cholesterol

Ö. Norrgård, K.-A. Ängquist, and O. Johnson (Univ. of Umeå, Sweden)

Br. J. Surg. 72:113–116, February 1985 6–36

Aggregation of abdominal aortic aneurysms (AAAs) in some families has been observed. The present study included 51 patients treated for AAA in northern Sweden between 1969 and 1982. The 38 men and 13 women had a mean age at diagnosis of 64 years. Eighteen patients had a family history of AAA, in first-degree relatives in 12 instances. No family history of hereditary connective tissue disease was obtained. Control subjects were 51 participants in a population study of serum lipids. Coronary disease was present in 20 AAA patients, 10 of whom had had myocardial infarction. Eight patients had intermittent claudication, and 2 had transient ischemic attacks. Significantly more patients than controls were smokers.

Serum triglyceride concentrations were higher in patients than in controls, as were concentrations of very low-density lipoprotein plus low-density lipoprotein (VLDL + LDL)-cholesterol. Serum high-density lipoprotein (HDL)-cholesterol concentrations were lower in the patient group. Total cholesterol concentrations were comparable. Serum concentrations of triglyceride, cholesterol, HDL-cholesterol, and (VLDL + LDL)-cholesterol were similar in patients who had first-degree relatives with AAAs and those without a family history of AAA. Serum lipid values were also similar in patients with and those without evidence of other atherosclerotic disease.

Low serum HDL-cholesterol concentrations were found in patients with AAA in this study. About half the patients had other manifestations of atherosclerotic disease. Serum lipid and lipoprotein values were similar in the patients with first-degree relatives who had AAA and in the others.

Congenital Abdominal Aortic Aneurysms: Report of a Case and Review of the Literature

William A. Darden, J. Timothy Fulenwider, Robert B. Smith III, and C. Whitaker Sewell (Atlanta)

Surgery 96:567–573, September 1984 6–37

Congenital abdominal aortic aneurysms in children are extremely rare even in groups with inherited disorders of connective tissue metabolism such as Ehlers-Danlos syndrome or Marfan's syndrome. A child with a congenital abdominal aortic aneurysm is described and a review of the literature is presented.

Boy, 2½, was first seen at age 5 days with multiple congenital cardiac anomalies, including postductal aortic coarctation (50 mm Hg gradient), patent ductus arteriosus, and massive mitral regurgitation. The aortic coarctation was successfully repaired at Henrietta Egleston Hospital for Children. The defective mitral valve was replaced at age 9 months. At age 1 year a left temporo-occipital hemorrhage was found to be caused by a congenital arteriovenous malformation. The lesion was successfully resected after evacuation of the hematoma.

At age 2½ years an attempt at cardiac catheterization through a right femoral approach was unsuccessful. Flush aortography demonstrated a 2.5 cm saccular aneurysm at the aortic bifurcation in addition to total occlusion of the right common iliac artery with well-developed collateralization of the external iliac and hypogastric arteries. Transperitoneal resection of the abdominal aortic aneurysm was accomplished with revascularization of the patent left common iliac artery with a 6.0-mm woven Dacron prosthesis that originated from the terminal aorta. The right common iliac artery was oversewn to preserve natural collateral flow. Cultures of the aneurysm were sterile. Histologic sections showed an occasional unorganized mural thrombus overlying fibrotic areas of intimal surface. Calcifications were occasionally present in the poorly organized tunica media. No characteristic lesions of cystic media necrosis were identified. Patient died of acute pneumonitis at age 35 months.

Most reported cases of abdominal aortic aneurysms in childen have been associated with inherited disorders of metabolism of connective tissues, such as in Ehlers-Danlos syndrome and Marfan's syndrome. Ehlers-Danlos syndrome type IV is the most common subtype associated with aneurysmal degeneration of single or multiple peripheral arteries; however, this type usually lacks most of the classic phenotypic changes associated with the syndrome. Arterial lacerations, arteriovenous fistulas, and pseudoaneurysms are frequently observed after angiography in these patients and problems of wound healing and integrity of arterial suture lines should be anticipated before operation.

At least 6 cases of abdominal aortic aneurysms associated with Marfan's syndrome have been reported; all the patients were male. Pathologic examinations in these cases suggested cystic medial necrosis with irregularity and fraying of elastic fibers consistent with changes noted in Marfan's syndrome. Other causes of abdominal aortic aneurysms include trauma or infection. Such aneurysms have also been reported in infants with tuberous sclerosis.

The rarest subgroup is the congenital idiopathic subgroup. Howorth described a case of idiopathic abdominal aneurysm that was detected in the early neonatal period. The aneurysm described in the present case is considered idiopathic in origin based on the histologic features of the aneurysm wall and absence of any definable connective tissue disorder. Although infection of the aneurysm would have been easy in this patient, there were no signs that suggested such an infection. Congenital aneurysms of the peripheral and visceral arteries have been reported to coexist with aneurysmal degeneration of the aorta.

Arterial Manifestations of Behçet Disease

Jae H. Park, Man C. Han, and Michael A. Bettmann (Harvard Med. School)
AJR 143:821–825, October 1984 6–38

Behçet disease, an uncommon systemic process that occurs most often in the third or fourth decade of life, is characterized clinically by recurrent orogenital ulcers and ocular and cutaneous inflammatory lesions. Arthralgias, vascular disease, involvement of the central nervous system, gastrointestinal symptoms, and epididymitis may also be seen. Cardiovascular involvement can include both arteries and veins. The authors describe 3 new cases of Behçet disease seen at Brigham and Women's Hospital and present a review of the arterial manifestations of this disorder that have been reported in the literature. One of the new cases is described below.

Woman, 25, presented with an acute onset of aphasia, right hemiplegia, and left facial palsy. Because of a 2-year history of recurrent oral and genital ulcerations and bilateral knee arthralgias, a diagnosis of Behçet disease was made. Her blood pressure on admission was 120/80 mm Hg. Physical examination revealed a pulsating mass, $4 \times 4 \times 5$ cm, at the base of the neck on the right side and a pulsating mass, $2 \times 3 \times 3$ cm, at the left side of the base. A third mass, $3 \times 3 \times 4$ cm, was

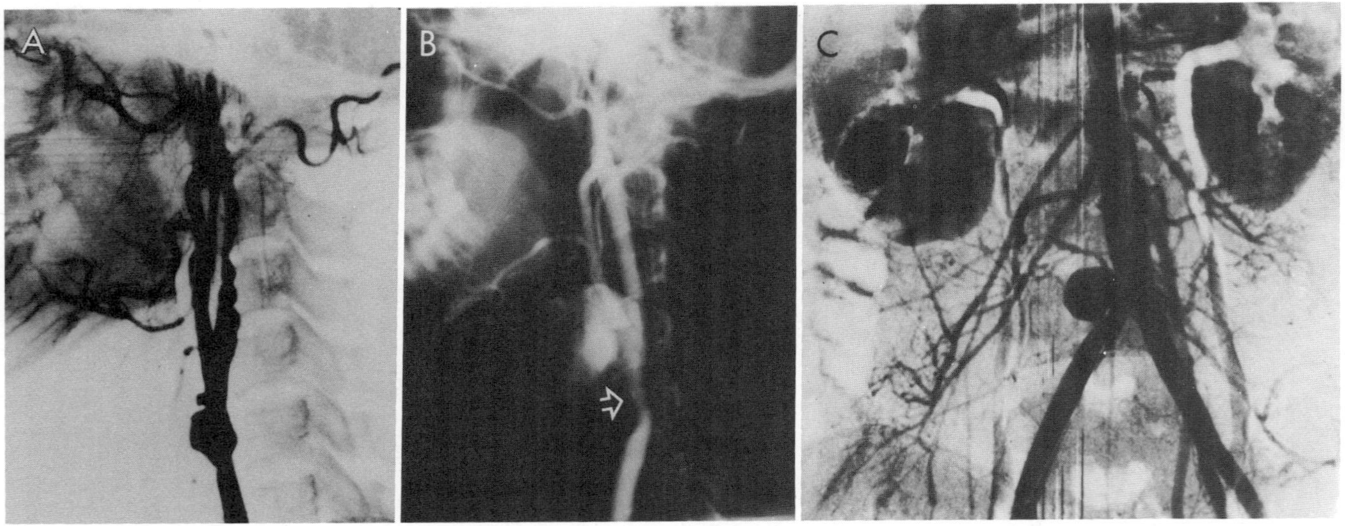

Fig 6–12.—A, selective left common carotid arteriogram shows small aneurysm of distal common carotid artery and marked irregular narrowing of proximal internal carotid artery. **B,** right common carotid arteriogram. Large, partly thrombosed aneurysm is seen originating just proximal to bifurcation of common carotid. Lumen of common carotid is compressed by unopacified part of aneurysm *(arrow)*. **C,** protruding aneurysmal sac, by appearance pseudoaneurysm, originating from right side of distal abdominal aorta just proximal to aortic bifurcation. (Courtesy of Park, J.H., et al.: AJR 143:821–825, October 1984.)

found in the midabdomen; bruits were audible over all three masses. The erythrocyte sedimentation rate was markedly elevated. Arteriography of the left common carotid artery revealed a small aneurysm just proximal to the bifurcation and marked, irregular narrowing of the proximal internal carotid artery (Fig 6–12). The right common carotid artery was markedly narrowed, with what appeared to be a pseudoaneurysm originating just proximal to the bifurcation (Fig 6–12, *B*). An abdominal aortic aneurysm, which had a similar appearance, was observed just proximal to the aortic bifurcation (Fig 6–12, *C*). Because no specific medical or surgical intervention was believed to hold promise, the patient was discharged on a conservative medical regimen.

When it is limited to mucocutaneous manifestations, Behçet disease has a relatively indolent course. However, when there is vascular or cerebral involvement, the prognosis is grim. The incidence of cardiovascular involvement in this disorder ranges from 7% to 29%, according to reports in the literature. The aorta is the most commonly affected artery, followed by the pulmonary, femoral, subclavian, popliteal, and common carotid arteries. Although almost every major artery has been reported to be affected, large vessel involvement is most common. Sixty-one of 94 arterial lesions (65%) previously reported involved aneurysms, with the most common site of formation being the abdominal aorta. The most common site of occlusion was the pulmonary artery.

To date, Behçet disease is the only vasculitis known to lead to aneurysms of the pulmonary artery. Arterial repair in Behçet disease is often unsuccessful and there is a tendency to disruption of grafts, accompanied by progression of the disease.

▶ Evidence is accumulating that atherosclerosis is not the single most important cause of aortic aneurysms. Familial occurrence of such aneurysms has been commented on by several groups, and Norrgård's paper is important in this documentation. Serum lipid abnormalities seem to be unrelated to the development of aneurysms in such families. In the search for arterial wall abnormalities that may result in aneurysm formation, one must take into consideration aortic aneurysms appearing in the newborn and the infant. Such congenital aneurysms are usually associated with connective tissue diseases, but this particular report of idiopathic aneurysm formation is interesting and calls attention to the fact that congenital arterial wall abnormalities may be found in the future to be an important cause of aneurysms in infants.

In the third abstract, we find that Behçet disease, which is an autoimmune disorder in which antibody is directed against endothelium and immune complex destruction of arterial wall occurs, progresses through pseudoaneurysms and finally rupture of such aneurysms. In fact, Behçet disease is not as rare as once thought. Vascular surgeons must be aware of this important entity. What do you think about the wisdom of not operating upon a patient with a pseudoaneurysm of the abdominal aorta as suggested in this article?

7 Occlusive Lesions of the Arteries

Cerebrovascular Ischemia

The Contribution of Spectral Analysis to the Diagnosis of Carotid Artery Disease

Martin Thomas, Shirley M. Otis, Mike M. Rush, Jack Zyroff, Ralph B. Dilley, and Eugene F. Bernstein (Scripps Clinic and Research Found., La Jolla, Calif.)

J. Vasc. Surg. 2:270–277, March 1985 7–1

New methods of spectral analysis of the Doppler velocity signal permit modest carotid arterial lesions to be detected more accurately than was previously possible. Noninvasive studies for extracranial carotid disease at the authors' institution include B-mode imaging with pulsed Doppler velocity analysis and continuous-wave (CW) Doppler imaging. Both the pulsed and CW Doppler signals are subjected to on-line spectral analysis. A total of 258 carotid arteries in 220 patients clinically suspected of having carotid disease were evaluated with both techniques and later examined angiographically.

The complete assessment was 85% sensitive for total occlusion and 90% sensitive for 50%–99% stenosis. The overall accuracy rate was 86%. The prevalence of disease in the study population was 70%. The positive predictive value for 50%–99% stenoses was 90%, and the negative predictive value for 0%–19% stenoses was 89%. A severe lesion was present in all vessels in which spectral analysis suggested stenosis exceeding 50% and the periorbital Doppler study was abnormal. Spectral analysis alone distinguished arteries with more than 50% stenosis and occlusions from arteries with lesser stenosis, including normal vessels, with a sensitivity of 89%.

Direct ultrasonographic assessment of the carotid artery is the best noninvasive means of diagnosing carotid disease. Measurements of peak frequency alone are useful in distinguishing vessels with hemodynamically significant stenoses from those with lesser stenoses and normal vessels. Addition of spectral analysis increases diagnostic accuracy, mainly among vessels with non-flow-limiting stenoses. Whereas it is useful in studies of carotid disease, it may be unnecessary for screening programs.

B-Mode Real-Time Ultrasonic Carotid Imaging: Impact on Decision-Making and Prediction of Surgical Findings

R. Farber, M. Bromer, D. Anderson, R. Loewenson, D. Yock, and D. Larson (Minneapolis)

Neurology (Cleveland) 34:541–544, April 1984 7–2

To evaluate the role of B-mode real-time ultrasonic carotid imaging (USI) in making endarterectomy decisions and to determine the predictive value of USI and carotid angiography (CAG), retrospective analysis was made of USI and CAG data collected prospectively for 100 carotid systems in 50 patients. The surgical findings served as a standard against which the USI and CAG results were compared.

The prediction of more than 50% stenosis or complicated ulceration by both techniques led to endarterectomy in 21 of 25 nonoccluded carotid systems. When CAG alone predicted surgical disease, endarterectomy was performed in 5 (62.5%) of 8 nonoccluded carotid systems. When USI alone indicated surgical disease, endarterectomy was performed in 10 (48%) of 21 systems. Accuracy in demonstrating high-grade stenoses was identical for the 2 methods, but USI overestimated 8 of 13 low-grade stenotic lesions. Overall, CAG correctly predicted high-grade or low-grade stenosis in 27 (84%) of 32 systems and USI in 20 (63%) of 32 systems. In 29 carotid systems, CAG correctly predicted the presence or absence of plaque ulceration in 12 (41%), as did USI in 11 (38%). The inclusion of prediction of superficial ulceration and plaque irregularity increased the accuracies of both methods to 72% (21 of 29). Adequate surgical data were available for 3 of the 5 carotid systems operated on based on CAG findings only. High-grade stenosis predicted by CAG was confirmed in 2 systems. In the third, a predicted high-grade stenosis proved to be of low grade. In the 10 vessels operated on according to USI data only, predicted high-grade stenosis was confirmed surgically in only 2 of 8 systems, but ulceration was confirmed in all 5 systems in which it was predicted. Of 3 carotid systems in which endarterectomy was performed despite unimpressive findings on CAG or USI, 2 had high-grade stenosis and all 3 had ulceration. Apparently CAG is a more accurate predictor of stenosis than USI is, but both methods are limited in predicting ulceration.

Role of Carotid Duplex Scanning in Surgical Decision Making

D. Preston Flanigan, James J. Schuler, Mary Vogel, Philip G. Borozan, Billie Gray, and Kim R. Sobinsky (Univ. of Illinois, Chicago)

J. Vasc. Surg. 2:15–25, January 1985 7–3

Eighty-one patients suspected of having cerebrovascular disease had a total of 157 carotid arterial systems evaluated by both duplex ultrasonography and contrast arteriography within a 2-week period. More than two thirds of the patients were men. All but 15% had focal carotid territory symptoms, and 5% had vertebrobasilar symptoms. Duplex scanning was done with a Diasonic model DS-10 duplex scanner. The findings were interpreted in blind by 2 surgeons, 1 operating only on symptomatic lesions and the other on both symptomatic and asymptomatic lesions.

Agreement was obtained between the two studies on the need for carotid artery operation in about 90% of cases by both surgeons. Forty percent of scans and 46% of arteriograms were considered to be of poor quality. Agreement of about 94% was achieved when poor-quality scans were eliminated from analysis. Duplex scanning was 81% accurate in detecting disease in comparison with angiography. It was 90% accurate for detecting ulceration, 83% accurate in detecting critical stenosis, and 99% accurate in detecting total occlusion. The positive predictive value of duplex scanning in diagnosis of total occlusion was 100%, and its negative predictive value was 98%.

These findings suggest a possible role for routine duplex ultrasonography, with the selective use of arteriography, in making surgical decisions in patients evaluated for cerebrovascular occlusive disease. This approach is in accord with current trends toward wider use of less expensive and outpatient diagnostic procedures to minimize costs.

Spontaneous Progression and Regression of Small Carotid Atheroma

Michael Hennerici, Wolfgang Rautenberg, Ursula Trockel, and Rolf G. Kladetzky (Univ. of Düsseldorf)

Lancet 1:1415–1419, June 22, 1985 7–4

Carotid atherosclerotic plaques removed at endarterectomy show evidence of a dynamic process of deterioration and repair within the arterial wall. An attempt was made, using B-mode ultrasonography, angiography, and histologic study, to evaluate the severity and composition of plaques semiquantitatively. Forty-three nonstenotic atheromatous carotid plaques were obtained from 31 patients, 21 men and 10 women with a mean age of 59 years. Eighteen patients had had stroke and 4, transient ischemic

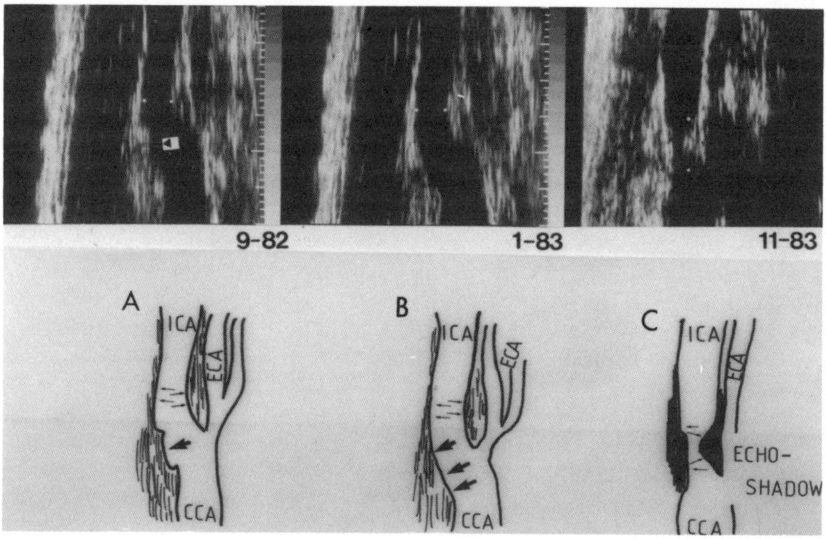

Fig 7–1.—High-resolution B-mode images of extracranial carotid system in woman, 49. During follow-up, large (about 10 mm in length) ulcerative lesion was demonstrated in posterior common carotid artery (*CCA*, **A**). There was reendothelialization (*small open arrow:* normal intimal surface; *small solid arrow:* regenerated intimal surface) at 3-month reexamination (**B**), and flat mural fibrosis *(large open arrow)* was demonstrated at 6-month reexamination, when new fibrous plaque was seen to be developing on anterior wall (**C**). Large solid arrows indicate floor and margin of ulcer crater. *ECA*, external carotid artery; *ICA*, internal carotid artery. (Courtesy of Hennerici, M., et al.: Lancet 1:1415–1419, June 22, 1985.)

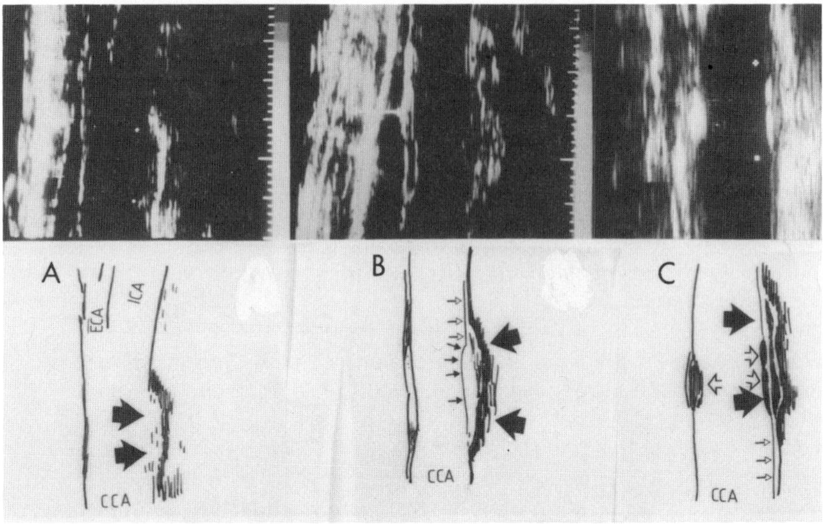

Fig 7–2.—High-resolution B-mode images of extracranial carotid system in man, 69, during follow-up. Initially (September 1982, **A**) there was soft plaque on inner wall of proximal internal carotid artery *(ICA) (small arrows)* and small ulcerative crater on anterior wall of bifurcation *(large arrow)*. During follow-up (January 1983, **B**) the latter disappeared. Note similar shadows of external carotid artery *(ECA)*, indicating identical sections imaged. Fourteen months later (**C**) severe stenosis had been produced by encroachment of posterior wall plaque and atheromatous degeneration of anterior wall near proximal ICA and distal common carotid artery *(CCA)*. (Courtesy of Hennerici, M., et al.: Lancet 1:1415–1419, June 22, 1985.)

attacks. Eighteen patients had 30 carotid arteries in which plaques appeared to produce no symptoms. Follow-up lasted 18 months.

Ultrasound duplex analysis showed progression of 30% of the plaques, regression in 19%, and no change in 51%. Progression was frequent in already complicated soft and hard plaques; it consisted of enlargement, calcification, or both. Fibrous plaques tended to persist unchanged. Some soft plaques regressed, and ulcerative lesions tended to heal by reendothelialization. The follow-up changes in 2 cases are shown in Figures 7–1 and 7–2. No patient had symptoms ascribed to atherosclerosis during follow-up. The course of carotid lesions could not be related to risk factors. Angiography confirmed many of the ultrasonographic findings but failed to demonstrate some flat or circular plaques and provided no morphological information.

These findings support the occurrence of dynamic progression and repair in carotid atherosclerotic plaques at an early stage of development. The course of these lesions may depend on various factors including lipid alterations. The observations agree with experimental findings in primate models of carotid atherosclerosis.

Ultrasound Characteristics of Recurrent Carotid Disease: Hypothesis Explaining the Low Incidence of Symptomatic Recurrence

Thomas F. O'Donnell, Jr., Allan D. Callow, Gregory Scott, Alexander D. Shepard, Paula Heggerick, and William C. Mackey (Tufts Univ.)
J. Vasc. Surg. 2:26–41, January 1985 7–5

Reported rates of recurrence of carotid stenosis based on symptoms average 1.5%, and the incidence of symptomatic recurrent stenosis when noninvasive hemodynamic studies are used is about 2%–2.5%. Real-time B-mode ultrasound imaging was used to evaluate 276 carotid arteries 1–180 months (mean, 38) after endarterectomy.

Recurrent stenosis was detected ultrasonographically in 12% of vessels and mild plaque disease in 15%. Known lipid disorder was associated with restenosis, as was evidence of other organ involvement by atherosclerosis. Ulcerated plaque in the operative specimen was more frequent in cases of restenosis. About 60% of patients in all groups took aspirin after operation. Most restenotic internal carotid arteries were detected 73–84 months after endarterectomy. Only 12% of patients with restenosis had recurrent symptoms. Soft plaque was much more frequent than hard plaque in the area of the endarterectomy. Restenosis in the common carotid artery, in contrast, was more often associated with hard or calcific plaque. Hyperplastic plaque was found in 2 of the 3 patients who were reoperated on.

Plaque hemorrhage or ulceration, or both, is unusual in recurrent stenosis (table), in contrast with primary atherosclerosis. The low incidence of plaque features associated with symptomatic disease may help explain the low frequency of symptomatic disease associated with recurrent carotid stenosis. Blood lipid abnormalities may predispose to recurrent stenosis. Recurrences are more frequent in women, suggesting a host hormonal or anatomical factor.

▶ The high accuracy of B-mode scan in conjunction with frequency analysis should make this type of examination a standard test for carotid artery disease. Direct carotid artery examination is now able to provide information such as progression and regression of atheroma and characteristics of the plaque and their surgical implication. None of this information can be furnished by indirect carotid artery examination such as oculoplethysmography.

Comparison of Carotid Plaque Characteristics of Primary Atherosclerosis and Recurrent Carotid Stenosis as Determined by B-Mode Image

Plaque characteristics	*Recurrent stenosis (n = 26)*	*Primary atherosclerosis*[21] *(n = 79)*
Ulcer	1 (4%)	27 (34%)
Hemorrhage	1 (4%)	29 (37%)
Either	2 (8%)	49 (62%)

(Courtesy of O'Donnell, T.F., Jr., et al.: J. Vasc. Surg. 2:26–41, January 1985.)

The Practice of Carotid Endarterectomy in a Large Metropolitan Area

Thomas Brott and Karen Thalinger (Univ. of Cincinnati)

Stroke 15:950–955, Nov.–Dec. 1984 7–6

Carotid endarterectomy presently is used to treat transient ischemic attacks related to carotid artery stenosis, and it also is done in asymptomatic carotid stenosis cases at some centers. Data were reviewed on experience with 431 endarterectomies done at 16 general hospitals in the Cincinnati area in 1980. The procedures were done on 371 patients. Endarterectomy was done for transient ischemic attacks in one third of the cases and for ipsilateral cerebral infarction in 17% of the cases. Asymptomatic carotid bruit and asymptomatic carotid stenosis were each the indications in about 15% of cases.

The rate of stroke after endarterectomy was about 9%. Stroke was more frequent in patients with previous ipsilateral symptomatic disease than in asymptomatic patients. There were no brain stem strokes. More than half the strokes followed a neurologically intact postoperative interval. Technical problems or hypotension were implicated in only three instances. One fifth of the strokes were fatal; most of the others produced a persistent focal deficit. Eight of 12 deaths were in patients with perioperative stroke. Three cardiac deaths complicated combined cardiac bypass operation. Morbidity could not be related to use of a shunt at endarterectomy. The severity of stenosis also was not a significant factor in perioperative morbidity or mortality.

Some late strokes in this series occurred without evidence of cardiac embolism or hemorrhage, suggesting a thrombogenic-embologenic operative site and raising the question of adjunctive perioperative medical treatment. Perioperative strokes may be underestimated in endarterectomy studies. Recent studies of patients with asymptomatic carotid bruit or stenosis have failed to support the need for prophylactic endarterectomy before major surgical procedure or coronary artery bypass graft operation.

Review of a Community Hospital Experience With Carotid Endarterectomy

Lydia G. Slavish, Gary G. Nicholas, and William Gee (Allentown, Pa.)

Stroke 15:956–959, Nov.–Dec. 1984 7–7

In 1977 Easton noted a combined permanent stroke-mortality of 21.1% for carotid endarterectomy performed in a community hospital. To determine whether carotid endarterectomy can be performed safely in such a hospital, data were reviewed on 743 carotid endarterectomies performed by 24 surgeons at Lehigh Valley Hospital Center from September 1977 to May 1982.

Ninety-four percent of procedures were performed for symptomatic disease or lesions of hemodynamic consequence. After operation, a new neurologic deficit was noted in 39 patients (5.3%); it was temporary in 26 (3.5%) and permanent in 13 (1.8%). Twenty deaths occurred (2.7%); 15

Mortality and Morbidity After Carotid Endarterectomy

Frequency of procedure (per year)	>24	24 or Less
Number of surgeons	4	20
Temporary deficit	19 (4.2%)	7 (2.4%)
Permanent deficit	9 (2.0%)	4 (1.4%)
Mortality	12 (2.6%)	8 (2.8%)
Total procedures	456	287

There was no statistically significant difference in parameters measured for 2 groups.
(Courtesy of Slavish, L.G., et al.: Stroke 15:956–959, Nov.–Dec. 1984; by permission of the American Heart Association, Inc.)

were attributable to neurologic causes and 5 to cardiac conditions. Thus, overall permanent stroke-mortality was 4.4%. The combined permanent stroke-mortality did not appear to be influenced by the frequency with which the surgeon performed such operations (r = 0.93) (table).

It appears that carotid endarterectomy in a community hospital is a safe procedure, with an overall permanent stroke-mortality of less than 5%. This margin of safety is not dependent on the frequency with which a given surgeon has performed the procedure, but it appears to be directly related to the adequacy of initial training under a wide variety of circumstances. Careful evaluation of such training should insure good surgical judgment and technical expertise.

▶ The report of a high stroke rate (21%) of carotid endarterectomy done at a community hospital has prompted several other hospitals to report their experience. The Springfield experience by Easton and Sherman (*Stroke* 8:565–568, 1977) has not been duplicated by these other reviews. Carotid endarterectomy is a safe surgical procedure whether performed in a university or a community hospital.

Training and judgment probably play a more important role than frequency of operation in preventing complications following carotid endarterectomy.

Complications of Intravenous DSA Performed for Carotid Artery Disease: A Prospective Study

Jannice O. Aaron, John R. Hesselink, and Robert Oot, R. L. Jones, Kenneth R. Davis, and Juan M. Taveras (Massachusetts Gen. Hosp.)
Radiology 153:675–678, December 1984 7–8

Complications of intravenous digital subtraction angiography (DSA) were examined in a prospective cost-benefit study of 102 patients examined for coronary artery disease. A 5.5 F Teflon catheter was introduced into the superior vena cava with fluoroscopic monitoring, and 40 ml of Renografin 76 was delivered at the rate of 15 ml per second. Two 65-degree

NEUROLOGIC COMPLICATIONS

Complaint	Type	No.
Dizziness	minor-transient	9
Confusion	major-transient	1
Seizures	major-transient	2
Visual disturbance*	major-transient	1
Stroke*	major-permanent	1
T.I.A.	major-transient	2
Headache	minor-transient	1
Total		17

*Symptoms developed after patient left radiology department.

(Courtesy of Aaron, J.O., et al.: Radiology 153:675–678, December 1984.)

oblique views of the carotid bifurcations were routinely obtained. If symptoms were present, an off-lateral view of the carotid siphons was also obtained, and an anteroposterior view of the head was included if the routine views showed significant stenosis in the neck. Average patient age was 66 years. Three outpatient studies were incomplete.

A total of 55 complications occurred in 37 patients. Six of the 17 CNS complications (table) were major and transient, and 1 was major and permanent. The latter patient developed hemiparesis in relation to complete occlusion of the vessel; partial recovery followed emergency endarterectomy. Two of the 35 systemic complications were major and permanent. Major complications were most frequent in patients aged 60 to 69 years. No relation with the number of injections or the amount of contrast used was apparent. No major complications occurred in the 25 patients who had received full anticoagulation therapy. Renal failure did not occur, but patients with a creatinine value of more than 2.5 were not examined. There were no severe allergic reactions. The incidence of complications could not be related to more severe carotid stenosis.

Intravenous DSA may be simple and safe in most patients, but risks are inherent in examining patients suspected of having carotid atherosclerotic disease. Patients with multisystem disease and those with a history of angina may be at relatively high risk of complications of DSA.

Hybrid Intravenous Digital Subtraction Angiography of the Carotid Bifurcation

Fred H. Burbank, Dieter Enzmann, Gary S. Keyes, and William R. Brody
Radiology 152:725–729, September 1984 7–9

Preliminary reports of hybrid intravenous digital subtraction angiography of the carotid bifurcation indicated promise; however, there has been no systematic clinical comparison of hybrid and temporal subtraction. Fifty consecutive patients with possible disease that involved the carotid bifurcation were evaluated with a hybrid digital subtraction angiography technique and a noise-reduction algorithm to determine whether hybrid subtraction offers any advantage over the conventional temporal subtraction. Temporal, hybrid, and reduced-noise hybrid images were obtained in right and left anterior oblique projections; both single- and multiple-frame images were created with each method. The resulting images were graded on a scale of 1 to 5 by experienced neuroradiologists.

When temporal subtraction was used alone, 4 images of the carotid bifurcation were considered nondiagnostic on the ipsilateral or contralateral projections, 32 were considered diagnostic on only one projection, and 64 were diagnostic on both projections. With the addition of hybrid subtraction, only 1 nondiagnostic image was viewed, and the number of diagnostic images increased to 87.

Analysis of variance showed that the method effect, reader-method interaction, and patient variation significantly affected image quality. Inter-reader correlation averaged 0.73. However, each reader expressed a preference for a given method. Temporal images were preferred over hybrid images (average scores, 3.2 and 2.4, respectively). Integrated temporal images were judged best (average score, 3.29) and single-frame, low-noise hybrid images were judged worst (average score, 2.23). There was significant preference for integrated over single-frame hybrid images but not for multiple-frame rather than single-frame temporal images. Images of female patients tended to be scored higher than those of male. Image quality deteriorated with age and improved with increasing dose of radiation.

All 3 neuroradiologists graded temporal images higher than hybrid images and multiple-frame higher than single-frame images, indicating that the observers gave the highest scores to the images with the maximum signal-to-noise ratios. However, in terms of diagnostic quality, the number of bifurcations seen on both ipsilateral and contralateral projections rose when hybrid and temporal subtraction were obtained, suggesting that hybrid subtraction offers a second view in a significant number of cases.

These results are open to criticism because only 3 readers participated in the study and their conclusions cannot reflect the views of radiologists in general. Furthermore, each reader obviously preferred one method over another.

In clinical use the authors recommend hybrid intravenous digital subtraction angiography of the carotid bifurcation in cases in which the temporal image is nondiagnostic and limiting hybrid postprocessing to one or two regions of interest to retain proved temporal subtraction quality for most of the image.

Carotid Digital Subtraction Angiography: Comparative Roles of Intra-Arterial and Intravenous Imaging

L. M. Reilly, W. K. Ehrenfeld, and R. J. Stoney (Univ. of California at San Francisco)

Surgery 96:909–917, November 1984 7–10

To determine the optimal role of intravenous digital subtraction angiography (IV DSA) and intra-arterial digital subtraction angiography (IA

DSA) in the diagnosis and management of carotid artery disease, 148 patients who underwent carotid endarterectomy were assessed preoperatively by IV DSA (54 patients), IA DSA (41 patients), or conventional angiography (CA) (53 patients). Special attention was given to the technical adequacy of the studies, extent of carotid visualization, volume of contrast fluid required, incidence of complications, and need for further angiography. The endarterectomy specimen was used to determine the accuracy of each imaging modality.

Sixty percent (39/65) of the IV DSA images, 96% (51/53) of the IA DSA images, and 100% of the CA images were technically adequate. The accuracy of IA DSA (94%) in demonstrating the degree of stenosis was significantly greater ($P < .0005$) than that of IV DSA (68%) and comparable to that of CA (97%). Also IA DSA consistently required less contrast material than did IV DSA (88 ml and 144 ml, respectively ($P < .0005$), but demonstrated carotid circulation to a greater extent. The complication rates associated with IA DSA and IV DSA were similar, but lower than with CA ($P < .05$).

The use of IA DSA is the optimal method for visualizing the carotid artery in most clinical settings. It provides an image quality equivalent to that of CA, resulting in the same degree of technical adequacy and overall accuracy. Also, IA DSA definitively visualizes the entire extracranial and intracranial cerebral circulation from its origin to the terminal intracranial branches. It is likely to become the most frequently used method of arteriography in evaluation of carotid artery disease.

Impact of Digital Subtraction Angiography on Carotid Evaluation

David C. Anderson and Gregory G. Fischer

Stroke 16:23–28, Jan.–Feb. 1985 7–11

The method of digital subtraction angiography by intravenous injection (DSAV) is based on the use of computer technology and subtraction to enhance contrast differences after the visualization of intravenously injected arteries containing relatively low iodine concentrations. The impact of DSAV was examined in a private neurology clinic where several of the neurologists have been interested in noninvasive technologies. Two 3-month periods, before and after the introduction of DSAV, were compared.

The use of ultrasonography declined when DSAV became available. Noninvasive tests were used in 36% of patients compared with their universal use before DSAV. Conventional arteriography was used in 29% of patients in the first period and in 4% after DSAV was introduced. The average interval from the first study to operation increased somewhat in the post-DSAV period, but preparations for DSAV were not responsible. No distinct change in management policies was observed. Patients presenting with more compelling symptoms generally had DSAV initially. The average cost of work-up was slightly higher in patients managed medically but was markedly reduced for those who had an operation.

Conventional noninvasive studies appear to have retained a screening role in cases with "soft" indications, whereas DSAV is used as a primary test in patients with "hard" indications. Conventional arteriography is being done on compelling indications and when DSAV is negative or inadequate. The risk of performing conventional angiography before endarterectomy in all candidates must be compared with the risk of missing pathology by performing DSAV instead.

▶ The role of intravenous digital subtraction angiography (DSA) in diagnosis of carotid artery disease continues to be questioned. The new hybrid form may or may not resolve the problem. Nevertheless, it would appear that intra-arterial DSA is a better technique. Whereas intravenous DSA has been touted as a simple outpatient procedure, this prospective study reveals a rather surprisingly high complication rate, including even transient ischemic attacks. Advocates of DSA must take into consideration the complication and diagnostic accuracy of intravenous DSA. Based on our experience and these studies, DSA is not a noninvasive procedure and it should not be used as a screening test.

Positron Imaging in Ischemic Stroke Disease

Robert H. Ackerman, Nathaniel M. Alpert, John A. Correia, Seth Finklestein, Stephen M. Davis, Roger E. Kelley, Geoffrey A. Donnan, Joseph G. D'Alton, and Juan M. Taveras (Massachusetts General Hosp., Boston)

Ann. Neurol. 15(Suppl.):S126–S130, 1984 7–12

Positron emission tomography (PET) is particularly suited to the study of ischemic stroke disease. It has the potential to demonstrate pathophysiologic changes in brain function, differentiate viable from nonviable tissue, and provide a more rational basis for developing specific therapies for ischemic lesions. In ischemic stroke disease, early-stage PET can demonstrate changes that are not initially seen on computed tomography (CT). It also can show that cerebral blood flow and oxygen metabolism can be uncoupled during the initial stages of stroke. Thus, useful information is obtained as disturbances in oxygen metabolism correlate better with events in the development of infarction than do disturbances in cerebral blood flow.

Other parameters such as oxygen extraction fraction, blood volume, and glucose metabolism can provide important interpretive data. However, the different tracer and scanning strategies that may be used in the study of ischemic disease all have relative limitations that may be related to the physical or biologic determinants of the tracer distributions, tracer half lives, or methods required for data quantitation. Nonetheless, the potential for PET to play a significant role in decreasing the morbidity of stroke is real. The ultimate success of the application of PET scanning to ischemic stroke disease depends on the comprehensiveness with which the physiologic information provided by PET is correlated with the clinical data and pathoanatomical data provided by CT.

Vertebral-Basilar Posterior Cerebral Territory Stroke: Delineation by Proton Nuclear Magnetic Resonance Imaging

J. P. Kistler, F. S. Buonanno, L. D. DeWitt, K. R. Davis, T. J. Brady, and C. M. Fisher (Massachusetts Gen'l. Hosp.)

Stroke 15:417–426, May–June 1984 7–13

Newly developed therapies for ischemic stroke in the vertebral-basilar posterior cerebral circulation depend on precise in vivo documentation of the extent and location of the infarct. Three-dimensional proton nuclear magnetic resonance (NMR) imaging was performed in 16 cases to study ischemic infarction in this territory. Three radiofrequency pulse sequences were used: inversion recovery (IR), saturation recovery (SR), and a Carr-Purcell-Meiboom-Gill (CPMG) spin echo (SE). Documentation of the pathophysiologic nature of the stroke was supported by transfemoral angiography in 7 cases, digital subtraction angiography in 6, and clinically in 3. All patients underwent cerebral computed tomography (CT) scanning for purposes of comparison.

Five of 7 patients with larger artery occlusive disease had basilar insufficiency with retrograde flow due to proximal basilar occlusion (1 subject), proximal to midbasilar stenopsis (2), and bivertebral occlusive disease (2). The other 2 had proximal posterior cerebral artery occlusions. Presumably 9 patients had small vessel disease, either thrombotic or embolic.

In 15 cases the location of the infarct could be detected by NMR scanning, particularly when using IR and SE pulse sequences that accentuate changes in T_1 and T_2 relaxation times, respectively. In 1 case, with a midbrain subthalamic infarct, motion artifact resulted in a blurred image.

In 4 of 8 cases described in detail, proton NMR scanning showed that the ischemic infarctions resulted from large vessel occlusive disease in the posterior cerebral circulation. Two of these 4 showed that infarcted areas can either be small and discreet or can occupy widely separate locations in the arterial territory. The other 4 cases illustrated that the topography of lacunar infarctions resulting from small penetrating or branch vessel disease can be identified in the posterior fossa.

In 5 cases T_2-weighted images were obtained with the SF pulse sequence in the same NMR imaging session as the T_1-weighted studies; areas of infarction appeared as increased image intensity that persisted in later echoes using the CPMG sequence, signifying a prolongation of T_2 relaxation times. This indicated that the alterations in T_1 and T_2 relaxation times were the major factors in showing the abnormalities in IR and SE studies. The NMR images were obtained between 36 hours and 2 months after the onset of symptoms.

It appears that NMR imaging techniques hold great promise in the study of posterior fossa strokes and in differentiating between large and small vessel ischemic disease, which is important when assessing the rationale and efficacy of medical or surgical therapy. The additional advantages of the three-dimensional approach and the lack of bone artifact make NMR imaging superior to CT scanning in identifying areas of infarction in the territory of posterior cerebral circulation. The effectiveness of NMR imaging depends on the high sensitivity of ischemic infarction to changes in T_1 and T_2 relaxation times, which are highlighted in the IR and SE images, respectively. Although the selection of these cases did not allow comparative studies of the timing of the onset or evolution of NMR alterations vs. CT scan changes, previous experience suggests that changes in human ischemic infarction can easily be detected on IR images less than 24 hours after the onset of symptoms.

▶ There is no doubt that metabolic changes at the cellular level, and not hemodynamic alterations, are most important as determinants of ischemia. Positron imaging offers a new approach to understanding the pathogenesis of cerebral ischemia. A normal CT scan may not be truly representative of a normal cerebral hemisphere.

Objective diagnosis of vertebral-basilar ischemia is often difficult. The NMR technique is a welcome new addition to diagnostic techniques. We will learn a lot more diagnostic information from the PET-scan and NMR in forthcoming years.

Dual Isotope Scintigraphy of the Carotid Arteries in Stroke Patients

Ch. Kessler, R. Reuther, and H. Henningsen (Ruprecht-Karls Univ., Heidelberg)

VASA 13:354–359, 1984 7–14

A new dual isotope scintigraphic evaluation of the carotid arteries was performed in 29 stroke patients, aged 36–75 years. This technique consists of simultaneous injections of 111-In-oxine labeled platelets and 99m-Tc labeled erythrocytes. It also consists of the ensuing subtraction of the circulating blood pool and elimination of the overshadowing of circulating radioactivity. Seventeen patients had a transitional ischemic attack, 10 patients a complete attack with permanent neurologic breakdown such as hemiparesis or aphasia. In all 10 patients an infarct area could be proven in the medial cerebral artery. Two patients had an asymptomatic carotid stenosis. On the clinically affected side of 14 patients, the angiogram was normal or showed only slight arteriosclerotic irregularities. In 4 patients a stenosis between 30% and 50% was found, and in 8 patients a high degree of stenosis (>50%) was found. Three patients showed an occlusion of the symptomatic internal carotid artery. The authors found 17 pathologic platelet accumulations with the single isotope technique (13 on the side clinically affected).

The dual isotope scintigraphy was able to eliminate three false positive results and one false negative. With this new technique of visualization of thrombi activity, the difference between circulating and static activity seems especially important since the greater part of radioactive-labeled thrombocytes belong to the circulating blood pool and the smaller part contributes to the formation of a thrombus. Finally, 11 pathologic platelet accumulations on the side clinically affected could be demonstrated. On the other hand the authors' findings show that with single isotope scin-

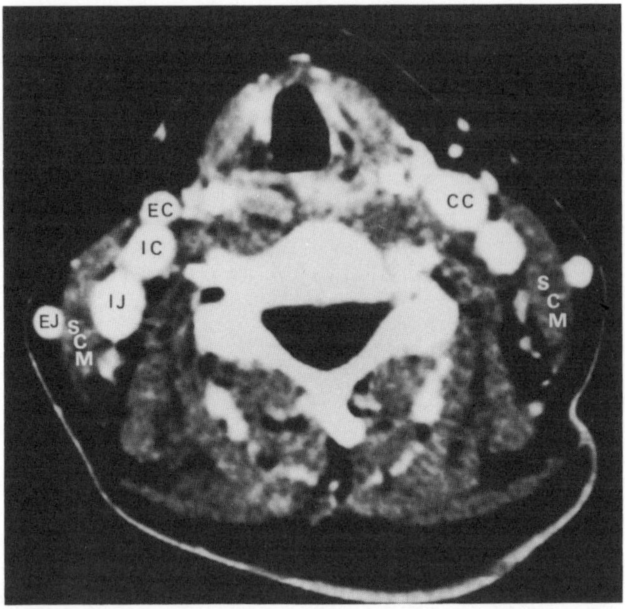

Fig 7–3.—Computed tomogram of cervical region at level of carotid bifurcation to show configuration of normal structures and their relations. Contrast fills lumina of neck vessels. *SCM*, sternocleidomastoid muscle; *IC*, internal carotid artery; *EC*, external carotid artery; *CC*, common carotid artery; *IJ*, internal jugular vein; and *EJ*, external jugular vein. (Courtesy of Culebras, A., et al.: Stroke 16:425–431, May–June 1985; by permission of the American Heart Association, Inc.)

tigraphy, the danger of a false positive result is greater than that of a false negative one. This means that, caused by anatomical characteristics of the circulation in the neck area, the evidence of platelet accumulation is not an indication of a thrombus formation but only a regional increase of the circulating platelet pool. It is demonstrated that in patients with low-grade carotid stenosis or normal angiogram, the dual isotope scintigraphy is frequently positive. Here two factors play a part: on the one hand the high speed flow in the sclerotic area hinders the attachment of thrombocytes and on the other hand thrombocytes play a domineering role in the development of arteriosclerotic changes, especially in the early phase.

These findings show that the dual isotope scintigraphy represents a significant refinement of the conventional platelet scintigraphy using one isotope only.

▶ Thrombotic activity of an ulcerating plaque is often difficult to determine. Dual-isotope scintigraphy may help to understand the pathogenesis of a transient ischemic attack in patients with otherwise normal arteriography.

Further work is needed to establish the validity of this test.

Computed Tomographic Evaluation of Cervical Carotid Plaque Complications

Antonio Culebras, Mark D. Leeson, Edwin D. Cacayorin, Charles J. Hodge, and Afif R. Iliya (SUNY, Upstate Med. Center)
Stroke 16:425–431, May–June 1985 7–15

A high incidence of intramural hemorrhage has been found in carotid artery specimens from patients undergoing endarterectomy for cerebral ischemic manifestations. The value of computed tomography (CT) in detecting intramural hemorrhage and other plaque complications was assessed in 25 patients with clinical evidence suggesting carotid disease who also had angiography. High-resolution CT scans of the carotid region were obtained with a GE 8800 scanner, in conjunction with bolus injection and drip infusion of Conray 60. Nine of the patients had transient ischemic attacks (TIAs), 8 had stroke, 7 had a reversible ischemic deficit, and 1 had unlocalized symptoms.

The normal CT appearances are shown in Figure 7–3. Histologic study of 15 endarterectomy specimens from patients with CT findings of discrete lucent defects in carotid plaques showed subintimal hemorrhage in 13 and focal necrosis and excessive subintimal thickening in one each. The angiographic and CT findings in 1 patient, with TIAs, are shown in Figures 7–4 and 7–5. Lucent defects were frequently associated with calcium deposits and luminal compromise.

Cervical CT is a relatively noninvasive means of assessing carotid plaque complications in vivo, particularly mural hemorrhage. It also permits serial study of asymptomatic carotid lesions and may demonstrate plaque com-

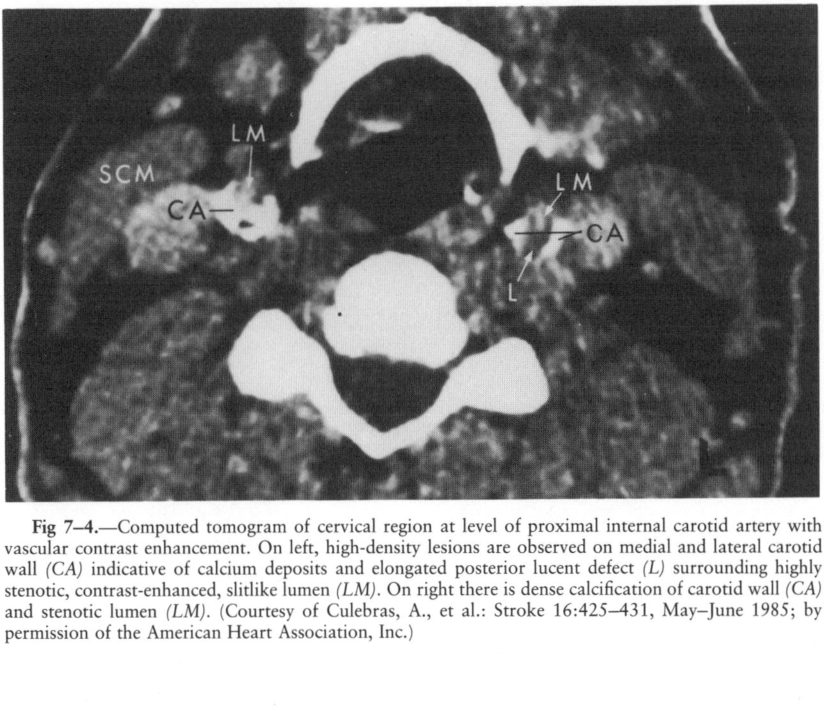

Fig 7–4.—Computed tomogram of cervical region at level of proximal internal carotid artery with vascular contrast enhancement. On left, high-density lesions are observed on medial and lateral carotid wall *(CA)* indicative of calcium deposits and elongated posterior lucent defect *(L)* surrounding highly stenotic, contrast-enhanced, slitlike lumen *(LM)*. On right there is dense calcification of carotid wall *(CA)* and stenotic lumen *(LM)*. (Courtesy of Culebras, A., et al.: Stroke 16:425–431, May–June 1985; by permission of the American Heart Association, Inc.)

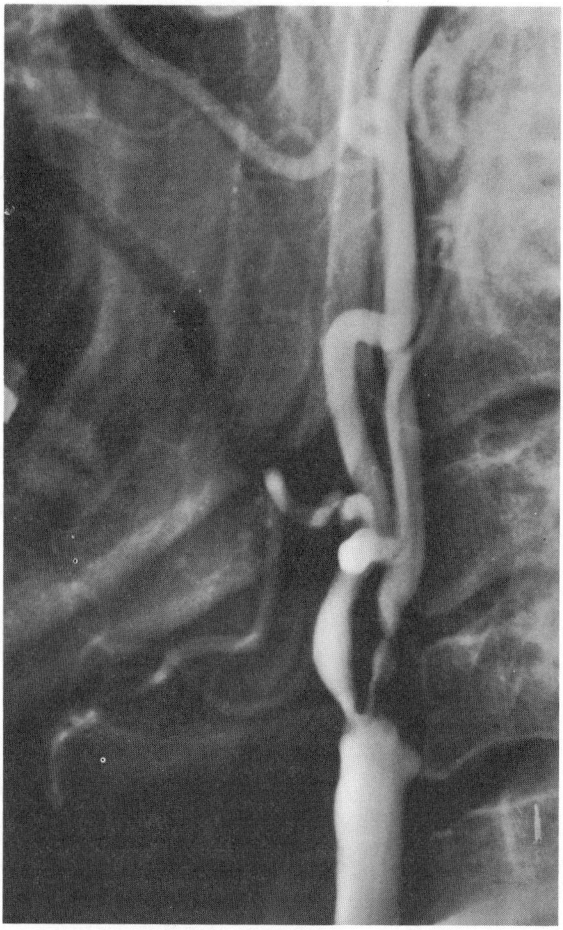

Fig 7–5.—Left carotid conventional arteriogram shows severe stenosis of proximal 1-cm segment of internal carotid artery. (Courtesy of Culebras, A., et al.: Stroke 16:425–431, May–June 1985; by permission of the American Heart Association, Inc.)

plications before symptoms are present. Lucent lesions in asymptomatic carotid arteries likely represent mural hemorrhages, focal necrosis, or excessive thickening.

Diagnostic Errors Discovered by CT in Patients With Suspected Stroke

Mona Britton, Tomas Hindmarsh, Veronica Murray, and Sven Anders Tydén (Stockholm)

Neurology (Cleve.) 34:1504–1507, November 1984 7–16

That many stroke patients are seen where computed tomography (CT) is unavailable makes it important to know how often CT diagnoses conflict with those obtained by other methods. A total of 256 unselected patients admitted with a sudden focal neurologic deficit were evaluated between 1978 and 1980 after installation of a CT scanner at a university hospital. Technically satisfactory examinations were obtained in 197 patients. Contrast enhancement was usually employed. The baseline and CT diagnoses agreed in 96% of 192 evaluable cases, but 8 patients had incongruent diagnoses. In 3 a diagnosis of hemorrhage was not confirmed by CT. Hematomas were found in 2 patients with pre-CT diagnoses of cerebral thrombosis. Antiplatelet therapy was made possible in the former cases and was avoided in the latter. Single patients were found to have subdural hematoma, hydrocephalus, and suspected tumor.

Few significant diagnostic errors were revealed by CT in this series of patients with presumed stroke. Computed tomography is mainly indicated if chronic subdural hematoma is suspected or if it is difficult to distinguish intracerebral hemorrhage from subarachnoid hemorrhage or meningitis. Patients who are candidates for acute intravenous heparin treatment should have CT if possible, since cerebrospinal fluid findings may be normal in patients with hemorrhage. The risk of diagnostic error may be less than 5% where CT is unavailable, provided strict criteria are applied for suspected stroke.

▶ A computed tomography scan is an integral part of an examination of patients with cerebral ischemic symptoms. In addition to information from within the hemisphere, infusion high-resolution CT scan now offers information about the extracranial carotid artery. Some have found CT scans to be helpful in determining even minimal patency and operability in patients with angiographic evidence of total occlusion of the internal carotid artery. The surgical equivalent of transforming dross to gold.

Persantine Aspirin Trial in Cerebral Ischemia: Endpoint Results
The American-Canadian Cooperative Study Group
Stroke 16:406–415, May–June 1985 7–17

The Persantine Aspirin Trial was a 15-center study of the efficacy of combined aspirin-dipyridamole (Persantine) treatment in lowering the incidence of cerebral or retinal infarction or death, in comparison with aspirin alone, in subjects who had transient ischemic attacks (TIAs) in the carotid territory, with or without persistent minor deficit. A total of 890 subjects were randomized to receive 325 mg of aspirin plus placebo or 75 mg of dipyridamole four times daily. All but 2% of subjects were followed for 1 year or longer and many for 4 to 5 years. Patients with hemispheric and monocular TIAs were included in the trial. Aspirin alone was given to 442 subjects and both drugs to 448. The series included mainly white males. Mean age was 63 years. Fifty-seven patients continued taking the study drugs.

Life-table analysis showed overall endpoint rates to be the same for the

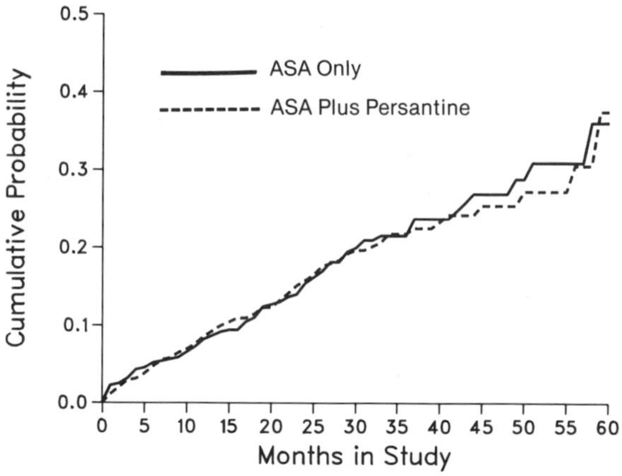

Fig 7–6.—Cumulative probability of any end point for aspirin *(ASA)* only and ASA plus Persantine groups by time in study. (Courtesy of American-Canadian Cooperative Study Group: Stroke 16:406–415, May–June 1985; by permission of the American Heart Association, Inc.)

aspirin-only and aspirin-diyridamole groups. The absolute endpoints were stroke, retinal infarction, and death from any cause. Cumulative probabilities of any endpoint are compared in Figure 7–6. Deaths from all causes were essentially equally divided between the two treatment groups. Recurrent TIAs were also similarly frequent in the two groups. There were 11 deaths from myocardial infarction in each group. No marked group differences in hemorrhagic complications were found.

Addition of dipyridamole to the use of aspirin in patients with TIAs had no advantage with respect to subsequent stroke, retinal infarction, or death from any cause. The French study also indicated that nothing is gained from adding diyridamole to aspirin in this setting.

▶ Aspirin has been demonstrated to be an effective antithrombotic agent. There is, however, concern about thrombotic effect at very high doses. In a recent editorial by J. Hirsh (*Arch. Int. Med.* 145:1582, 1985), it was emphasized that the thrombogenic effect is unlikely to occur in the usual therapeutic dose (350 mg–1 gm/day). Whether smaller doses of aspirin are equally effective as 1300 mg/day in the American–Canadian cooperative study remains to be seen.

Nevertheless, additional Persantine administration did not show any effect and the combined use of Persantine and aspirin should be discouraged. Similar results have also been observed in the French study. Until more information becomes available, patients with transient ischemic attacks should be treated with an aspirin dose of approximately 1 gm/day.

Coronary Artery Disease in Patients With Cerebrovascular Disease: A Prospective Study

Roxann Rokey, Loren A. Rolak, Yadollah Harati, N. Kutka, and Mario S. Verani (Houston)
Ann. Neurol. 16:50–53, July 1984 7–18

Coronary artery disease (CAD) is the leading cause of death in most patients who recover from transient ischemic attacks or stroke. However, such patients seldom are evaluated for CAD. A prospective examination was made of 50 consecutive patients with transient ischemic attacks or mild stroke to determine the prevalence and importance of CAD. All patients were examined by a cardiologist, as well as by exercise ^{201}thallium scintigraphy and exercise radionuclide ventriculography.

Sixteen patients were suspected to have CAD on the basis of clinical evaluation (group 1). The remaining 34 patients had no history, physical findings, or electrocardiographic (ECG) changes indicative of CAD (group 2). Patients in groups 1 and 2 did not differ significantly with regard to age, sex, prevalence of risk factors for CAD or cerebrovascular disease, and number and severity of lesions demonstrated by cerebral angiography. In 15 of the 16 group 1 patients, abnormalities were seen on cardiac scans indicative of CAD. Cardiac imaging demonstrated exercise-induced ischemia in 11 of these patients: the exercise ECG disclosed exercise-induced ischemia in only 5. Cardiac catheterization, performed in 13 of the 15 patients, revealed significant CAD in 10 and severe cardiomyopathy in 2. In 14 of the 34 group 2 patients, evidence of CAD was seen on 1 or both radionuclide scans. Cardiac imaging demonstrated exercise-induced ischemia in 13 of these 14 patients; and the exercise ECG showed ischemia in only 6. Of 9 patients who underwent cardiac catheterization, 8 were found to have significant CAD, 4 with multivessel disease. Overall, 29 of the 50 patients had abnormal results on exercise radionuclide cardiac imaging, including 14 with no clinical suspicion of CAD. Identification of CAD led to changes in management in 13 patients, 4 in group 1 and 9 in group 2.

Coronary artery disease can be easily, safely, and accurately evaluated noninvasively in patients with cerebrovascular disease. The long-term benefits of detecting CAD in patients with transient ischemic attacks or stroke have yet to be ascertained.

Natural History of Carotid Arterial Disease in Asymptomatic Patients With Cervical Bruits

G. O. Roederer, Y. E. Langlois, K. A. Jager, J. F. Primozich, K. W. Beach, D. J. Phillips, and D. E. Strandness, Jr. (Univ. of Washington)
Stroke 15:605–613, July–Aug. 1984 7–19

Management of asymptomatic patients with cervical bruit or carotid artery disease is controversial. A prospective study was initiated in January 1980 to follow with duplex scanning a consecutive series of 162 asymptomatic patients with mild cervical bruits to determine the stability of arterial lesions at the carotid bifurcation, the occurrence and type of neurologic symptoms during follow-up, and the possible role of risk indicators on disease changes. Patients were seen at 6-month intervals during the first year and yearly thereafter for 3 years. Based on duplex scanning assessment, disease of the carotid bifurcation is classified as normal, 1%–15% diameter reduction, 16%–49% reduction, 50%–79% reduction, 80%–99% stenosis, and occlusion.

Patients were aged 27–86 years (mean, 63.6). Duplex scanning showed 8 internal carotid arteries to be normal, 96 (29%) in the 1%–15% category, 106 (33%) in the 16%–49% class, 93 (29%) in the 50%–79% group, 9 (3%) in the 80%–99% category, and 12 (4%) occluded. During follow-up, 10 patients became symptomatic; 6 had transient ischemic attacks (TIAs), and 4 had strokes. The development of symptoms was accompanied by disease progress in 8 patients. Life table analysis showed an annual rate of occurrence of symptoms of 4%. The mean annual rate of disease progress from a less than 50% to a greater than 50% stenosis was 8%. When progress in all categories were considered, 60% of the sides would have progressed after 3 years. The presence of or progression to a greater than 80% stenosis was highly correlated (P = .00001) with development of total occlusion of the internal carotid artery or new symptoms. Most events occurred within 6 months of the finding of an 80%–99% stenosis, with mean interval to the event of 4.9 months. The major risk factors associated with disease progress were cigarette smoking (P = .04), diabetes mellitus (P = .04), and age younger than 65 years (P = .02). Hypertension and treatment with aspirin or dipyridamole did not correlate with disease progress.

A close relation exists between disease progression and appearance of ischemic neurologic deficits or subsequent internal carotid artery occlusion. Of 4 patients who had spontaneous strokes, 3 occurred without warning TIAs for an overall unpredictable stroke rate of 1.8%. Although 90% of the spontaneous symptoms were associated with a more than 80% stenosis at the time the symptoms occurred, 40% occurred on sides that were narrowed by less than 50% initially. Eighty-nine percent of the symptoms were preceded by disease progress to a greater than 80% stenosis. Therefore, progress of a lesion to a more than 80% stenosis is an important warning observation, since it carries a risk of ischemic symptoms or ipsilateral occlusion within 6 months and a 46% risk at 12 months.

The findings strongly suggest that it is safe to follow noninvasively at 6-month intervals asymptomatic patients with a less than 80% diameter-reducing lesion of a carotid artery. Angiography and surgical treatment can be delayed until the first appearance of TIAs or disease progress to a greater than 80% stenosis.

Incidental Asymptomatic Carotid Bruits in Patients Scheduled for Peripheral Vascular Reconstruction: Results of Cerebral and Coronary Angiography

Norman R. Hertzer, Edwin G. Beven, Jess R. Young, Patrick J. O'Hara, Robert A. Graor, and William F. Ruschhaupt III (Cleveland Clinic Found.)
Surgery 96:535–543, September 1984 7–20

Management of incidental asymptomatic carotid bruits in patients scheduled for other cardiovascular operations is still uncertain. Such bruits have been found to be an indication of synchronous heart disease. From 1978 to 1982 routine preoperative coronary angiography was performed in a series of 1,000 patients under consideration for elective peripheral vascular reconstruction, including 295 who were selected primarily because of recognized extracranial cerebrovascular disease.

Incidental asymptomatic carotid bruits were discovered in 144 (20%) of the remaining 705 patients who primarily were scheduled for such procedures as aortic replacement, lower extremity revascularization, or visceral artery bypass. Cerebral angiography and cardiac catheterization were performed in 139 of the 144 to assess the incidence of severe stenotic lesions among patients with asymptomatic carotid bruits, as well as the perceived value of asymptomatic bruits as an indication of synchronous coronary artery disease.

Incidental asymptomatic carotid bruits were more prevalent among patients with disease of a lower extremity and visceral occlusive disease than among those with aortoiliac aneurysms. Incidence of carotid stenosis that exceeded 50% of diameter of the lumen in patients with diabetes and hypertension, or both, was nearly identical to that for all patients with asymptomatic carotid bruits. Carotid stenosis that exceeded 50% of diameter of the lumen was documented by biplanar angiography in 39 (58%) of 67 patients with unilateral bruits and in 54 (75%) of 72 patients with bilateral bruits; greater than 75% stenosis was present in 42% and 46% of these subsets, respectively.

A total of 102 (71%) of 144 patients with carotid bruits had either advanced but compensated or severe CAD, compared with 322 (57%) of the 561 patients without bruits. Severe, surgically correctable coronary artery disease (CAD) was present in 29% of patients with incidental carotid bruits and in 24% of those without bruits, as well as in 32% of patients who had documented carotid stenosis and in 22% of those who did not. The incidence of severe, correctable CAD was significantly higher among patients suspected of having CAD by standard clinical criteria (33% to 38%) than among those who were not (13%), irrespective of whether carotid bruits were present or absent.

Elective myocardial revascularization was performed in 153 (22%) patients with an early mortality of 5.2%. Prophylactic carotid endarterectomy was performed in 54 patients with incidental asymptomatic carotid bruits (38%) with one death and one postoperative stroke (1.6%). Postoperative strokes occurred in 3 of 714 other peripheral vascular revascularizations (0.4%). Overall operative mortality was 2.7%. Thus, in the attempt to improve surgical risk and to reduce late morbidity caused by stroke and myocardial infarction, there were 4 neurologic deficits

(0.4%) and 28 deaths (3.0%) after 930 elective cardiac, extracranial, and peripheral vascular procedures.

Although this study does not resolve the controversy concerning management of incidental asymptomatic carotid bruits in patients scheduled for other operations, it confirms the assumption that patients with carotid bruits are more likely to have advanced coronary artery disease than those without bruits, although the clinical cardiac status is more closely related to incidence of severe, correctable CAD than is the presence of carotid bruits alone.

These conclusions are further confirmed by the findings that more patients have severe, correctable CAD (174 patients) than had incidental carotid bruits (144) and three times as many patients underwent elective myocardial revascularization (153) than had prophylactic endarterectomy (54), suggesting that management of incidental asymptomatic carotid bruits in patients who require other peripheral vascular operations should be redirected to address the critical problem of simultaneous severe CAD.

Combined Carotid and Coronary Operations: When Are They Necessary?

Ellis L. Jones, Joe M. Craver, Richard A. Michalik, Douglas A. Murphy, Robert A. Guyton, David K. Bone, Charles R. Hatcher, and Norman A. Riechwald (Emory Univ.)

J. Thorac. Cardiovasc. Surg. 87:7–16, January 1984 7–21

The study population comprised 3 groups of patients operated on since 1973. Group 1 (132 patients, 73% men, mean age 62 years) had combined carotid and coronary operations; they were compared with 167 patients without evidence of extracranial carotid vascular disease who had elective coronary artery bypass (CAB). Group 2, comprising 51 patients, had a stroke following isolated CAB; they were compared with 52 nonstroke patients who were operated on during the same time, so as to identify factors that favor the development of stroke as a complication of elective CAB. Group 3, 169 patients having asymptomatic cervical bruit, high-risk neurologic symptoms, or prior carotid endarterectomy and undergoing CAB alone, was retrospectively studied to determine the extent of carotid vascular obstruction and frequency of perioperative stroke.

Hypertension was significantly more prevalent in group 1 than in the elective CAB control group (67% vs. 47%), whereas there was no difference in incidence of unstable angina, history of congestive heart failure, or history of diabetes. Asymptomatic bruit was the reason for combining carotid and coronary operations in the majority of patients. Significant (75% or greater reduction in cross-sectional area) unilateral or bilateral obstructive disease was present in 89% of patients. The incidence of left main coronary artery obstruction (equal to or greater than 50% reduction in cross-sectional area) was 15% in the combined carotid group and 10% in patients having CAB alone.

Hospital mortality and perioperative stroke rate in group 1 were 4 of 132 (3%) and 2 of 126 (1.6%), respectively. These rates were not significantly different from those of the control group having CAB alone. The rehospitalization rate for group 1 patients was 2.3%, not statistically greater than for patients without extracranial cerebrovascular obstruction undergoing CAB alone. Overall incidence of postoperative stroke in 5,676 patients having CAB alone was 0.9% (51 patients).

Patients in group 3 with asymptomatic cervical bruit had postoperative stroke at a rate of 3.3% (2 of 60); those with a history of stroke or transient ischemic attacks and those who had carotid endarterectomy prior to elective CAB had postoperative stroke rates of 8.6% (6 of 70) and 5.1% (2 of 39), respectively.

Most strokes following CAB are embolic in origin and not related to flow states through the extracranial carotid vascular circulation.

It is suggested that simultaneous carotid and coronary operations should be performed in patients with bilateral carotid disease and symptomatic carotid vascular disease associated with unstable angina, left main obstruction, or diffuse multivessel disease. Staged procedures are suggested for patients with stable angina and symptomatic carotid lesions and for difficult carotid revascularization procedures. Coronary artery bypass alone may be performed for most patients with asymptomatic cervical bruit, moderate or mild carotid artery obstruction, and unstable angina associated with prior stroke, although in the latter case postoperative risk of neurologic injury may be increased.

▶ In reviewing the results of carotid surgery or peripheral vascular reconstruction, the ultimate cause of death is always myocardial infarction, a result of coronary artery disease. Therefore, awareness of severity of coronary artery disease and that of all three arterial beds singularly or in combination must be appreciated.

At present, there is no clear-cut approach to which patients should be subjected to combined carotid and coronary surgery. A cooperative study among major centers may help to solve this important dilemma.

Intraluminal Clot of the Carotid Artery Detected Radiographically

L. Caplan, R. Stein, D. Patel, L. Amico, N. Cashman, and B. Gewertz (Michael Reese Hosp., Chicago)

Neurology (Cleveland) 34:1175–1181, September 1984 7–22

Recognized thrombi of the carotid artery include flat plaques; ulcerated plaques with superimposed nidi of agglutinated platelets, fibrin, and thrombin; and complex stenotic lesions. A review was made of the radiologic and pathologic findings and clinical course in 9 patients with intraluminal filling defects angiographically identifiable as a free clot within the internal carotid artery.

The thrombus was unilateral in 8 patients and bilateral in 1. Eight clots were attached to atheromatous plaques, some of which were calcified. Three patients had serious concurrent illness, including pancreatic cancer with widespread venous and arterial occlusions, active rheumatiod vasculitis, and chronic pulmonary disease with polycythemia. All patients had risk factors for atherosclerosis: 7 were hypertensive, 3 had coronary artery disease, and 1 had symptomatic peripheral vascular occlusive disease. In some patients, repeat angiography showed total occlusion of the internal carotid artery, which had previously contained free clot. Thus, in most cases, a floating, radiographically visible clot merely represents a stage in the atherosclerotic process that eventually leads to complete occlusion of the vessel lumen. The clot was related to severe atherosclerosis in 3 patients. Fresh hemorrhage was identified beneath a plaque in 2 patients. In 3 younger patients, the thrombi remained unexplained, even though 2 had coagulation abnormalities. Sudden onset of cerebral hemisphere signs was the most common stroke syndrome, occurring in 5 patients. Two patients had both transient ischemic attacks (TIAs) and a fixed deficit, and 2 had TIAs alone. In 3 patients, the neurologic deficit developed gradually and progressively for hours or days. Sudden-onset fixed deficits were often associated with radiologically confirmed distal embolization to the middle cerebral artery and its branches. No patient had a new stroke after surgical or anticoagulant treatment.

Management of Patients With Symptomatic Extracranial Carotid Artery Disease and Incidental Intracranial Berry Aneurysm

Paul M. Orecchia, George Patrick Clagett, Jerry R. Youkey, Robert A. Brigham, Daniel F. Fisher, Richard F. Fry, Paul T. McDonald, George J. Collins, and Norman M. Rich

J. Vasc. Surg. 2:158–164, January 1985 7–23

Removal of a significant stenosis proximal to a berry aneurysm may increase the risk of rupture, but prophylactic aneurysm clipping might predispose to perioperative stroke from symptomatic carotid bifurcation disease. Ten patients with symptomatic extracranial carotid occlusive disease and asymptomatic intracranial berry aneurysms were seen in a 4-year period. The 5 men and 5 women had a mean age of 63 years. Nine patients had transient ischemic attacks, amaurosis fugax, or hemispheric stroke, and 1 had severe nonfocal symptoms. Thirteen berry aneurysms were recognized. Seven patients had aneurysms 6 mm or more in diameter. Most aneurysms were in the intracranial internal carotid, middle cerebral, or posterior communicating artery. Three patients had correction of hemodynamically significant carotid stenosis, 2 ipsilateral to anterior circulation aneurysms. Nine patients had 10 standard carotid endarterectomies.

No perioperative aneurysm leakage or rupture was evident in any of the 12 carotid artery operations. Two patients had neurologic complications, both transient. Two underwent aneurysm clipping after carotid endarterectomy. One patient died suddenly, presumably by aneurysm rupture, 3 months after a second endarterectomy. Six other patients remained without carotid or intracranial symptoms during a mean follow-up of 13 months. Two patients have died of unrelated problems.

Carotid artery operations appear to be safe in patients with asymptomatic intracranial aneurysms of less than 10 mm in diameter. Elective clipping, if indicated, can be done after carotid operation. Clipping may be reasonable before carotid operations in patients with larger aneurysms and a high risk of spontaneous rupture, but it is not of proved benefit.

Carotid Artery Surgery in Diabetic Patients

David R. Campbell, Carl S. Hoar, Jr., and Frank C. Wheelock, Jr. (Boston)

Arch. Surg. 119:1405–1407, December 1984 7–24

Preoperative patient characteristics and postoperative outcomes were analyzed in 191 carotid artery operations performed on 156 patients at the New England Deaconess Hospital. Because of the hospital's association with the Joslin Clinic, most (62.3%) of the patients had diabetes. Overall, 79.5% of the patients were operated on because of transient ischemic attacks and 10.9% because of previous strokes; 9.6% were asymptomatic. Patients with hemispheric transient ischemic attacks had the best results. Complete relief of symptoms was obtained in 90.4% of the diabetic patients and in 96% of the nondiabetic patients. Of diabetic and nondiabetic patients operated on because of a recent stroke, approximately 33% reported relief of symptoms, 33% experienced significant improvement, and the remainder had no change. Of the 18 patients with nonhemispheric transient symptoms, 50% reported no change in symptoms and the others were divided between those claiming relief of symptoms and those noting significant improvement. Almost 20% of the patients were lost to long-term follow-up observation (range, 2–10 years). The most striking finding at follow-up examination in the remaining patients was the increased mortality from myocardial infarction among diabetic patients. Of the nondiabetic patients, 14.2% died of myocardial infarction, 4.1% died of other causes, 4.1% died of a stroke, 6.1% died of unknown causes, and 71.4% were still alive. Among the diabetic patients, 38.1% died of myocardial infarction, 5.3% died of other causes, 2.6% died of a stroke, 1.3% died of unkown causes, and 52.6% were still alive. When only those patients followed for more than 4 years were considered, the differences between the 2 groups was even more pronounced, with 55.8% of the diabetic patients dying of myocardial infarction, compared with only 25% of the nondiabetic patients. This is especially significant as the incidence of symptomatic heart disease preoperatively, and perioperative morbidity and mortality, were similar in both groups. Asymptomatic heart disease appears to be more common in diabetic patients, and seems to progress more rapidly.

The Lucid Interval in Stroke Following Carotid Endarterectomy

William H. Prioleau, Jr., L. Dieter Voegele, and Peter Hairston (Charleston, S.C.)

Am. Surg. 51:114–115, February 1985 7–25

The use of an indwelling shunt during carotid endarterectomy remains controversial, although the occurrence of a stroke after a lucid interval suggests that inadequate cerebral protection during surgery was not a factor. Review was made of 789 carotid endarterectomies performed in a community where surgeons were divided in their views regarding use of a shunt.

Thirty-nine neurologic deficits (7.1%) occurred in 543 cases where a shunt was used, and 9 (3.7%) occurred in 246 cases where no shunt was used. Seven of the latter strokes occurred after a lucid interval. Mortality associated with deficits occurring after a lucid interval was 44% compared with 13% in cases of immediate deficit. Lucid intervals in 8 patients were interrupted in the first 12 hours after operation, 6 after 3–6 days and 2 subsequently. Lucid intervals in the latter 2 patients lasted until another major operation was performed, at which time severe stroke developed.

This analysis of stroke by the presence of a lucid interval provides evidence that thrombosis and embolism, rather than ischemic injury, are the chief problems in carotid surgery. The high mortality associated with deficits that follow a lucid interval supports a policy of immediate surgery when a delayed stroke is detected.

Chronic Ocular Ischemia

G. D. Sturrock and H. R. Mueller (Basel, Switzerland)

Br. J. Ophthalmol. 68:716–723, October 1984 7–26

Chronic ocular ischemia probably is sometimes missed or its recognition is delayed. Seven patients aged 50 to 77 years with severe carotid artery disease and ocular changes of chronic ischemia were evaluated by Doppler sonography at the University Eye Clinic. One case is described below.

Woman, 59, without symptoms, was found on routine examination to have forward new vessels on the left disc. Results of a glucose tolerance test were negative. Acuity was normal in both eyes. A prominent vascularized glial veil arose from the left optic disc. Microaneurysms, telangiectases, and areas of vascular closure were seen peripherally, and there was focal constriction of the superotemporal artery. Bilateral carotid bruits were noted. Brachial blood pressure was 80/65 mm Hg on the right and 120/80 mm Hg on the left. Doppler sonography showed a brachiocephalic steal syndrome, and angiographic study confirmed total occlusion of the brachiocephalic trunk and retrograde flow down the right vertebral artery to supply the subclavian and common carotid arteries. The middle third of the left common carotid artery was occluded, so that cerebral perfusion depended totally on the left vertebral artery. A brachiocephalic endarterectomy was carried out, and subsequent Doppler sonography showed physiologic flow in the right vertebral and common carotid arteries. The capillary network at the tip of the fibrovascular frond on the left disc shrunk as the amount of glial tissue increased (Fig 7–7). Normal vision in the left eye persisted.

The presentation of chronic ocular ischemia includes a picture of neovascular glaucoma, asymptomatic retinal hemorrhages, and new disc vessels. Any part of the eye may be involved, but it is uncommon for both eyes to be affected. A clinical diagnosis of chronic ocular ischemia implies the presence of severe carotid artery

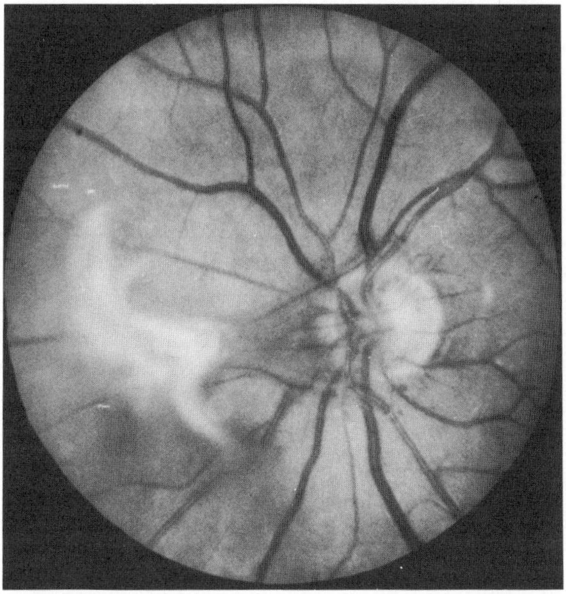

Fig 7–7.—Partial fibrosis of new disc vessels 2 years after brachiocephalic endarterectomy. (Courtesy of Sturrock, G.D., and Mueller, H.R.: Br. J. Ophthalmol. 68:716–723, October 1984.)

disease. The diagnosis alone probably does not call for major vascular surgery, but carotid bypass surgery should be considered for safeguarding cerebral perfusion. Recognition of chronic ocular ischemia can lead to the diagnosis and operative relief of a compromised cerebral blood supply.

▶ Both intracranial aneurysm and intraluminal clot are surprising arteriographic findings. In the presence of intraluminal clot, exposure of the carotid artery must be done with extreme care to prevent embolization. Carotid endarterectomy is a safe procedure, and fear of rupture of intracranial aneurysm during and following carotid endarterectomy is unjustified.

With the exception of higher incidence of myocardial infarction in diabetes, there appears to be no difference in morbidity between diabetics and nondiabetics.

In addition to understanding amaurosis fugax, surgeons must know that carotid artery stenosis plays a significant role in producing chronic ocular ischemia.

Does Contralateral Carotid Occlusion Influence Neurologic Fate of Carotid Endarterectomy?

Stephen M. Sachs, J. Timothy Fulenwider, Robert B. Smith III, William A. Darden, Atef A. Salam, and Garland D. Perdue (Emory Univ.)

Surgery 96:839–844, November 1984 7–27

Opinions vary regarding the operative risks and late prognosis for patients undergoing endarterectomy for carotid stenosis with contralateral carotid occlusion. In a review of experience from January 1978 through December 1982, outcomes were compared in 54 patients who underwent carotid endarterectomy (CEA) with contralateral carotid occlusion (group 1) and in 410 demographically similar patients without contralateral carotid occlusion (group 2) who underwent 503 CEAs.

The indications for CEA in group 1 were hemispheric transient ischemic attacks in 22 patients, asymptomatic stenosis in 12, nonhemispheric symptoms in 11, previous cerebral infarction in 8, and vascular tinnitus in 1. General anesthesia, routine intraluminal shunting, systemic heparinization, and arteriotomy closure without patch were routinely used in both groups. Permanent postoperative neurologic deficits developed in 3 patients in group 1 (5.6%) and in 10 patients in group 2 (2%). Transient postoperative neurologic deficits with complete recovery occurred in 2 patients in group 1 and in 10 patients in group 2. These differences in transient and permanent neurologic deficit rates did not differ significantly between groups. Operative mortality was 0% and 0.8% in groups 1 and 2, respectively (not significantly different). Two patients in group 1 (3.8%) and 13 patients in group 2 (3.6%) sustained late postoperative ischemic brain infarctions; again, the difference between groups was not significant. The results of Kaplan-Meier survival analyses were virutally the same in both groups, with cardiac disease being the usual cause of death.

The findings indicate that patients with carotid stenosis and contralateral carotid occlusion may undergo CEA with a risk of morbidity or mortality similar to that in patients without contralateral occlusion. The presence of contralateral carotid occlusion does not necessarily imply an unfavorable early or late prognosis after CEA.

Surgical Treatment of Patients With a Carotid Artery Occlusion and a Contralateral Stenosis

E. R. Hammacher, B. C. Eikelboom, T. J. Bast, R. De Geest, and F. E. E. Vermeulen (Niewegein, The Netherlands)

J. Cardiovasc. Surg. 25:513–517, Nov.–Dec. 1984 7–28

Patients with carotid occlusion and hemodynamically significant contralateral stenosis are at increased risk for stroke, and the proper management of their conditions remains uncertain. Severe symptoms of cerebrovascular disease often are present. Review was made of data on 33 such patients seen since 1972 who had undergone endarterectomy of the nonoccluded carotid artery. Six patients had a history of transient ischemic attacks, and 11 had had a stroke. One patient had symptoms of vertebrobasilar insufficiency. Symptoms were located on the side of stenosis in 4 cases. Fifteen patients were operated on prophylactically. Seven of them required other major surgery. A shunt was used intraoperatively in 9 patients.

No new permanent neurologic symptoms occurred within 30 days after operation. During follow-up periods averaging 29 months, there were 3 fatal cerebrovascular accidents. In 1 case, the symptoms suggested a stroke on the side of occlusion. Angiography of the extracranial arteries, performed in 20 patients an average of 1½ years after operation, showed all vessels to be patent and no restenosis.

Patients with hemodynamically significant carotid lesions who require major surgery should have carotid endarterectomy. Although the risk of carotid surgery is increased by contralateral occlusion, no postoperative neurologic deaths occurred in this series, and there were no new permanent neurologic deficits in the postoperative period. Patients who continue to have transient ischemia on the occluded side after endarterectomy of the stenotic side should be considered for extracranial-intracranial bypass.

▶ If untreated, a high stroke rate (20%) is observed in patients with carotid artery occlusion and a contralateral stenosis. It is reassuring to note there is no increased morbidity in this group of patients compared to those without contralateral occlusion. In patients with a totally occluded artery, even the contralateral stenotic artery may be asymptomatic. Carotid endarterectomy should be considered if such stenosis is severe as it can be done safely.

Benefits, Shortcomings, and Costs of EEG Monitoring

Richard M. Green, William J. Messick, John J. Ricotta, Maurice H. Charlton, Richard Satran, Margaret M. McBride, and James A. DeWeese (Univ. of Rochester)

Ann. Surg. 201:785–792, June 1985 7–29

The efficacy of electroencephalogram (EEG) monitoring was reviewed in a series of 562 patients who had carotid endarterectomy under continuous monitoring since 1979. Operation was usually performed with normocapnic general anesthesia. The need for temporary shunting during clamping was based on EEG findings and the surgeon's preference.

Electroencephalographic changes were observed in 18% of the patients who were operated on, including 37% of those with completed stroke and 21% of asymptomatic patients. More than one third of patients with contralateral carotid occlusion had EEG changes. Nine of the 15 perioperative strokes were associated with technical problems, and these were more frequent when shunts were used. Patients with stroke before endarterectomy were at greater risk of perioperative stroke. The EEG was unchanged in 3 patients who had lacunar infarcts before operation and awoke with a worse deficit. A shunt was used in 91 of 102 patients with EEG changes.

This experience failed to show that routine EEG monitoring is advantageous in carotid endarterectomy. It is expensive, and not all cases of ischemia will be detected. Use of a shunt may involve a greater risk of stroke from technical error than is associated with hemodynamic ischemia. The use of EEG monitoring may reduce the incidence of shunting where the record remains normal after clamping, but the decision to shunt where dysfunction is observed should be based in part on the clinical and computed tomographic findings. Selective shunting is not demonstrably beneficial unless a stroke has occurred before endarterectomy.

Correlation of Cerebral Blood Flow and EEG During Carotid Occlusion for Endarterectomy (Without Shunting) and Neurologic Outcome

Richard B. Morawetz, H. Evan Zeiger, Holt A. McDowell, Jr., Robert D. McKay, Pam D. Varner, Simon Gelman, and James H. Halsey (Univ. of Alabama Medical Center)

Surgery 96:184–189, August 1984 7–30

The use of indwelling shunts during carotid endarterectomy intended to prevent ischemic infarction of neural tissue remains controversial. The authors analysed prospectively 129 consecutive carotid endarterectomies performed for atherosclerotic ulcerative stenosis without the use of intraoperative shunting to determine the significance of intraoperative ischemia. Patients were graded according to the Mayo Clinic classification of preoperative risk factors based on major medical and angiographically determined risks as described by Sundt et al. Continuous 16-channel electroencephalogram (EEG) monitoring and intermittent regional cerebral blood flow (rCBF) measurements with ^{133}Xe were used to monitor these patients intraoperatively. Complications were divided into death, major morbidity that interfered with normal daily living, minor morbidity that did not interfere with daily living, and transient neurologic dysfunction that cleared at the time of discharge.

The overall mortality was 2.5%, major morbidity was 2.5%, minor morbidity was 1.7%, and rate of transient neurologic dysfunction was 1.7%. Complications were confined to patients judged to be Mayo Clinic class III and IV. There was no association between blood flow during carotid occlusion and either the development of complications ($P = .27$) or presence of new deficits when the patients awoke, ($P = .54$). None of 8 patients with an rCBF of less than 9 ml 100 gm^{-1} $minute^{-1}$ during carotid occlusion suffered a complication or developed a new or delayed deficit; this implies that 20 to 30 minutes of ischemia at this level can be tolerated by uninjured brain tissue. Seven of these patients showed flat EEG during carotid occlusion but none experienced an increase in neurologic deficit. Three of 10 patients with neurologic complications showed EEG changes during occlusion, but only 1 awoke with a new deficit.

The authors conclude that preoperative assessment of medical and angiographic risk factors as described by Sundt et al. was more useful in identifying patients who are likely to develop neurologic complications than was the use of intraoperative EEG and rCBF monitoring. Currently, the authors are considering selective shunting for patients with identifiable preoperative acute ischemic brain injury; however, these patients will continue to be at great risk during carotid endarterectomy.

▶ Intraoperative EEG monitoring should not be the sole determining factor in making a decision for or against the use of a shunt. The electroencephalogram should be used primarily for monitoring nothing else. A change in EEG monitoring may occur because of a change in blood pressure, the effect of anesthetics, or malfunction of an indwelling shunt. The EEG details these changes and allows proper treatment to be instituted appropriately.

The Performance of Endarterectomy for Disease of the Extracranial Arteries of the Head

Mark L. Dyken (Indiana Univ.) and Robert Pokras (National Center for Health Statistics)

Stroke 15:948–950, Nov.–Dec. 1984 7–31

The performance of endarterectomy on extracranial vessels of the head and neck in the United States was estimated from data collected from the National Hospital Discharge Survey, VA hospitals, and armed forces hospitals. The number of endarterectomies done has increased steadily from 1971 through 1982. An estimated 15,000 such operations were done in nonfederal hospitals in 1971. In 1982, the procedure was done about 82,000 times in nonfederal hospitals and about 3,000 times in federal

NUMBER OF ENDARTERECTOMIES OF VESSELS OF HEAD AND NECK*

	National Hospital Discharge Survey (Estimated to Nearest 1000)	Army and Air Force (% Navy)	VAH†
1971	15,000	170	
1972	16,000	186	
1973	22,000	211	
1974	23,000	282	
1975	34,000	246 (359)	
1976	34,000	370 (530)	
1977	41,000	381 (539)	
1978	42,000	387 (559)	2,077
1979	54,000	503 (654)	2,037
1980	55,000	772	2,076
1981	73,000	800	3,070
1982	82,000	854	3,424
Death Average %	2.8%	2.1%	2.5%

*Boxed areas include endarterectomies other than those for vessels of the head and neck.

†VA hospitals

(Courtesy of Dyken, M.L., and Pokras, R.: Stroke 15:948–950, Nov.–Dec. 1984; by permission of the American Heart Association, Inc.)

facilities, representing 4.7- and 2.9-fold increases, respectively (table). An estimated 2.8% of patients operated on in nonfederal hospitals during the 12-year survey period were discharged dead. This was slightly higher than the percentage of deaths in federal hospitals.

The marked increase in endarterectomies in recent years is difficult to understand in view of the lack of objective, double-blind, prospective studies showing that the procedure is clearly advantageous over medical treatment. Surgeons must feel that the operation has considerable value, but data are not available to either refute or support this belief. It is possible that many deaths occur after a procedure that many physicians may not agree was indicated and that many other patients had strokes.

▶ The number of carotid operations is on the rise, probably due to better detection of carotid stenosis by noninvasive tests. Carotid endarterectomy, even performed in a community hospital, is a safe procedure. The Easton-Sherman Report is grossly exaggerated and has been refuted by other reports. The concern expressed by Dyken, based on estimation, is unjustified. The increase in carotid endarterectomies in the United States is in the best interests of a rapidly aging population.

The Effect of Unilateral Carotid Endarterectomy on Neuropsychologic Test Performance in 53 Patients

Robert S. Bennion, Milton L. Owens, and Samuel E. Wilson (Los Angeles)
J. Cardiovasc. Surg. 26:21–26, Jan.–Feb. 1985 7–32

The relationship between carotid disease and dementia remains uncertain, but a growing number of surgeons and neurologists have found that endarterectomy for extracranial atherosclerotic disease significantly improves neuropsychologic test performance. Six psychomotor tests were used to assess the conditions of 53 patients before, 3–7 days after, and 3 months after unilateral carotid endarterectomy. The operative technique included general anesthesia and use of a Javid shunt. The Ravens progressive matrices, spatial orientation, vocabulary, arithmetic, short-term memory, and finger-tapping tests were carried out. Eighty-one percent of patients had a more than 50% reduction in carotid diameter on angiography. More than half of the patients also had 50% or greater stenosis of the contralateral carotid artery.

No patient had a postoperative neurologic deficit or significant complications from endarterectomy. Psychometric test scores did not change postoperatively in 18 patients with previous stroke. The patients with high-grade stenosis, who had a 75% or greater reduction in luminal diameter, had significantly increased early postoperative test scores (Fig 7–8), which returned to baseline by 3 months. Improved scores were correlated with increased intraoperative carotid flow.

Psychometric test performance increased after unilateral carotid endarterectomy in patients with high-grade stenosis in this study, but baseline

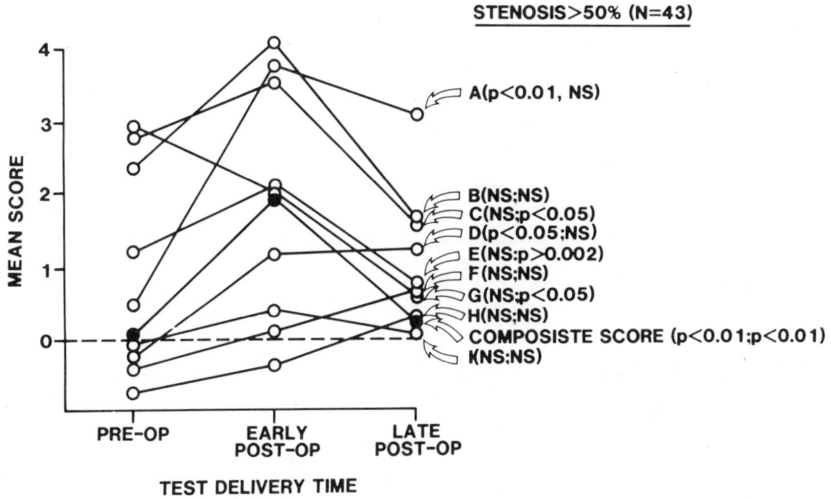

Fig 7–8.—Psychometric test performance in 43 patients with greater than 50% carotid stenosis preoperatively. *A:* spatial orientation (SOP = R); *B:* contralateral finger tap; *C:* ipsilateral finger tap; *D:* arithmetic; *E:* short-term memory; *F:* vocabulary (SOP = R); *B:* contralateral finger tap; *G:* spatial orientation (SOP = L); *H:* vocabulary (SOP) = L; *I:* Ravens. (Contribution by Bennion, R.S., et al.: J. Cardiovasc. Surg. 26:21–26, Jan.–Feb. 1985).

performance was present 3 months postoperatively. Either an autoregulatory process or progression of atherosclerotic change may be responsible for a gradual return of cerebral perfusion to preoperative levels in these cases.

Late Survival After Carotid Endarterectomy for Transient Ischemic Attacks
Reginald S. A. Lord (Sydney)
J. Vasc. Surg. 1:512–519, July 1984 7–33

The value of carotid endarterectomy in the management of patients with transient ischemic attack (TIA) is not universally accepted, since it is believed that survival after operation is shortened by high incidence of myocardial infarction. The authors used life-table analysis to compare the longevity of 266 consecutive patients with carotid TIAs who were treated by 310 carotid endarterectomies with that of an age- and sex-matched population from the same geographic region. Patients with abnormal ECG, history of cardiac disease, or severe hypertension were supervised by the cardiologist. Patients judged to be at excessively high risk for general anesthesia because of recent myocardial infarction, poor ventricular contraction, poorly controlled ventricular rhythm, or severe renal or respiratory failure were not treated by carotid reconstruction until the risk had diminished to an acceptable level. Coronary artery grafting was done on patients with concomitant coronary artery disease before, after, or combined with carotid reconstruction. Endarterectomy was undertaken for carotid stenosis narrowing the lumen by 50% or more in any diameter. The patients were followed from 30 months to 12 years.

Mean survival rate at 5 years was 78% and 64% at 10 years. Compared with an age- and sex-matched group, the survival rate was virtually identical at 6 years and was not significantly different up to 8 years. Mean survival rate of 119 patients with only cardiac risk factors was not significantly different from the matched cohort. The survival rate of 65 patients with other risk factors, including diabetes, lower limb ischemia, malignant disease, chronic respiratory disease, chronic renal failure, and previous stroke was 69% at 5 years and 51% at 10 years. The difference compared with the matched group was significant ($P = .05$), amounting to an increased mortality rate between the fourth and eighth years. Bilateral carotid endarterectomies were carried out in 44 patients, whose 81% survival rate at 5 years was not significantly different from the matched group.

The results indicate that survival is not impaired when carotid lesions are surgically corrected, and other risk factors are controlled. The virtually normal survival statistics are mainly due to a comprehensive holistic approach in which correctable risk factors were actively investigated and treated before and after operation. In particular, coronary artery disease and hypertension were aggressively treated. The decreased survival among patients with diabetes, respiratory and renal disease, malignancy, and symptomatic lower limb ischemia shows that these risk factors that cannot be controlled or that are naturally progressing limit survival. Caution is indicated in recommending carotid endarterectomy to treat TIAs in patients with such risk factors.

▶ The Australian long-term follow-up again demonstrates that carotid endarterectomy is a durable procedure. Only 1.5% of patients in this study suffered a late stroke. This figure contrasts with 30% to 40% liability to stroke in patients with untreated carotid TIAs reported by Millikan (*Stroke* 2:201–208, 1971). Neurologists should take note of this study.

Could mental functions be improved by performance of carotid endarterectomy? This question has attracted interest in the past. The difficulty in answering this question definitely lies in the fact that there is no reliable quantitative analysis of the human mind.

Recurrent Carotid Stenosis: A 5-Year Series of 65 Reoperations

Mohan B. Das, Norman R. Hertzer, Norman B. Ratliff, Patrick J. O'Hara, and Edwin G. Beven (Cleveland Clinic)

Ann. Surg. 202:28–35, July 1985 7–34

Recurrences were analyzed in a series of 1,726 carotid endarterectomies performed between 1979 and 1983. Sixty-one patients required 65 corrective procedures for recurrent carotid stenosis. The 39 men and 22 women had a mean age of 60 years. Three patients had bilateral recurrences, and 1 had a second recurrence after reoperation on the same side. Thirty-three recurrent lesions were associated with neurologic symptoms, most often transient ischemic attacks (TIAs). Restenosis occurred a mean of 42 months after initial operation. Only 6 endarterectomies had been performed by the patch angioplasty method.

Reoperations for recurrent stenosis comprised 4% of all carotid endarterectomies during the 5-year review period. Earlier lesions represented myointimal hyperplasia, whereas atherosclerotic restenosis more often was associated with neurologic symptoms occurring later during follow-up. Stroke was more commonly related to atherosclerotic restenosis. Two patients died within a month of reoperation, for an operative mortality of 3%. Two others had neurologic deficits. Only 1 of 59 operative survivors followed for a mean of 22 months had a completed stroke, and this may have been unrelated to extracranial disease. Patients reoperated on for TIAs or vertebrobasilar symptoms did better than those with completed stroke.

Earlier carotid restenosis after endarterectomy is associated with myointimal hyperplasia, and later, clinically more serious cases are associated with atherosclerosis. The authors recommend noninvasive testing annually for 3 years after carotid endarterectomy and then every other year. Restenosis is adequately managed by patch angioplasty, and this procedure might be considered more often for primary endarterectomy.

Carotid Endarterectomy: Relationship of Outcome to Early Restenosis

Stephen C. Nicholls, David J. Phillips, Robert O. Bergelin, Kirk W. Beach, Jean F. Primozich, and D. Eugene Strandness, Jr. (Univ. of Washington)

J. Vasc. Surg. 2:357–381, May 1985 7–35

Restenosis has occurred more frequently than expected after carotid endarterectomy, raising the question of whether the procedure may produce a worse lesion in asymptomatic patients. A prospective study was carried out in 134 patients having a total of 145 procedures since 1980. Ultrasonic duplex scanning was performed and patients were followed clinically for a mean period of 18 months and for as long as 4 years. Mean age was 65 years. Thirty-three patients were operated on prophylactically; 20 others had had stroke.

Operative mortality was 0.7%, and the perioperative stroke rate was 1.3%. Two of 9 late deaths were stroke-related. Twelve patients had ipsilateral focal symptoms, 6 of them strokes. Two of 7 patients with transient ischemic attacks referable to the operated side had recurrent high-grade stenosis. Such stenosis was seen in 22% of all patients during follow-up. Lesions regressed in 7 patients. The incidence was greater in women. Most restenoses were seen within 2 years of operation. No consistent association with symptoms was noted. Three patients were operated on again for recurrent disease, all with good clinical results.

Restenosis occurs frequently after carotid endarterectomy, especially in women, and regresses in a significant proportion of cases. There is no reason to think that surgery will improve focal ipsilateral symptoms, and operation probably should be reserved for patients whose nonhemispheric symptoms can be relieved through compensation for inadequate contralateral circulation. Restenosis can recur after reoperation.

▶ There is a discrepancy in the incidence of recurrent carotid stenosis in these two reports (4% vs. 22%), probably due to the type of noninvasive test used. In the Cleveland series, periorbital Doppler or carotid compression tomography was used. Both are indirect tests and are less accurate than direct tests, such as the Duplex scan.

In most instances, patch angioplasty, using either a vein or prosthetic material, is required in treating myointimal hyperplasia because a cleavage plane in the arterial wall is often absent.

The Rationale for Patch-Graft Angioplasty After Carotid Endarterectomy: Early and Long-Term Follow-Up

Giovanni P. Deriu, Enzo Ballotta, Luigi Bonavina, Franco Grego, Simonetta Alvino, Lorenza Franceschi, Giorgio Meneghetti, and Aldo Saja (Univ. of Padua, Padua Italy)

Stroke 15:972–979, Nov.–Dec. 1984 7–36

Experience with carotid endarterectomy (CE) closed with patching to delay and prevent recurrent stenosis was reviewed in 74 patients who had 86 endarterectomies for atherosclerosis of the carotid bifurcation from March 1980 to July 1983. Thirty patients were asymptomatic at the time of CE. The 61 men and 13 women had respective mean ages of 62 and 56 years. New neurologic symptoms during follow-up were usually evaluated by Doppler sonography.

Surgery was done under general anesthesia with pharmacologic hypertension and systemic heparinization. The EEG was monitored and "stump pressures" were measured. A shunt was used in only 17 patients in whom changes were seen on EECs. Carotid arteriotomies were extended into the internal carotid artery. The arteriotomy was routinely closed by a PTFE patch graft angioplasty.

No patient had transient or permanent neurologic deficit after CE. None died after operation of causes related to surgery. In 192 case-control patients who had 204 CE procedures in 1970 through 1979 without shunt protection and with patch closure of the arteriotomy, 2.5% had neurologic deficits and early mortality was 1.5%.

Fifty one of the present patients were followed for 6 to 36 months after operation. The endarterectomized carotid artery was patent in all cases. There were no pseudoaneurysms and no patch infections.

Patch grafting at CE enlarges the lumen at the level of possible myointimal fibroplasia or new plaque formation. The patch could, by serving as a source of cells for rapid reendothelialization of the endarterectomized segment, decrease the occurrence of proliferative lesions in the walls of the operated vessel. Routine patch graft angioplasty after CE is recommended. Direct closure of the endarterectomized carotid artery is considered the chief cause of recurrent stenosis.

▶ A more critical review of the results of carotid endarterectomy, as assessed by the Duplex scan, will change the minds of those surgeons who never use patch for closure of the arteriotomy.

Results of Extracranial-Intracranial Arterial Bypass for Intracranial Internal Carotid Artery Stenosis: Review of 105 Cases

Philip R. Weinstein, R. Rodriguez y Baena, and Norman L. Chater (Univ. of California at San Francisco)

Neurosurgery 15:787–794, December 1984 7–37

The results of extracranial-intracranial arterial bypass (EIAB) were reviewed in 105 patients who had transient ischemic attacks (TIAs) or mild stroke with a fluctuating deficit and who were operated on in a 10-year period. All had at least 60% narrowing of the petrous, cavernous, or supraclinoid level of the internal carotid artery from atherosclerotic disease and either delayed delivery of contrast distal to the stenosis or inadequate collateral filling from the opposite carotid or vertebral artery. The superficial temporal artery was anastomosed to a cortical branch of the middle cerebral artery. Heparin is now used in low doses during operation in selected patients, after two operative strokes and one operative bypass occlusion occurred in early patients. Further, larger recipient vessels are chosen.

Mean follow-up is 54 months. Operative complications led to failure in 5 patients. Operative mortality was 1%, and 2% of patients had permanent surgical morbidity. Two of three stroke-related deaths that occurred during follow-up were ipsilateral to the bypass. Eighty-nine percent of 82 patients had no further TIAs or stroke. The late mortality from neurologic causes was 0.4% per year.

The EIAB operation is reasonably safe for symptomatic intracranial carotid stenosis. The long-term bypass patency rate is satisfactory, and bypass did not appear significantly to increase the risk of stroke in this series. Care is needed to prevent perioperative hypotension. Shorter occlusion times and low-dose heparin therapy will limit the occurrence of operative stroke, as will improved microanastomotic techniques. The procedure may not be suitable where many small cortical arteries are involved by diffuse atherosclerosis.

Microanastomosis of Temporal External Artery (TEA) to Middle Cerebral Artery (MCA) Branch in 150 Cases of Cerebrovascular Occlusive Disease

R. Mrówka (Katowice, Poland)

Zentralbl. Neurochir. 45:233–244, 1984 7–38

The results of microneurosurgical anastomosis of the superficial temporal artery to the cortical branch of the MCA were assessed in 150 patients seen between 1980 and 1983 with signs of ischemia in the internal carotid artery territory. The largest group had completed stroke and evidence of generalized atherosclerosis. Ten percent of patients had traumatic occlusion of the cerebral arteries. A stabilizing hemostatic clamp was used for end-to-side anastomoses and for continuous-suture anastomosis. Operation was performed with the operating microscope and 10–0 Ethilon or Prolene suture material.

The anastomosis was correctly performed in 91% of cases. Three failures were technical. Overall mortality was 14%. Most patients with transient ischemic attacks (TIAs) or prolonged reversible ischemic neurologic deficit (PRIND) improved clinically after operation. Less improvement was evident in those with completed stroke. One-year follow-up indicated clinical improvement in 58% of patients, most of whom had TIAs or PRIND. Improvement continued over the next year in a majority of patients. Early control angiography showed patent anastomoses in 79% of studies and later control in 86%. Clinical improvement was more frequent where an anastomosis was visible at angiography.

Microsurgical anastomosis of the superficial temporal and middle cerebral arteries has a greater prophylactic than therapeutic role in patients with cerebrovascular disease. "Spasm" of the anastomosis may represent passive adaptation to altered hemodynamic conditions, rather than an active process in the vessel wall.

Results, Complications, and Follow-up of 415 Bypass Operations for Occlusive Disease of the Carotid System

Thoralf M. Sundt, Jr., Jack P. Whisnant, Nicolee C. Fode, David G. Piepgras, and O. Wayne Houser (Mayo Clinic)

Mayo Clin. Proc. 60:230–240, April 1985 7–39

A total of 415 carotid-middle cerebral artery bypass procedures was carried out over 8 years in 403 patients with acute or persistent ischemic symptoms related to occlusion or inaccessible stenosis of the internal carotid or middle cerebral artery. The primary indication was transient ischemic attacks, and the most frequent pathologic feature was internal carotid occlusion. Antiplatelet drugs and anticoagulants were used by many patients preoperatively. A branch of the superficial temporal artery was joined to a middle cerebral branch. The occlusion time for the anastomosis was about 25–30 minutes in most cases. The anterior branch of the superficial temporal artery was used in 216 operations, the posterior branch in 166, and both in 33.

Operative mortality was about 1%; 3 of the 5 deaths were cardiogenic. Five patients had a permanent deficit from occlusion of the arterial pedicle or damage to cortical vessels. Neurologic function 6 months after operation was as good as or better than at baseline in 95% of surviving patients.

The bypass pedicle was patent in nearly all patients evaluated. Six patients died of ischemic stroke during follow-up. Strokes were eightfold more likely to occur within 6 months of surgery than subsequently. The actuarial risk of stroke 6 months to 3½ years after surgery was 0.23% per month.

A high rate of patency was found in this series of temporal artery-middle cerebral artery bypass procedures. Neurologic function was preserved or improved in 95% of patients who remained alive 6 months after operation. The results compare favorably with those of carotid endarterectomy performed at the same center.

▶ In well-selected cases, extracranial-intracranial bypass appears to be an effective revascularization procedure. This is evident in the Mayo Clinic series where results are comparable to carotid endarterectomy.

Elective Carotid Resection for Squamous Cell Carcinoma of the Head and Neck

Donald P. Atkinson, Lloyd A. Jacobs, and Arthur W. Weaver (Detroit)
Am. J. Surg. 148:483–488, October 1984 7–40

The prognosis for patients with squamous cell carcinoma adherent to the carotid artery is very poor, although some patients can be salvaged by aggressive surgical resection. Data are reported on the surgical management of 12 patients with squamous cell carcinoma adherent to the bifurcation or internal carotid artery who were technically resectable for cure. Before operation special attention was given to the possibility of concurrent cerebrovascular disease and to the degree of patency of the carotid and vertebral vessels that carry the collateral circulation after resection.

One patient developed an acute neurologic complication and died and another had a stroke several months after resection but survived, for a neurologic morbidity secondary to carotid resection of 16.7% and mortality of 8.3%.

The patient who died was neurologically intact after operation but had a cerebral infarction on the first postoperative day. Reconstruction was not carried out because the somatosensory-evoked cortical potential was normal after clamping, even though the stump pressure was 36 mm Hg. Inadvertently, this patient did not receive subcutaneous heparin after operation. The patient who had a stroke developed aphasia 3 months after carotid resection. Although the stump pressure was 64 mm Hg, reconstruction had been advised and a Goretex graft was placed. Infection of the wound developed and thrombosis of the graft and embolization most likely accounted for the stroke (Fig 7–9).

Two patients with stump pressures of less than 50 mm Hg had a potential for cerebral ischemia and were considered to be candidates for reconstruction after resection. However, analysis of somatosensory-invoked cortical potential indicated that electric responsiveness was not affected by carotid occlusion, and reconstruction was not performed in either patient.

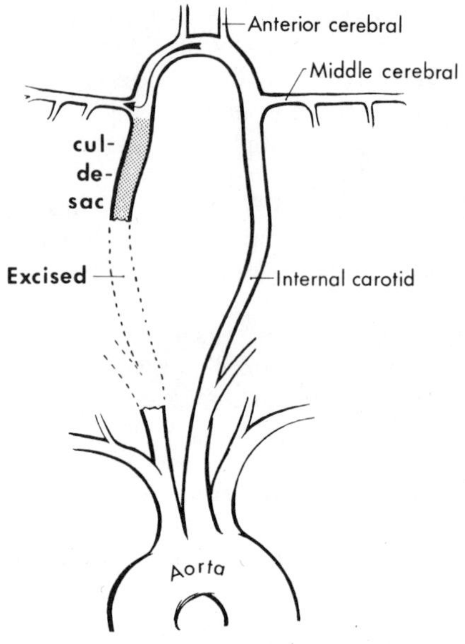

Fig 7–9.—Possible cause of delayed stroke. Propagation of thrombus from carotid stump into circle of Willis. (Courtesy of Atkinson, D.P., et al.: Am. J. Surg. 148:483–488, October 1984.)

Six of the 12 patients are alive, 5 without evidence of disease; however, only 2 have been followed long enough (31 and 68 months) to be regarded as long-term survivors.

Preoperative four-vessel arteriography with intracranial views is mandatory to detect coexisting arteriosclerotic disease that may limit collateral perfusion. Preoperative Matas-type tests are potentially dangerous and do not provide the information that can be obtained with intraoperative measurement of stump pressure of the internal carotid artery. Carotid reconstruction is unnecessary if stump pressure is 50 mm Hg or greater. If the stump pressure is less than 50 mm Hg, reconstruction is indicated if the pharynx has not been entered during resection. If mucosal entry is necessary and stump pressure is less than 50 mm Hg, resection should not be performed because of the increased risk of graft complications. Somatosensory-evoked potentials are predictive of cerebral tolerance to temporary interruption of blood flow but not necessarily of tolerance to permanent interruption of flow. The grafting material of choice for reconstruction is the autogenous vein. In patients who do not undergo reconstruction, administration of low-dose heparinization started before operation and continued for 10 days may diminish the chances of delayed stroke.

▶ Occasionally, vascular surgeons will be asked by oncologic surgeons to provide opinion on how to manage tumor invasion of the carotid artery. This article outlines the proper approach to this problem. Intraoperative measurement of stump pressure, in conjunction with somatosensory evoked cortical potential, provides objective information. These facts may be used to determine whether arterial reconstruction is needed. Although 50 mm Hg stump pressure has been recommended by the author, others have found that 70 mm Hg is optimal (Ehrenfeld et al.: *Surgery* 93:299–305, 1983). The use of evoked potential may help to solve this dilemma in the future.

Subclavian Steal: Treatment With Percutaneous Transluminal Angioplasty
William J. Bean, Bruce A. Rodan, and Dennis A. Franqui (Jupiter, Fla.)
South. Med. J. 77:1044–1046, August 1984 7–41

Subclavian steal is characterized by diversion of blood flow from the basilar artery with retrograde flow through the ipsilateral vertebral artery due to narrowing or occlusion of the subclavian artery. Surgical bypass has been the usual treatment for symptomatic patients. An alternative approach, percutaneous transluminal angioplasty, was used in 3 cases treated at Palm Beach-Martin County Medical Center.

A patient with stenotic disease localized to a single vessel did well after angioplasty. A second patient had associated vascular lesions but also did well. Endarterectomy can be done after subclavian angioplasty in these cases if a significant or symptomatic carotid plaque is present. In the third patient the proximal arterial supply to the arm was opened, but problems related to carcinoma-induced coagulopathy and chemotherapy necessitated amputation of the extremity.

Subclavian steal can be accurately diagnosed by the Dopscan method. Percutaneous transluminal angioplasty was used successfully to treat subclavian steal in 3 patients in this study, 1 of them 3 times, without complications in the CNS. Screening by Doppler ultrasound can identify associated carotid disease. Angioplasty should provide a more acceptable treatment for subclavian steal. Steal in 3 left subclavian arteries has been managed by angioplasty more recently without complications.

Surgical Reconstruction of the Proximal Vertebral Artery
Fernando G. Diaz, James I. Ausman, Raul A. de los Reyes, Jeffrey Pearce, Carl Shrontz, Hooshang Pak, and Jean Turcotte (Detroit)
J. Neurosurg. 61:874–881, November 1984 7–42

The value of anticoagulant therapy never has been confirmed in a randomized study of patients with proved lesions causing vertebrobasilar insufficiency (VBI), and advances in microvascular operation have allowed a more aggressive approach to these patients. Data were reviewed on fifty-five patients seen in 1980–1983 with symptoms of VBI and associated proximal vertebral artery stenosis or occlusion. Mean age was 63 years. Five of 48 patients with multiple episodes and 4 of 7 with a single event had a permanent deficit. Most patients had multiple angiographic abnormalities, and most had associated internal carotid artery lesions. Thirty-seven patients had received antiplatelet agents, and 15 had received anticoagulants. Forty-eight patients underwent transposition of the vertebral artery to the ipsilateral carotid artery, 18 in conjunction with ipsilateral carotid endarterectomy. Seven patients had a vertebral artery endarterectomy before the transposition was completed. Vertebral-to-carotid transposition was completed simultaneously with carotid endarterectomy in 7 patients.

Symptoms resolved completely in all but 2 patients. Complications included vocal cord paralysis with temporary hoarseness in 3 patients, and diaphragmatic elevation without apparent respiratory difficulty in 2 patients. Only 4 patients had a permanent Horner's syndrome. There were no deaths. Only 1 of 55 anastomotic sites was occluded on postoperative angiography in 52 patients.

Angiography is necessary to make a specific diagnosis in patients presenting with VBI. Anticoagulation fails to solve the primary hemodynamic problem, and surgical reconstruction warrants further attention in the management of these cases. The procedure used should be individualized. Transposition of the vertebral to the carotid artery is a useful approach to proximal lesions in the first and second parts of the vertebral artery.

Revascularization of the Extracranial Vertebral Artery at any Level Without Cross-Clamping

Howard J. Senter, Sami M. Bittar, and Edwin T. Long (Pittsburgh)
J. Neurosurg. 62:334–339, March 1985 7–43

Vertebrobasilar transient ischemic attacks are believed to be due chiefly to hemodynamic insufficiency secondary to extracranial vertebral artery stenosis or occlusion. Exposure of the artery distal to the stenosis is difficult, and cross-clamping for vein grafting or carotid artery transposition is hazardous. Four patients with confirmed posteriorfossa transient isch-

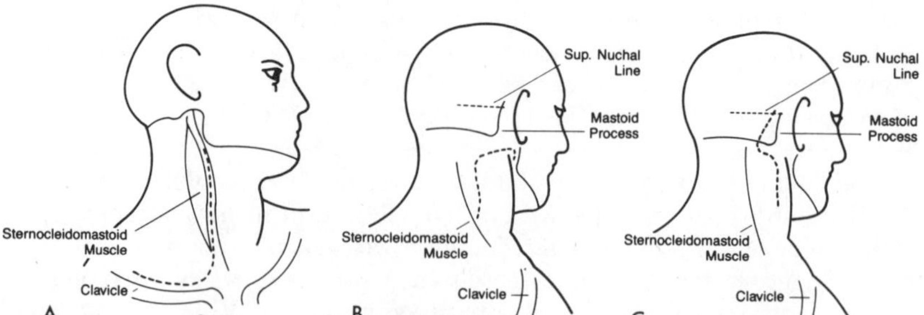

Fig 7–10.—Schematics of skin incisions for exposure of vertebral artery, as described for each of its 3 segments. **A,** incision to expose the vertebral arteries from C4 through C7 anteriorly. **B,** incision to expose the vertebral artery at its lateral C2 to C4 segment. **C,** incision to expose the vertebral artery from the third, or C1, segment to the foramen magnum segment. (Courtesy of Senter, H.J., et al.: J. Neurosurg. 62:334–339, March 1985.)

emic attacks underwent a subclavian-to-vertebral artery bypass vein graft procedure. The patients, with a mean age of 67 years, were followed for a mean period of 1 year after operation. All patients had experienced at least one attack per week, and their conditions had failed to respond to aspirin-dipyridamole therapy (plus warfarin, in one instance). The most common initial symptoms were diplopia, vertigo, ataxia, and sudden drop attacks.

The operative exposure is shown in Figure 7–10. After exposure of the vertebral artery at the appropriate level and exposure of the subclavian artery, an intraluminal shunt was placed in the vein graft, and distal and then proximal end-to-side anastomoses were performed. The shunt then was removed. One postoperative death resulted from ischemic bowel disease. Another patient had a transient C5 motor deficit from a brachial plexus stretch syndrome, and one had mild Horner's syndrome from surgical injury of the anterocervical sympathetic chains. The 3 surviving patients had no further transient ischemic attacks.

This procedure provides an immediate high-flow bypass. Blood flow to the brain stem is maintained by the shunt during graft placement, and complete occlusion of the vertebral artery does not contraindicate extracranial reconstruction. The subclavian-to-vertebral artery vein graft procedure warrants further consideration in the management of cases of symptomatic extracranial vertebral artery atherosclerosis that are refractory to medical measures.

Surgical Repair of Vertebral Artery Stenoses

André Thevenet and Carlo Ruotolo (Cedex, France)

J. Cardiovasc. Surg. 25:101–110, Mar.–Apr. 1984 7–44

One of the most frequent manifestations of transient ischemic attacks is vertebrobasilar insufficiency. Stenotic lesions at the origin of the vertebral artery are equally as frequent, although not always responsible for symptoms. Data are reported on surgical correction of 325 obstructive lesions at the origin of the vertebral arteries in 290 patients operated on from January 1973 to September 1980.

The lesions included atheromatous stenosis within the subclavian artery at the vertebral origin in 283 arteries, kinking that involved the first few centimeters of the vertebral artery in 25, and extrinsic compression on the first segment of the vertebral artery or within the transverse foramina in 17.

The operative procedures, most of which were supraclavicular, involved ostial endarterectomy in 111 cases, subclavian-vertebral endarterectomy in 153, subclavian-vertebral endarterectomy with patch in 17, reimplantation in the subclavian artery in 14, subclavian-vertebral anastomosis in 6, and subclavian resection-anastomosis in 5. Supra-aortic trunk reconstruction was performed in 9 cases. Carotid endarterectomy and vertebral repair were performed simultaneously in 36 cases, and staged reconstructions were performed in 72 cases, with carotid endarterectomy as the initial procedure in 51 cases and as the second procedure in 21.

Two deaths (0.6%) occurred within 30 days of surgery; postoperative neurologic deterioration was noted in 4 patients (1.2%). Almost 50% of patients showed Horner's syndrome of different degrees, but the symptoms persisted in only 4% of cases. Thirteen local reoperations were performed in the immediate postoperative period, 2 for hemostases, 2 for chylothoraxes, and 9 for distal subclavian thrombosis. Postoperative arteriograms, available for 95 patients 1 month to 6 years after surgery, showed excellent anatomical results in 81%, poor results in 14%, and total occlusion of the vertebral artery in 5%. Follow-up for 2 to 9 years showed that 68% of the patients were asymptomatic, 11% were markedly improved, 9% had persisting symptoms, and 12% had died.

Although obstructive lesions of the vertebral artery are often responsible for vertebrobasilar insufficiency, they are often neglected. Their frequency is suggested by the fact that 1,382 vascular reconstructions of the carotid artery, 789 of the supra-aortic trunk, and 683 of the vertebral arteries were performed over a 20-year period at the authors' hospital. The findings in this series indicate that transsubclavian vertebral ostial endarterectomy is a simple and safe procedure, providing satisfactory long-term results.

Vertebrobasilar Transient Ischemic Attacks in Internal Carotid Artery Occlusion or Tight Stenosis

Julien Bogousslavsky and Franco Regli (Vaudois Univ.)

Arch. Neurol. 42:64–68, January 1985 7–45

It has been suggested that hemodynamic sequelae of carotid obstruction may have an important role in the development of vertebrobasilar insufficiency (VBI). The potential hemodynamic or emboligenic role of the internal carotid artery was assessed in 9 patients with internal carotid occlusion and in 3 with high-grade stenosis of the extracranial segment and VBI. No patient had more than 30% stenosis of the vertebral or the subclavian artery. Control patients without VBI were matched with the study group for age, sex, and degree of internal carotid obstruction. Follow-ups averaged 21 months in the study group and 39 months in the control group.

The occurrence of VBI correlated with an infarct on computed tomography, poor collateral circulation, and bilateral carotid atherosclerosis. There were no significant differences in emboligenic lesions, but posterior-to-anterior flow through the posterior communicating arteries was seen only in patients with VBI. All study patients who were not operated on had vertebrobasilar transient ischemic attacks during follow-up.

The findings suggest hemodynamic disorder in patients with VBI but significant disease in the carotid system only. A condition of "steal VBI" appears to develop. These patients require close follow-up, since their functional prognosis and probably their life expectancy are worse than that for patients with carotid occlusion and no VBI. Patients with the most extensive extracranial carotid disease have the most severe infarcts and the most disability.

Long-Term Results of Direct Vertebral Artery Operations

George J. Reul, Denton A. Cooley, Susan K. Olson, Grady L. Hallman, O. H. Frazier, David A. Ott, J. Michael Duncan, and James J. Livesay (Houston)

Surgery 96:854–862, November 1984 7–46

Vertebral artery lesions combined with carotid lesions entail a potentially greater risk of stroke. Only 40 of more than 3,200 cerebrovascular operations done between 1971 and 1983 at the Texas Heart Institute were direct vertebral artery operations. Only patients with arteriosclerotic lesions were included. The 22 women and 18 men had a mean age of 62 years. Dizziness and limb weakness were the most frequent symptoms. Completed stroke occurred in 14 (35%). Twenty-one patients were hypertensive, and 22 had significant carotid disease, 9 having totally occluded carotid arteries. There were 24 with significant stenosis of both vertebral arteries. If possible, other extracranial cerebrovascular lesions were repaired first. In 21 patients, transection of the vertebral artery and reimplantation to the apical part of the subclavian artery were done after resection of the stenotic segment. Six also had endarterectomy. Fifteen patients had patch grafting with double-velour Dacron or polytetrafluoroethylene, 4 with vertebral endarterectomy. Two patients had bilateral vertebral artery surtery.

There were no operative deaths. One patient had a transient ischemic attack postoperatively and sustained another stroke, which was fatal, 6 years later. Four of 5 repeat angiograms showed graft patency. The 12-year actuarial survival rate was 76%. The 8 patients who died were without symptoms. Twenty-one of 30 survivors followed were asymptomatic, 7 did not improve, and 2 had recurrences. One asymptomatic patient had a stroke 7 years postoperatively.

Direct vertebral artery surgery led to significant long-term symptomatic relief and prevented transient ischemic attacks and strokes in this group of patients with severe disease. More patients may benefit from this surgery with the availability of better noninvasive diagnostic methods and more complete angiographic studies with digital subtraction.

► Direct vertebral revascularization has now received more attention. The preceding six articles represent some new thoughts on this subject. Not all vertebral-basilar ischemic symptoms are relieved after correction of concomitant high-grade carotid artery stenosis. Most U.S. surgeons favor reimplantation of the vertebral artery to the carotid artery rather than transsubclavian endarterectomy of the vertebral artery ostium. The most difficult part of vertebral artery surgery is reconstruction at the level of C1-C2. Percutaneous transluminal balloon dilation appears to be an alternative procedure in patients with vertebral-basilar symptoms in the presence of "subclavian steal."

Upper Extremity Ischemia

Evaluation of Upper Extremity Vasculature With High-Resolution Ultrasound

L. Andrew Koman, M. Gene Bond, Ralph E. Carter, and Gary G. Poehling
(Bowman Gray School of Medicine, Winston-Salem, N.C.)
J. Hand Surg. 10A:249–255, March 1985 7–47

A real-time 10-MHz B-mode ultrasonographic technique was used to evaluate 29 vascular and perivascular lesions of the upper extremity in 21 patients. Most lesions were arterial repairs, but perivascular masses and thrombosed or occluded arteries also were examined.

Patency of arterial repairs was accurately assessed in all 16 instances. Known alterations in arterial anatomy and pathways were well-demonstrated. Stenosis and dilatation could be quantified distal and proximal to anastomotic sites, which were characterized by increased intimal reflections, relatively increased near- and far-wall thicknesses, and altered vessel-wall mobility during the cardiac cycle. The appearances of a vein graft are shown in Figure 7–11. The degree of vascular compression or involvement was accurately predicted by sonography in all 7 operated patients with perivascular masses. Arteriography was avoided in at least 2 patients who

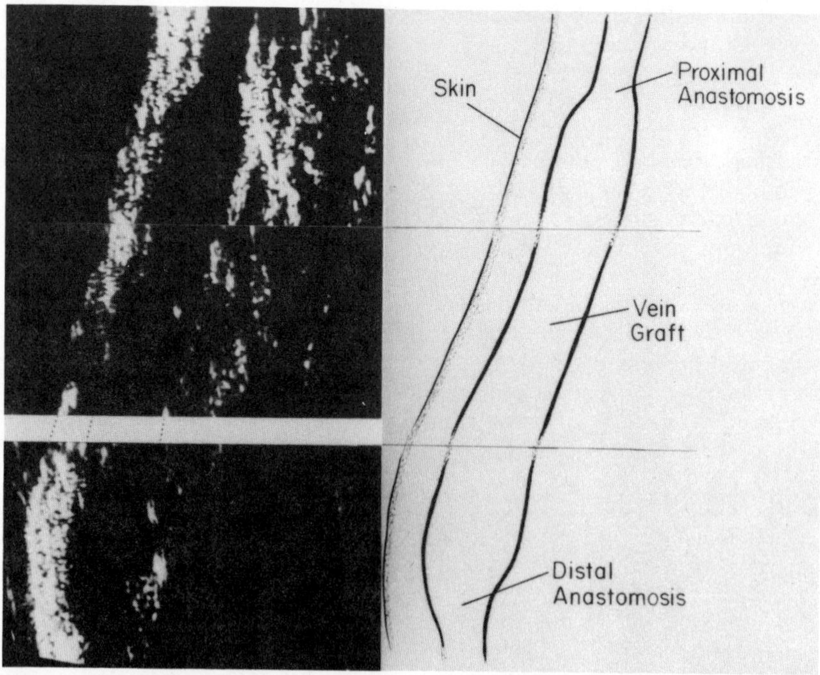

Fig 7–11.—Full-length, composite longitudinal sonogram of vein graft in Case 1, including proximal and distal anastomoses. Echoes are bright or white, and sonolucent (or homogeneous) structures are dark or black. Dynamic imaging showed differences in arterial wall motion and reversed the interposition vein-graft wall motion. (Courtesy of Koman, L.A., et al.: J. Hand Surg. 10A:249–255, March 1985.)

had clinical evidence of vascular compromise. Five arteries with thrombosis or occlusion unrelated to adjacent masses of vascular repair were imaged in 3 patients; all 3 of these explorations confirmed the sonographic impression.

Real-time ultrasonography is an accurate means of evaluating vascular and perivascular lesions in the upper extremity. Preoperative ultrasonography can rule out aneurysmal dilation and determine the site of a mass and its effect on adjacent vascular structures. Postoperative studies can also show the size of an anastomosis and the presence of pre- and post-anastomotic dilatation.

Raynaud's Phenomenon Progressing to Gangrene After Vincristine and Bleomycin Therapy

Inkeri Elomaa, Marjo Pajunen, and Pekka Virkkunen (Univ. of Helsinki)
Acta Med. Scand. 216:323–326, 1984 7–48

Raynaud's phenomenon has been described in patients with testicular cancer given vinblastine and bleomycin therapy and in those with head-neck tumors given cisplatin, vincristine, and bleomycin. A smoker, who had had Raynaud's phenomenon for 2 years before developing non-Hodgkin's lymphoma, had symptoms of vertebral artery insufficiency and gangrene in the fingers after a second course of chemotherapy including vincristine and bleomycin.

Woman, 50, with a 30-year history of frostbite injury in the fingers and toes,

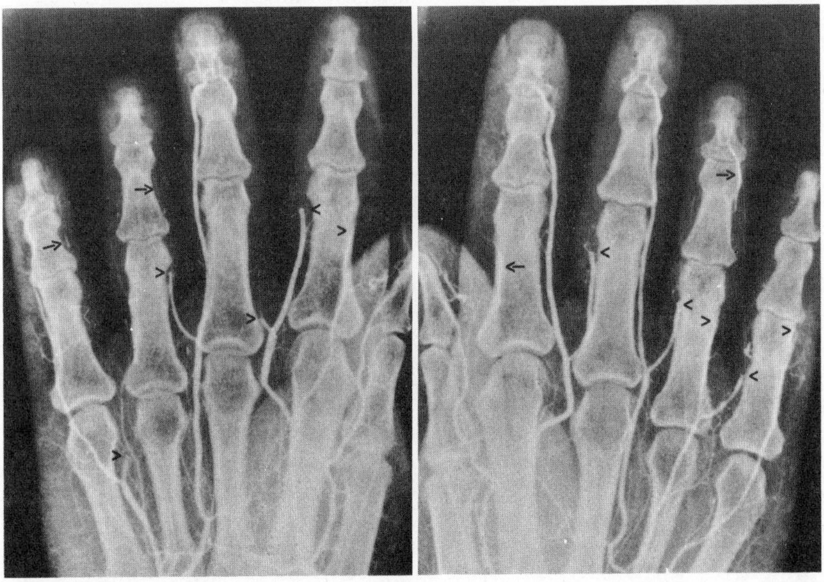

Fig 7–12.—Arteriograms of left and right hands 10 seconds after contrast injection into brachial arteries. Note arterial occlusions *(arrowheads)* and poor distal arterial filling partly through collateral circulation *(arrows)*. (Courtesy of Elomaa, I., et al.: Acta Med. Scand. 216:323–326, 1984.)

had had typical Raynaud's phenomenon for 2 years, with attacks only in the winter. No symptoms suggested scleroderma, and screening tests for collagen disease were negative. Cervical and inguinal node enlargement led to a diagnosis of non-Hodgkin's lymphoma of the large-cleaved cell type. Chemotherapy included bleomycin and CHOP (cyclophosphamide, doxorubicin, vincristine, and prednisone). Dysarthria, dysphagia, vertigo, and nystagmus developed after a second course of treatment, and the patient could not walk without aid. Symptoms resolved within 1 week, but Raynaud's phenomenon progressed, and cutaneous gangrene developed in two fingers, despite anticoagulation and intra-arterial vasodilator therapy. Angiography showed arterial occlusions, collateral circulation, and poor distal arterial filling in both hands (Fig 7–12). Thoracic sympathectomy was done on the left side, but the painful second and third fingertips had to be amputated. Lymphoma escaped control during the vascular episodes. Treatment excluding vincristine and bleomycin led to no new vascular complications, but the lymphoma is not in remission.

Raynaud's phenomenon appears to be a common complication of treatment with vinca alkaloid plus bleomycin, but there is only one previous report of gangrene. This treatment should be used cautiously in patients with a history of vascular disorder. Schedules excluding this combination may be advisable in such patients.

Nifedipine-Induced Fingertip Vasodilation in Patients With Raynaud's Phenomenon

Mark A. Creager, Kenneth M. Pariser, Eileen M. Winston, Helen M. Rasmussen, Kenneth B. Miller, and Jay D. Coffman (Boston)

Am. Heart J. 108:370–373, August 1984 7–49

It has been previously shown that nifedipine, a calcium channel blocking agent, causes vasodilation in the forearm resistance vessels; its vasodilating properties have not been demonstrated in the blood vessels of the finger. The authors investigated the effect of nifedipine on fingertip hemodynamics in 10 patients with Raynaud's phenomenon. Fingertip blood flow was determined in a 20 C environment by venous occlusion air plethysmography. Fingertip vascular resistance was calculated as the ratio of mean blood pressure to fingertip blood flow. Nifedipine was administered sublingually as gel in a 10 mg-dose. Seven patients participated in a double-blind crossover clinical trial assessing the efficacy of nifedipine in patients with Raynaud's phenomenon. Each patient received nifedipine, 10–20 mg orally, 4 times daily for a minimum of 3 weeks, and then placebo at the same dosages for 3 weeks.

Nifedipine increased fingertip blood flow in 8 patients. Excluding 2 patients with the largest baseline blood flows, average fingertip blood flow increased 56%, from 3.3 ± 1.0 to 5.2 ± 1.6 ml 100 ml^{-1} $minute^{-1}$ ($P < .01$). Fingertip vascular resistance for the 10 patients decreased 40%, from 40.7 ± 10.8 to 24.2 ± 6.1 units ($P < .05$). The frequency and severity of Raynaud's phenomenon was less in all 7 patients when taking nifedipine as compared to placebo. Three of 4 patients with fingertip ulcers showed healing of the ulcers while taking nifedipine. Adverse effects included indigestion, constipation, and leg edema.

The pathophysiology of Raynaud's phenomenon is still not well understood. Increased sympathetic nervous system activity, or pathology in the digital arterial wall, or both, may be responsible for digital vasospasm. Several short-term clinical trials reported that nifedipine reduced the frequency of Raynaud's phenomenon. Nifedipine inhibits norepinephrine-induced vasoconstriction in isolated blood vessel strips. In addition, it attenuates the increase in coronary vascular resistance that occurs with the cold pressor test.

The authors conclude that nifedipine-induced fingertip vasodilation may contribute to clinical improvement in some patients with Raynaud's phenomenon. Long-term clinical trials and a larger volume of patients will be needed to conclude that nifedipine will be effective in all patients with Raynaud's phenomenon.

Nifedipine in the Treatment of Raynaud's Phenomenon: Evidence for Inhibition of Platelet Activation

Raymond Malamet, Robert A. Wise, Walter H. Ettinger, and Fredrick M. Wigley (Johns Hopkins Med. Inst.)

Am. J. Med. 78:602–608, April 1985 7–50

Platelet activation has been demonstrated by increased plasma concentrations of β-thromboglobulin in patients with Raynaud's phenomenon. The effect of nifedipine, a calcium channel blocker used effectively for treatment of Raynaud's phenomenon, on platelet activation was examined in 13 patients. The patients were participating in a double-blind study of nifedipine and dazoxiben. Mean age was 35 years. Fifteen normal subjects with a mean age of 30 years were also studied. The mean duration of Raynaud's phenomenon was 11 years. Eight of 9 evaluable patients had associated connective tissue disease. Nifedipine was given in a dosage of 20 mg three times daily and dazoxiben in a dosage of 100 mg four times daily for 2-week periods.

Study patients had elevated plasma β-thromboglobulin concentrations while taking placebo. Platelet factor 4 levels were not abnormal. Nifedipine administration was associated with significantly lower β-thromboglobulin and platelet factor 4 concentrations. No such changes occurred with dazoxiben administration. Raynaud episodes were significantly less severe during nifedipine therapy than during placebo periods. No such effect was apparent with dazoxiben.

Nifedipine inhibits platelet activation in patients with Raynaud's phenomenon and is associated with subjective improvement. The thromboxane synthetase inhibitor dazoxiben does not have similar effects. The findings support a role for platelet activation in the pathogenesis of Raynaud's phenomenon, either as a primary event or secondary to intrinsic vascular abnormality. It has been suggested that in vivo platelet activation may mediate both vasoconstriction and the development of fixed anatomical vascular disease.

Hemorrheologic Effects of Prostaglandin E_1 Infusion in Raynaud's Syndrome

G. S. Lucas, M. H. Simms, N. M. Caldwell, S. J. C. Alexander, and J. Stuart (Univ. of Birmingham)

J. Clin. Pathol. 37:870–873, August 1984 7–51

Prostaglandin E_1 (PGE_1) is a potent vasodilator that has been reported to improve red blood cell deformability and to benefit clinically patients with Raynaud's syndrome. The rheological effects of a 72-hour infusion of PGE_1 were examined in 18 patients who had severe, chronic Raynaud's syndrome and were admitted for central venous catheterization. Either PGE_1 or placebo was infused, the former in a dose of 10 ng kg^{-1} $minute^{-1}$ in ethanol-normal saline solution. The 9 PGE_1-treated and 9 placebo patients were similar in age, sex, and type of Raynaud's syndrome.

Mean baseline index of erythrocyte filtration was significantly higher than in healthy subjects. No significant change occurred after PGE_1 infusion during the 4-week study, but a significant increase in the index of filtration occurred in the placebo group 2 weeks after infusion. The PGE_1 infusion was followed by an acute-phase response, with significant increases in leukocyte numbers and serum C-reactive protein and plasma fibrinogen concentrations. Hyperproteinemia was the likely cause of plasma hyperviscosity at weeks 2 and 4. Platelet numbers fell significantly immediately after the infusion and rebounded at week 2. The placebo group showed only a rise in plasma viscosity immediately after infusion. The PGE_1 infusion caused an acute-phase response in the 3 patients with Raynaud's syndrome secondary to systemic sclerosis, as well as in the 6 with primary Raynaud's syndrome.

Infusion of PGE_1 did not improve red blood cell filterability in these patients with severe Raynaud's syndrome, but it did produce an acute-phase response with hyperproteinemia and leukocytosis. Prostaglandin E_1 could act as a mediator of both the chronic and the acute stress responses in patients with extensive vascular disease.

▶ After arterial reconstruction, most patients will refuse arteriography because of unpleasant experience with the preoperative study. The B-mode scan offers an alternative means of evaluating the status of the operation. Also, arteriography may be avoided in some of the cases preoperatively by using ultrasound imaging in conjunction with finger systolic pressure.

Now the multiple factors responsible for Raynaud's phenomenon are joined by chemotherapy for testicular cancers! Some objective evidence is now available regarding the effect of calcium channel blockers in treatment of Raynaud's phenomenon. The waxing and waning nature of the disease, however, makes it difficult to evaluate the true value of any medical therapy, including prostaglandin infusion.

Visceral and Renal Ischemia

Transcutaneous Doppler Ultrasound Measurement of Celiac Axis Blood Flow in Man

M. I. Qamar, A. E. Read, R. Skidmore, J. M. Evans, and R. C. N. Williamson (Bristol, England)
Br. J. Surg. 72:391–393, May 1985 7–52

The transcutaneous Doppler ultrasound technique has been used to measure blood flow reproducibly in the carotid arteries and in fetal vessels. The method has now been used to measure flow in the superior mesenteric artery in 23 women and 19 men aged 19 to 68 years. Thirty-six were healthy subjects, and 6 were outpatients in whom cardiovascular and gastrointestinal disease had been excluded. Mean resting celiac axis blood flow (CABF) was 703 ml per minute, with no sex difference and no correlation with age. Ten subjects had a 38% increase in CABF after ingesting a liquid meal. A 24% increase over baseline flow persisted at 10 minutes.

Noninvasive measurement of CABF by the Doppler ultrasound method is a relatively simple and reproducible means of detecting postprandial changes in CABF. The test appears to be useful in physiologic and clinical studies. The mean coefficients of variation were 7.8% in a 1-day test and 9.2% in a 2-day test.

Noninvasive Diagnosis of Intestinal Angina
K. A. Jäger, G. S. Fortner, B. L. Thiele, and D. E. Strandness (Univ. of Washington)
J. Clin. Ultrasound 12:588–591, Nov.–Dec. 1984 7–53

Intestinal angina has no pathognomonic clinical features, and its confirmation has required contrast angiography. Ultrasonic duplex scanning

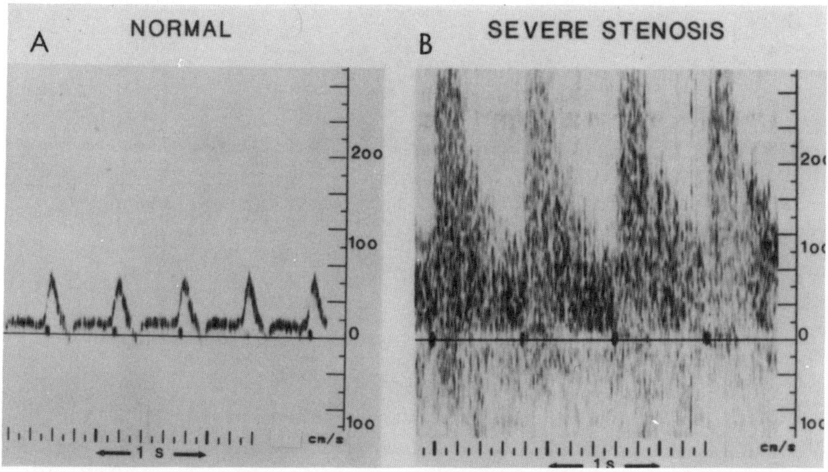

Fig 7–13.—**A,** normal superior mesenteric artery wave form in healthy subject. Peak systolic blood flow velocity is less than 10 cm per second. **B,** velocity spectra obtained from superior mesenteric artery of patient. Large increase in velocity (more than 300 cm per second) and spectral broadening throughout entire cardiac cycle at recording site just distal to stenosis indicate high-grade stenosis. (Courtesy of Jäger, K.A., et al.: J. Clin. Ultrasound 12:588–591, Nov.–Dec. 1984.)

can provide information on arterial luminal narrowing and quantitative data on blood flow velocity. It has been useful in the noninvasive diagnosis of extracranial cerebrovascular disease and in localizing peripheral arterial stenosis. The system combines real-time B-mode imaging with pulsed Doppler frequency analysis, the latter utilizing a fast Fourier spectrum analyzer.

Woman, 54, had had postprandial epigastric pain and diarrhea for 6 months, associated with smaller meals and loss of 30 lb. Withdrawal of conjugated estrogens was followed by slight symptomatic improvement. The postprandial pain was relieved by sublingual nitroglycerin but not by antacids. An abdominal bruit was heard, but abdominal ultrasonography, esophagoduodenoscopy, colonoscopy, and barium enema examination yielded normal results. The patient had a long smoking history. Duplex scanning showed extremely high peak velocities at the origins of the celiac and the superior mesenteric arteries, indicating severe stenoses (Fig 7–13). Spectral broadening was also observed. The pulsatile components of flow were markedly reduced at distal recording sites. Digital subtraction aortography confirmed the noninvasive findings. A high-grade stenosis of the celiac origin was repaired by vein patch angioplasty, and an aortomesenteric saphenous vein graft was used to bypass the superior mesenteric artery lesion. Symptoms were absent after operation, and the patient gained weight. A duplex scan 6 weeks after operation showed patent reconstructions with normal flow velocities and good pulsatile flow at recording sites distal to the graft.

Ultrasonic duplex scanning holds promise for simplifying the evaluation of patients suspected of having mesenteric vascular disease. If compromise of the splanchnic blood supply is documented, aortic angiography will confirm the diagnosis, and elective revascularization can be considered. Duplex scanning in conjunction with a test meal could provide a mesenteric circulatory stress test.

Computed Tomography of the Normal Mesentery

Paul M. Silverman, Frederick M. Kelvin, Melvyn Korobkin, and N. Reed Dunnick (Duke Univ.)

AJR 143:953–957, November 1984 7–54

The normal CT appearance of the mesentery and its vasculature was determined in 30 adult patients. The jejunal and ileal branches of the superior mesenteric system were well outlined by mesenteric fat. The right colic vessels were demonstrated in 26 patients and the middle colic branches of the transverse colon in 29. The superior left colic branches of the descending colon were visualized in 14 patients and the sigmoid branches (inferior left colic branches) in 23. The difficulty in demonstrating branches to the descending colon was related to the small amount of mesenteric fat surrounding these vessels. The ileocolic branches were seen in 27 patients. The superior mesenteric artery and vein were demonstrated in all patients and the inferior mesenteric artery was identified in 26. The more distal mesenteric branches coursed through the mesentery in an undulating manner. The ability to identify the peripheral mesenteric vessels

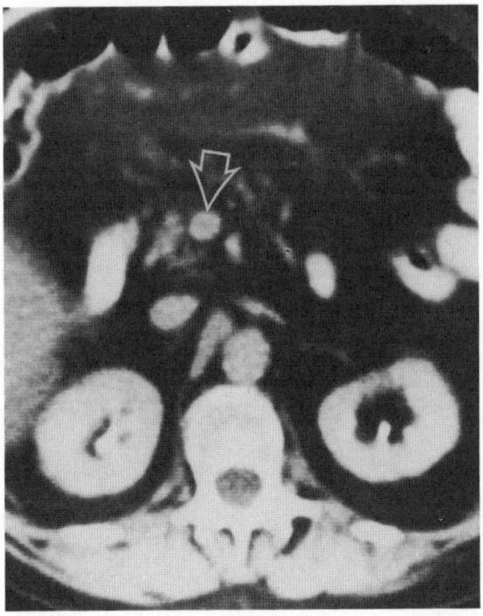

Fig 7–14.—The CT scan at the level of the superior mesenteric vein shows a central lucency *(arrow)* that at surgery was found to be a clot. (Courtesy of Silverman, P.M., et al.: AJR 143:953–957, November 1984.)

was not affected by the absence of intravenous contrast material, as identification depended directly on there being adequate amounts of surrounding low-attenuation fat. In all patients, the attenuation value of mesenteric fat averaged −117.4 Hounsfeld units.

Although the larger mesenteric vessels are readily identified on abdominal CT scans obtained with or without the use of intravenous contrast material, contrast enhancement of the vessels allows more precise evaluation of pathology involving them. Computed tomography may suggest the diagnosis of mesenteric arterial or venous occlusion by demonstrating a thin, dense, vascular wall surrounding a central low-density area representing clot (Fig 7–14). The CT diagnosis of mesenteric venous thrombosis may allow conservative management because of the extensive venous collaterals that are usually present, whereas acute arterial occlusion may need to be confirmed by angiography before surgical thrombectomy. Mesenteric lymph nodes usually are not demonstrated by CT, but they may become identifiable when enlarged and may displace the normal mesenteric vasculature. Various pathologic processes may infiltrate the mesenteric fat, alter its structure, and create an increase in its CT number. The margins of normal vessels coursing through infiltrated areas of the mesentery may be obliterated by the infiltrating process. Inflammatory disorders that may change the normally homogeneous low-attenuation appearance of mesenteric fat include pancreatitis, Crohn's disease, mesenteric abscesses, edema, and tumor infiltration.

▶ Diagnosis of mesenteric ischemia relies on arteriography. The use of a Duplex scan to assess mesenteric or celiac artery blood flow should prove to be useful as a confirmatory test in patients suspected of having mesenteric ischemia because of mesenteric arteriographic abnormalities. Infusion CT scan also helps to evaluate the status of the mesenteric artery.

Ischemic Colitis Complicating Reconstruction of the Abdominal Aorta
Torben Schroeder, Jens Krogh Christoffersen, Jørgen Andersen, Soren Bille, Erik Gravgaard, Hans-Henrik Kimose, Jørgen Lorentzen, Poul Ostri, and Hans Jørgen Buchardt Hansen
Surg. Gynecol. Obstet. 160:299–303, April 1985 7–55

Ischemia of the left colon is a rare but serious complication of abdominal aortic reconstruction. It carries a mortality of 75% and may account for up to one fourth of all deaths after aortic operations. The chief cause is ligature of a patent inferior mesenteric artery. Twenty-three cases, occurring in 3,092 aortic reconstructions performed between 1975 and 1981, were reviewed. Seventeen patients had full-thickness necrosis and 6, mucosal gangrene. Median age was 67 years. In all patients a synthetic aortic prosthesis was inserted, and 3 had aortic endarterectomy as well. No patient had mesenteric revascularization.

The incidence of full-thickness colonic necrosis was 0.5%. The celiac and superior mesenteric arteries were stenosed in 1 patient each, but only half the 23 patients were evaluable. A patent inferior mesenteric artery was occluded in 11 patients as a result of the operation. In 18 cases this vessel was occluded after operation. Diarrhea was the chief presenting feature; it often was bloody. Perforation was found in all but 1 of the 14 patients reoperated on. The sigmoid was involved in 19 cases, the descending colon in 8, and the rectum in 9. Patients underwent diverting colostomy on the transverse or sigmoid colon. Twelve patients with full-thickness necrosis (71%) and 1 of the 6 with mucosal gangrene died. Peritonitis caused half the deaths.

Ischemic colitis complicating abdominal aortic reconstruction is related to ligation of the inferior mesenteric artery, abolition of the collateral supply, a nonocclusive low-flow state, or more than one of these. The sigmoid should be closely inspected at the end of every aortic reconstruction. Angiography may be useful if the patency of the inferior mesenteric artery is in doubt.

▶ Recognition of colon ischemia following reconstruction of the abdominal aorta is difficult. Fortunately, the incidence is rather low, 0.5% in 3,092 reconstructions. As reported previously, the incidence increases in patients with ruptured abdominal aneurysms. Sigmoidoscopy should be the first step in the diagnostic work-up.

Flow Separation in the Renal Arteries
Hani N. Sabbah, Earl T. Hawkins, and Paul D. Stein (Henry Ford Hosp., Detroit)
Arteriosclerosis 4:28–33, Jan.–Feb. 1984 7–56

To characterize the nature of flow in the proximal portion of the renal arteries, a common site for the development of atherosclerosis, the authors conducted pulsatile flow studies in an exact, clear acrylic mold of a normal human aorta and renal arteries. The mold was made from a cast of a segment of the abdominal aorta and left and right renal arteries prepared in situ during autopsy of a woman, aged 27 years. The mold was incorporated into a pulse duplicating system and flow in the mold was visualized by illumination of buoyant particles, 100 to 300 μ in diameter, added to the glycerin-saline test fluid. The branch (renal) to trunk (aorta) flow ratio ranged from 0.053 to 0.350. Flow separation was considered to be present when particles near the vessel wall reversed direction.

Secondary flows (spiraling) were observed in both the left and right renal arteries at all flow rates studied. Secondary flows were very evident during systole but were markedly diminished or absent during diastole. Whenever flow separation occurred during systole, it was always observed near or at the origin of the renal arteries at the superior aspect of the wall. Flow separation was observed throughout systole at a branch-to-trunk flow ratio of 0.053. As the flow ratio increased, flow separation was observed only at peak systolic flow and during the deceleration phase of systole and only in the right renal artery. When the branch-to-trunk flow ratio was increased to 0.175, flow separation was observed only during the deceleration phase in the right renal artery. At a flow ratio of 0.35, flow separation was no longer present. Increasing the pulse rate from 65 to 98 strokes per minute had no influence on flow separation with regard to the frequency of its occurrence.

The results suggest that flow separation may occur near the renal ostia if renal flow diminishes appreciably while aortic flow remains elevated, as during exercise. Because low wall shear is involved in flow separation, mass transfer across the arterial wall may be adversely affected and possibly contribute to atheroma formation.

▶ Hemodynamic patterns play an important role in the development and distribution of atheroma. Similar to the observation by Zarins on carotid bifurcation atherosclerosis (*Circ. Res.* 53:502–114, 1983), low wall shear is responsible for the formation of atherosclerotic plaque in the renal artery, too.

Critical Perfusion Pressure for Renal Function in Patients With Bilateral Atherosclerotic Renal Vascular Disease

Stephen C. Textor, Andrew C. Novick, Robert C. Tarazi, Victor Klimas, Donald G. Vidt, and Marc Pohl

Ann. Intern. Med. 102:308–314, March 1985 7–57

An attempt was made to determine whether vascular stenosis affecting the entire renal mass can hemodynamically limit the adaptation of renal function to pressure changes within the clinical range. At the Cleveland Clinic Foundation, effective renal plasma flow and the glomerular filtration rate (GFR) were measured before and during graded reductions in blood pressure by means of nitroprusside infusion in 16 patients with hypertensive atherosclerotic renovascular disease. Mean age was 59 years. Antihypertensive drug treatment other than diuretics was discontinued for 48 hours before study as tolerated. The renal plasma flow was estimated using ^{131}I-iodohippurate, and the GFR was determined using ^{125}I-iothalamate. Nitroprusside was infused at rates of 0.2–3 $\mu g\ kg^{-1}\ minute^{-1}$ to produce a stable, graded reduction in blood pressure.

Patients with bilateral stenosis had more marked renal functional reduction than did those with unilateral stenosis. Renal venous renin values often lateralized to the more severely affected kidney regardless of whether bilateral or unilateral stenosis was present. Eight patients with unilateral disease tolerated blood pressure reduction from a mean of 205/103 mm Hg to 146/84 mm Hg with no change in total renal function. A similar pressure reduction in 8 patients with bilateral renal artery stenosis led to marked but reversible declines in plasma flow and GFR. Sensitivity of renal function to pressure reduction disappeared in 4 patients who were restudied after revascularization.

Vascular stenosis involving the entire renal mass may limit renal function, and this may provide a means of identifying patients at loss of renal function during antihypertensive therapy. The possibility that patients with bilateral stenosis but no demonstrable pressure sensitivity may not be at risk of renal parenchymal atrophy warrants further study. A central question is whether identification of a critical perfusion pressure for renal function constitutes an indication for renal revascularization.

Revascularization to Preserve Renal Function in Patients With Atherosclerotic Renovascular Disease

Andrew C. Novick, Stephen C. Textor, Barry Bodie, and Raja B. Khauli (Cleveland Clinic)

Urol. Clin. North Am. 41:477–490, August 1984 7–58

A significant number of patients with advanced atherosclerotic renovascular disease have their blood pressure controlled by medical treatment but are at a high risk of renal dysfunction and failure. Twenty-five patients seen in 1974–1983 with end-stage renal failure due to atherosclerotic renovascular disease had a mean age of 58 years at the time renal failure developed. Angiography showed high-grade stenosis or total occlusion involving both renal arteries or the artery to a solitary kidney in all cases. Eight patients had surgical revascularization, and 6 currently are alive after a mean of 58 months. Thirteen of 16 patients followed on maintenance dialysis died after a mean of 9 months.

Angiographic screening is considered for patients with generalized atherosclerosis, a decrease in size of one or both kidneys, and a serum creatinine above 1.5 mg/dl. Atherosclerosis is the most common cause of total renal artery occlusion. Revascularization can lead to significant recovery of function in some of these cases. Initial studies with the sodium nitroprusside infusion study suggest that the critical perfusion pressure for renal function can be defined in patients with arterial stenosis affecting the entire renal mass. The perfusion limit can lead to deteriorating function during antihypertensive therapy and can be reversed by revascularization. No such perfusion limit is found in patients with unilateral vascular disease.

Renal function improved postoperatively in 67% of 51 patients with advanced atherosclerotic renovascular disease who underwent revascularization for preservation of renal function in 1975–1981. Function deteriorated postoperatively in only 6% of patients. Dramatic improvement may be seen in patients with complete bilateral obstruction where renal viability is maintained by collateral flow. Actuarial patient survival has been nearly identical to that of a normal age-matched population.

Renal Revascularization in the Azotemic Hypertensive Patient Resistant to Therapy

Christopher Y. Ying, Charles P. Tifft, Haralambos Gavras, and Aram V. Chobanian

N. Engl.J. Med. 311:1070–1075, Oct. 25, 1984 7–59

Renal insufficiency is not a typical presenting factor of renovascular hypertension. The authors undertook a study of 106 consecutive patients admitted for diagnostic evaluation of severe hypertension to assess the frequency of renovascular hypertension in patients with azotemia and hypertension refractory to drug therapy and to determine the effects of renal revascularization on blood pressure and renal function in these patients. Diagnostic studies used were intravenous pyelography, renal vein renin sampling, and selective angiography.

Of the 106 patients, 39 (37%) patients proved to have renovascular hypertension. Of 21 patients with renal insufficiency, 10 had renovascular hypertension. Eight of these patients presented at a mean age of 65.3 ± 2.2 years, with hypertension lasting from 4 to 20 years (mean, 11.3 ± 2.1 years), and serum creatinine levels ranging from 1.8 to 6.1 mg/dl (mean, 2.8 ± 0.5 mg/dl). Intravenous pyelograms were not suggestive of renovascular disease in 3 of 6 cases. Renal vein renin levels did not lateralize in 3 patients. Arteriography showed severe bilateral atherosclerotic disease in 7 patients and unilateral renal artery stenosis in a solitary functioning kidney in 1 patient. Medical therapy in the hospital often induced further deterioration of renal function despite enhanced blood pressure control. Surgical revascularization (4 patients) and percutaneous transluminal angioplasty (3 patients) produced improvement or stabilization of renal function and control of blood pressure in these azotemic patients. Benefits of therapy persisted for 10 to 42 months of follow-up.

These studies indicate that refractory hypertension in association with renal insufficiency is a relatively common clinical presentation for renovascular hypertension and bilateral renal artery disease. Recognition of this clinical association is important in view of the potential for a beneficial therapeutic outcome. Intravenous pyelography and renal vein renin sampling have limited diagnostic value in these patients. In spite of notable incidence of acute tubular necrosis induced by radiographic contrast material, renal dysfunction was reversible. Selective arteriography is the diagnostic procedure of choice. The demonstration of severe renovascular disease in the azotemic hypertensive patient should prompt serious consideration of intervention like surgical revascularization, percutaneous transluminal angioplasty, or, if necessary, nephrectomy.

▶ The above three articles summarize current thoughts about renal revascularization in patients with renovascular hypertension and chronic renal failure. The use of antihypertensive drugs may cause a decrease in perfusion pressure and deterioration of renal function but only in patients with bilateral renal artery stenosis. Surgical revascularization or PTLA leads to an improvement of renal function and control of blood pressure in such patients. Identification of critical perfusion pressure is important, and the test suggested in article 7–57, may be useful in selecting patients for revascularization.

Extracorporeal Replacement of the Renal Artery: Techniques, Indications, and Long-Term Results

J. M. Dubernard, X. Martin, D. Mongin, A. Gelet, and F. Canton (Lyons, France)

J. Urol. 133:13–16, January 1985 7–60

Twenty-four patients who had complex lesions involving the renal artery branches and renal hypertension were managed by extracorporeal replacement of the renal artery by a branched vascular autograft. Ten had aneurysms, 9 dysplasias, and 5 atheromatous involvement. In 20 patients the renal artery and its branches were replaced by a hypogastric branched autograft and in the other 4, by a saphenous vein graft.

End-to-end anastomoses are preferred, but if the graft and the arterial diameters do not match, end-to-side reimplantation of a renal arterial branch on a limb of the graft can be carried out. Autotransplantation of the kidney is performed on the iliac vessels with end-to-end anastomosis.

The 14 females and 10 males, with respective mean ages of 36 and 44 years, were operated on chiefly for high blood pressure; the mean was 211/115 mm Hg. Four patients had progressive renal failure. Three partial nephrectomies were carried out. A total of 76 peripheral anastomoses were performed. Nineteen patients were cured of hypertension during a mean follow-up of 4½ years. Two others were improved, 2 had no change in blood pressure, and 2 had secondary nephrectomy for pelvicaliceal dilatation. Eight of the 76 distal anastomoses in 5 patients were thrombosed. Two patients with complete thrombosis of the renal artery that was operated on are doing well with moderate medical treatment. Renal function remained stable in all patients. Two of the 4 patients who initially had altered renal function were improved and the other 2 were stable during follow-up.

Extracorporeal repair is the only feasible surgical approach to intrarenal lesions of renal arterial branches. Lesions involving three or more renal artery branches are suitable for this procedure, regardless of their intrasinus or extrasinus location. Renal function can be preserved in patients who previously would have been managed by nephrectomy.

Concomitant Renal Revascularization in Patients Undergoing Aortic Surgery

Mark T. Stewart, Robert B. Smith III, J. Timothy Fulenwider, Garland D. Perdue, and James O. Wells (Emory Univ.)

J. Vasc. Surg. 2:400–405, May 1985 7–61

Renal artery stenosis is present in up to half of patients undergoing aortography for peripheral vascular disease, and it can progress to complete occlusion with loss of renal mass. The effects of concomitant renal revascularization and aortic surgery were assessed in 63 patients operated on between 1975 and 1982. Patients having nephrectomy only were not included. The 42 men and 21 women had a mean age of 60 years; and the average follow-up period was 23 months. Most patients had symptomatic aortoiliac occlusive disease or abdominal aortic aneurysms, or both. Seven patients were operated on solely for renovascular hypertension. Five patients who were not hypertensive were treated prophylactically because of severe renal artery stenosis. A total of 92 renal artery anastomoses were done. Thirteen patients underwent revascularization of a single kidney. The aorta was replaced or bypassed by a tube graft, an aortobi-iliac graft, or an aortobifemoral graft.

The operative mortality was 3%. Only 2 renal grafts were known to become occluded and another was moderately stenotic, for a graft failure rate of 3%. No patient required chronic dialysis, although 20 patients had moderate renal functional impairment at time of operation. Only 5 patients had an increase in serum creatinine level of more than 0.5 mg/dl. The average blood pressure fell from 198/99 to 143/83 mm Hg postoperatively. Blood pressure control was improved in nearly two thirds of surviving patients.

Renal revascularization can be achieved at the same time as aortic replacement or bypass in patients with diffuse atherosclerotic disease, with acceptable operative mortality and morbidity. A beneficial blood pressure response and improved renal function can be expected in properly selected patients.

Late Results After Surgical Treatment of Renovascular Hypertension: A Follow-up Study of 122 Patients 2 to 18 Years After Surgery

Linda Bardram, Ulf Helgstrand, Merete Holm Bentzen, Hans Jørgen Buchardt Hansen, and Hans Chr. Engell (Rigshosp., Copenhagen)

Ann. Surg. 201:219–224, February 1985 7–62

Good early results have been reported from the surgical treatment of atherosclerotic renovascular hypertension. Long-term results were evaluated in 122 patients operated on for correctable renal artery stenosis because of inadequate medical control of hypertension between 1963 and 1980. There were 67 males with a median age of 47 years and 55 females with a median age of 46. Ninety-five patients had atherosclerosis and 17 had fibromuscular hyperplasia. Operative mortality was 5%. Seventy-one percent of patients were normotensive at discharge, and another 18% were improved. Eighteen patients were operated on for persistent or recurrent hypertension. Five patients required supplemental operations on the contralateral kidneys.

The late results were evaluated in 69 patients followed for a median of 9 years. Eighty-seven percent of those with atherosclerotic disease were improved, and half were normotensive without medication. All but 7% of patients with fibromuscular hyperplasia and all those with other causes of stenosis benefited from operation. Seven of 10 patients who were reoperated on were improved at follow-up. Ten unimproved patients were reoperated on, with satisfactory results in 7. Eight of 11 patients with bilateral disease were improved at long-term follow-up.

These long-term results support the value of operation for renal fibromuscular hyperplasia and for atherosclerotic renovascular disease. Operation is much preferable to lifelong medical care in patients with fibromuscular hyperplasia. Nearly 90% of the patients with atherosclerotic disease in this study were cured or improved at follow-up. Postoperative mortality has been reduced in recent years in patients with bilateral renovascular disease.

Percutaneous Transluminal Angioplasty vs. Surgery for Renovascular Hypertension

G. Andrew Miller, Kerry K. Ford, Simon D. Braun, Glenn E. Newman, Arl V. Moore, Jr., Robert Malone, and N. Reed Dunnick (Duke Univ.)
AJR 144:447–450, March 1985 7–63

Percutaneous transluminal angioplasty (PTA) has a high initial success rate in hypertensive patients, but hypertension recurs in many instances within months after successful angioplasty. The results obtained in 63 hypertensive patients in whom 71 arteries were treated in a 4½-year period were evaluated. The 35 females and 28 males were aged 14 months to 72 years. The cause of stenosis was atherosclerosis in 46 cases, fibromuscular dysplasia in 15, and neurofibromatosis in 2. Dilation was with 5- or 6-mm polyvinyl chloride or polyethylene balloons in conjunction with systemic heparin therapy. Surgical bypass procedures were performed on 43 arteries in 39 patients in a 14-year period. Ten of these patients were operated on after PTA was begun at the authors' institution.

Six atherosclerotic lesions could not be passed by PTA at a time when less-sophisticated equipment was available. Two technical failures occurred in patients with neurofibromatosis. Eighty-three percent of technically successful dilations of renal lesions gave long-term benefit, compared with only 45% of procedures for ostial or mixed lesions of atherosclerosis. All patients with fibromuscular dysplasia continued to do well at 6 months. One death resulted from ischemic bowel after PTA in a patient with severe visceral arterial disease. Another patient required nephrectomy for delayed renal artery occlusion. Major complications of surgical bypass occurred in 20% of patients. Six nephrectomies were necessary for occluded bypass grafts.

Percutaneous transluminal angioplasty is the preferred procedure for hypertension secondary to fibromuscular dysplasia or renal arterial atherosclerotic lesions that are anatomically renal. Angioplasty can be repeated or operation performed if stenosis recurs, and initial PTA may prevent the need for surgical bypass. Angioplasty is less successful in treatment of ostial or mixed atherosclerotic lesions.

▶ Although good results have been achieved in surgical treatment of fibromuscular hyperplasia, PTLA appears to be the treatment of choice now. In atherosclerotic renal artery stenosis, especially ostial lesions or in calcified arteries, bypass grafting remains the most effective treatment. In occlusion involving branches of the renal artery, the French group has shown that extracorporeal repair yields good surgical results. These facts aid in deciding present day therapy.

The operative mortality of 3%, reported by the Emory group, suggests that concomitant renal revascularization in patients undergoing aortic surgery is now a safe procedure and, perhaps, should be performed more often.

Reports on reoperative surgery for renovascular hypertension are few. The experience reported by the Michigan group is welcomed. Their experience in surgical treatment of renovascular hypertension has always been respected.

Pediatric Digital Subtraction Angiography

Gary M. Amundson, Richard L. Wesenberg, Dagmar L. Mueller, and Robert H. Reid (Calgary, Alberta)

Radiology 153:649–654, December 1984 7–64

There is little information concerning the use of intravenous digital subtraction angiography (DSA) in children, even though its relative ease of performance, low complication rate, and diagnostic accuracy indicate that it has considerable potential. A review was made of the initial 10-month experience with 87 DSA examinations in 74 children 3 days to 19 years of age. The major routes for catheter placement were the external jugular vein in younger children and the superior vena cava in older children.

Seventy five of the 87 DSA studies were completed successfully, with imaging of all major organ systems. There were 1 major and 7 minor complications related to the procedure. The major complication was acute pulmonary edema developing secondary to administration of excessive

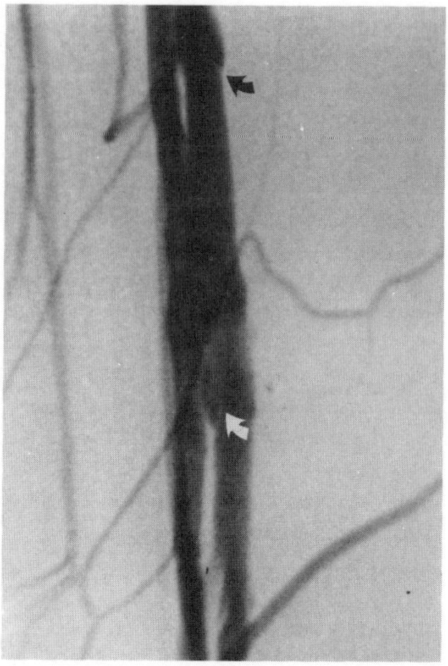

Fig 7–15.—Peripheral venogram in a child with a clinically suspected deep vein thrombosis. Only a 15% concentration of MD-76 (sodium and meglumine diatrizoate, 370 mg/ml of iodine) was used. (Courtesy of Amundson, G.M., et al.: Radiology 153:649–654, December 1984.)

contrast medium and fluid; six minor complications developed secondary to catheters placed in the external jugular vein with flow rates of more than 8 ml/second, and another was secondary to pressure injection through a Broviac catheter. Most patients underwent DSA for diagnostic purposes, usually in evaluation of the intracerebral circulation. The major intracerebral arteries, veins, and dural sinuses were particularly well demonstrated, and smaller branches (e.g., the posterior inferior cerebellar artery) also were imaged consistently. None of the 22 patients who underwent abdominal studies required standard arteriography, because the quality of the DSA was considered sufficient for diagnosis. The nonrenal studies were generally of superior quality. The major vessels arising from the aorta and their branches were easily demonstrated, and the intrarenal arteries and parenchyma were visualized in some instances. Although the renal veins were not seen, the portal venous system could be evaluated by examination of the venous redistribution of contrast medium. All examinations of the extremities were of diagnostic quality (Fig 7–15), with good visualization of not only the major vessels, but also the small vessels. Venous drainage of the extremity could also be evaluated during venous circulation. Gating was not available for the thoracic examinations, thus many were not of sufficient diagnostic quality when compared with the results obtained by standard angiocardiography. Radiation exposure was not a limiting factor in this series because of the low exposure used (2–38 mR per frame).

Digital subtraction angiography is widely applicable to many organ systems and is particularly useful in assessing intracranial disease and for preoperative evaluation of neoplasms. Further correlative studies are needed to establish more specific indications for the use of DSA in children.

Percutaneous Transluminal Angioplasty for Pediatric Renovascular Hypertension

Philip Stanley, Grant Hieshima, and Mark Mehringer (Los Angeles)

Radiology 153:101–104, October 1984 7–65

Percutaneous transluminal angioplasty (PTA) was attempted in 5 children, 22 months to 12 years of age, with severe renovascular hypertension. One child was comatose, and another had congestive failure. A third patient had an abdominal mass secondary to aortic aneurysm associated with bilateral renal artery stenoses. Preliminary angiography revealed a renovascular lesion on 1 side in 4 patients, 3 of whom had involvement of the mid or distal main renal artery. Concentric tubular stenosis was present in 1 child, a discrete weblike band in another, tubular stenosis with aneurysmal irregularity and poststenotic dilatation in a third child, and a discrete weblike band involving an upper pole branch at the bifurcation, as well as poststenotic dilatation, in a fourth child. The fifth child had received a Dacron aortic graft and underwent saphenous vein patch angioplasty for an aortic aneurysm, with the subsequent development of stenosis of the right artery at the site of patch angioplasty. In all 5 patients, PTA successfully dilated the stenosis without complication. All 5 were normotensive without medication within 48–72 hours. Hypertension recurred 10 months later in 1 child, and angiography showed stenosis of the main renal artery similar to that of the original lesion. The other 4 children remained normotensive after follow-up observation for 1–2 years.

▶ Diagnosis and treatment of pediatric vascular problems offer a challenge to vascular surgeons. Use of intravenous digital subtraction angiography and percutaneous balloon dilatation may be useful in this little population, too.

Renal Artery Dissection

Bruce M. Smith, George W. Holcomb III, Robert E. Richie, and Richard H. Dean (Nashville, Tenn.)

Ann. Surg. 200:134–146, August 1984 7–66

Dissecting aneurysms of the renal artery, or renal artery dissections, are stenotic or occlusive lesions that are most frequently encountered in hypertensive patients with underlying atherosclerotic or fibromuscular disease. Acute dissections may occur spontaneously as a complication of diagnostic or therapeutic angiography or as an agonal event associated with overwhelming systemic illness. Chronic dissections may result in renovascular hypertension or may be asymptomatic.

The authors describe their experience with 14 renal artery dissections in 9 patients seen over the past decade at Vanderbilt University Medical Center and review the findings in an additional 77 renal artery dissections in 72 patients reported in the literature.

In the present study 7 of the dissections were chronic and 4 were acute. Six of the 7 chronic dissections were functional and 1 was silent. Two of the acute dissections were spontaneous, and 2 occurred as complications of angiography. Postmortem examination revealed 3 agonal dissections in 2 additional patients; 1 was found at autopsy, and bilateral dissections were found at the time of cadaveric donor nephrectomy. Ten renal artery bypass procedures, including 5 complex branch reconstructions (3 of which were carried out ex vivo), were performed in 7 patients, resulting in 100% immediate patency and maintenance or improvement of renal function. Long-term follow-up has shown all 7 patients to have sustained patency of the reconstructed renal arteries, excellent control of blood pressure, and normal renal function. Nephrectomy has not been necessary and there have been no associated deaths.

Of the 72 patients with 77 renal artery dissections reported in the literature, 55 (76.4%) survived, although the kidney was preserved in only 26 (47.3%) of the 55 survivors in these earlier series. Renal failure was associated with 59% of the deaths in these patients.

The lethality of renal artery dissections and the success of revascularization, which preserves renal function and improves associated renovascular hypertension, underscore the need for an aggressive approach to the recognition and treatment of this condition. The aims of therapy should be arterial reconstruction and preservation of functioning renal tissue.

Acute Nontraumatic Obstructions of the Renal Artery

M. Lacombe (Clichy, France)

Presse Med. 10:2425–2428, November 1984 7–67

Acute obstructions of the renal artery are infrequent, and their diagnosis is frequently missed. In this study, 13 patients (17 kidneys at risk) with obstruction of the trunk of the renal artery underwent surgical treatment. Delay between onset of obstruction and surgical procedure ranged from 18 hours to 36 days (median, 8 days). Ten patients were anuric at the time of operation. Eleven kidneys (64.5%) were saved. Renal function, regardless of the period of obstruction, reappeared in all cases after surgical revascularization.

In one quarter of the cases, a total infarct ensued, whereas in two thirds of the cases the kidney's viability was conserved. Classically, renal lesions appear rapidly, achieving their maximum intensity within 1½ hours. After this if the kidney is still viable, the duration of the obstruction does not influence the degree of lesions, and time of the revascularization does not modify results. The persistence of definitive renal insufficiency is a sequela of ischemic lesions after arterial obstruction. Its degree depends on the quality of the collateral circulation and not on when the obstruction is removed.

Treatment of acute obstruction of the renal artery is essentially surgical. The risks of medical treatment alone are predictable in cases seen late, which are the rule or when there is an atheromatous stenosis of the renal artery. Medical care is blind therapy since no examination can reveal before operation the exact state of the kidney. Infarct of the kidney renders all medical treatment useless.

Indication for operation is absolute whatever the delay after onset of acute obstruction, even if several days elapse. Renal lesions ensue at the onset of obstruction. If the kidney has remained viable, time does not affect the outcome once the initial period is past.

▶ Diagnosis of acute renal artery occlusion is difficult and often delayed because of a lack of awareness of this condition. Quite often valuable time has elapsed before revascularization. Therefore, it is reassuring to know that revascularization is possible even after a delay of several days. Dissection of the renal artery is uncommon, and here again, the Vanderbilt group has contributed valuable information about this condition.

Reoperation for Complications of Renal Artery Reconstructive Surgery Undertaken for Treatment of Renovascular Hypertension

James C. Stanley, Walter M. Whitehouse, Jr., Gerald B. Zelenock, Linda M. Graham, Jack L. Cronenwett, and S. Martin Lindenauer (Univ. of Michigan)

J. Vasc. Surg. 2:133–144, January 1985 7–68

Patients who require reoperation after arterial reconstruction for renovascular hypertension are at an increased risk of nephrectomy. Reoperations necessary for complications of reconstruction were reviewed from 1961 to 1983, when 72 reoperations were carried out in 58 patients, who were among 373 who had 425 primary operations for renovascular hypertension. The reoperation rate was 15.5%. Thirty-seven pediatric patients were operated on primarily, as were 176 adults with fibrodysplastic disease and 160 with atherosclerotic renovascular lesions. The most frequent primary operation was autogenous saphenous vein grafting from the aorta or iliac vessels.

Nine children had 10 reoperations, most often for persistent or recurrent hypertension. Four operations were for acute thrombosis after primary operation. Six reoperations resulted in nephrectomy. All but 11% of children were cured or improved. Thirty-three adults required 44 reoperations after primary operations for fibrodysplastic disease. Twelve patients had early graft thrombosis or stenosis. Thirteen were reoperated on later for graft thrombosis, 17 for graft stenosis, and 2 for aneurysmal vein graft change. Nephrectomy was necessary in 39% of patients. Eventually 97% of patients were cured or improved. Sixteen patients with atherosclerotic disease had 18 reoperations, 93% for recurrent or persistent hypertension. Only one of six kidneys was reoperated on early but seven of 12 reoperated on later were removed. Eighty-one percent of patients were cured or improved.

Reoperation for complications of primary renal arterial reconstruction is a serious undertaking. Delay in recognizing the complication increases the chance that the kidney will have to be removed. Better results can be obtained by promptly evaluating patients with persistent or recurrent hypertension angiographically and by timely reoperation if necessary.

Aorto-Iliac Ischemia

Criteria From Intra-Arterial Femoral Artery Pressure Measurements Combined With Reactive Hyperemia to Assess the Aortoiliac Segment: A Prospective Study

P. F. Verhagen and Th. J. M. V. van Vroonhoven (St. Elizabeth Hosp., Tilburg, Netherlands)

Br. J. Surg. 71:706–708, September 1984 7–69

There have been no uniform criteria for direct measurement of femoral artery blood pressure (FAP) combined with postischemic reactive hyperemia (FAP study) for assessment of the aortoiliac segment, especially in multilevel disease. In a previous retrospective study criteria were established for detection of significant stenoses by comparing the results of FAP studies with 6-month postoperative clinical results in patients with angiographically proved multilevel disease.

From the results it was concluded that hemodynamically important aortoiliac disease existed when the femorobrachial systolic pressure index at rest (GA index at rest) was less than 70% or when the difference (index gradient) between the GA index at rest and the lowest index during reactive hyperemia (GA index) was more than 20%.

These criteria have now been used prospectively in FAP studies performed on 50 extremities of 45 patients with multilevel arterial occlusive disease of the lower extremities to assess the aortoiliac segment and to predict the outcome of vascular reconstruction. The common femoral and the radial or brachial arteries were cannulated under local anesthesia to obtain systolic pressures. Reactive hyperemia was achieved by placing a tourniquet around the thigh; 4-minute total arterial occlusion was caused by inflating the tourniquet.

Proximal reconstruction was performed in 27 extremities, including 16 aortofemoral and 4 aortoiliac reconstructions, 5 intraluminal angioplasties of the iliac segment, 1 femorofemoral bypass, and 1 thromboendarterectomy of the common iliac artery. Distal reconstruction was done in 23 extremities, including 21 femoropopliteal and 2 femorocrural bypasses.

At evaluation 6 months after operation results of the FAP study were positive in 19 of 27 extremities that had proximal reconstructions and negative in 8 (including 5 extremities that showed no improvement). All 20 femoropopliteal bypasses with a good crural runoff gave clinical improvement. Three distal reconstructions occluded in the immediate postoperative period, probably due to outflow disease and not because of undetected inflow disease.

Mean values of the GA index were 10.7% (range 1% to 23%) in the proximal group and 2.5% (range 0% to 8%) in the distal group. When the 3 distal reconstructions that occluded are omitted, the criteria used were 86% sensitive, 100% specific, and 93% accurate in predicting the postoperative hemodynamic result. Positive predictive value was 100%; negative predictive value was 89%. There were no complications from the FAP studies.

By using as criteria for significant aortoiliac disease a GA index at rest of less than 70% or, in case of a GA index at rest of more than 70%, an index gradient of more than 20%, the FAP study becomes an excellent way to assess the aortoiliac segment and to predict the outcome of reconstruction in multilevel arterial occlusive disease of the lower extremities. These criteria are similar to those of Brewster et al. and Flanigan et al.

▶ This seems to be a simple answer to a complex problem.

Use of Continuous-Wave Doppler Ultrasound Velocimetry to Assess the Severity of Coarctation of the Aorta by Measurement of Aortic Flow Velocities

R. K. H. Wyse, P. J. Robinson, J. E. Deanfield, D. S. Tunstall Pedoe, and F. J. Macartney (London)

Br. Heart J. 52:278–283, September 1984 7–70

Transcutaneous Doppler ultrasound velocimetry has been used successfully, with the Bernoulli equation, to estimate the fall in pressure across valve lesions. An attempt was made to determine whether this approach can add useful data in the noninvasive assessment of patients with coarctation of the aorta. Thirty patients, aged 8 days to 17 years, were examined; 13 were less than 6 years of age. Seven studies were done preoperatively; 24, a mean of 5½ years after repair. Doppler studies also were done in 13 control children without coarctation. Peak flow velocity in the ascending and descending aorta was measured using a combined pulsed and continuous-wave Doppler velocimeter.

Arm-leg systolic blood pressure gradients ranged from 22 to 75 mm Hg in patients with coarctation that had not been treated surgically. The peak flow velocity in the descending aorta was significantly higher in cases of coarctation than in control subjects, with no overlap. The flow velocity correlated with the arm-leg systolic pressure gradient at a level of 0.84, and the predicted and calculated pressure gradients correlated at a level of 0.85. More than 80% of peak flow velocities in the ascending aorta in study patients were above the control range. Two patients had significant aortic stenosis, and many others had known aortic valve abnormalities.

Continuous-wave Doppler ultrasound velocimetry is a rapid and accurate means of recognizing the presence or absence of coarctation or recoarctation of the aorta and of evaluating the severity of the lesion. The severity of obstruction can be quantified directly both at presentation and at follow-up.

▶ Follow-up of patients undergoing vascular reconstruction is terribly important, and this method allows accurate estimation of postcoarctation restenosis.

The Vasculitis of Atrophie Blanche (Livedoid Vasculitis) and Abdominal Aortic Pathology

A. L. Schroeter (Mayo Clinic) and R. B. Harris (Penticton, B. C.)

Cutis 34:298–302, September 1984 7–71

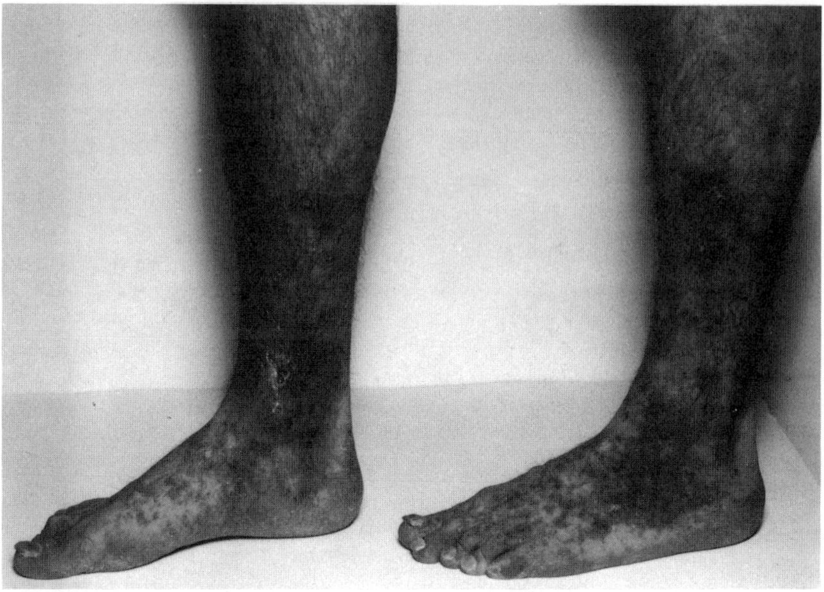

Fig 7–16.—Typical stellate "punched out" ulcers of livedoid vasculitis are seen on medial aspect of right ankle. (Courtesy of Schroeter, A.L., and Harris, R.B.: Cutis 34:298–302, September 1984.)

Livedoid vasculitis is a chronic, recurrent hyalinizing vasculitis of the small dermal vessels of the lower extremities. Like livedoid reticularis, it has been associated with systemic mesenchymal disorders including lupus erythematosus and rheumatoid arthritis, as well as some infectious, metabolic, cardiovascular, and carcinomatous diseases. Abdominal aortic disease was found in 7 of 42 cases of livedoid vasculitis seen at Mayo Clinic (16.6%). Calcification alone was seen in 4 cases, diffuse atherosclerosis in 1, aortoiliac occlusive disease in 1, and a 10-cm aneurysm with thrombus in 1. Three patients had surgery for aortic disease.

The clinical appearance of livedoid vasculitis is shown in Figure 7–16. Biopsy specimens showed segmental thickening, endothelial proliferation, and hyaline degeneration of the subintimal layer and focal thrombosis of dermal vessels. The vessel walls were not destroyed, and cholesterol crystals and clefting were not noted. Immunofluorescence studies showed deposits of IgG, IgM, Clq, or fibrin in hyalinized vessels. At roentgenographic study all 7 patients were found to have aortic calcification. Two of the 3 patients who had graft replacement of aneurysms continued to have lesions and problems with occlusive vascular disease below the level of replacement.

The diagnosis of livedoid vasculitis may serve as a harbinger of systemic disorder, notably disease of the abdominal aorta. Investigation is warranted because of the tendency of the atheromatous aorta to undergo aneurysmal change. Removal of all diseased tissue may reverse an otherwise poor prognosis.

Algodystrophy After Aortic Bifurcation Surgery
M. D. Churcher
Lancet 2:131–133, July 21, 1984 7–72

Algodystrophy may follow surgery at the aortic bifurcation. Patients present with pain, trophic changes, and cutaneous dysesthesia in one or both legs. The author presents 6 patients with symptoms and signs of an algodystrophy after aortic bifurcation surgery for leg ischemia.

Man, 53, was treated for claudication with a right lumbar sympathectomy and iliac bypass graft. He presented with pain over the right upper thigh, which developed after he was discharged from the hosptial. Further surgery at the aortic bifurcation was performed 14 months later. The symptoms of pain and dysesthesia on the upper thigh became worse. An aching and throbbing pain, extending from the iliac fossa to the ankle, was exacerbated by activity and relieved by rest. Examination revealed a cold limb with absent peripheral pulses and cutaneous dysesthesia over the thigh. A right paravertebral sympathetic injection with 15 ml of 0.25% bupivacaine warmed the foot and relieved both pain and cutaneous dysesthesia. Right-sided celiac plexus block with 15 ml of 45% alcohol was performed to produce a more extensive sympathectomy. Patient improved.

In all 6 patients, symptoms and signs of algodystrophy developed after aortic bifurcation surgery. The pain, cutaneous dysesthesia, and weakness were temporarily relieved by sympathetic block with local anesthetic. Celiac plexus or splanchnic injection in conjunction with bilateral surgical lumbar sympathectomy may achieve the more extensive sympathetic interruption necessary for pain relief in lower body quadrant disorders. As illustrated by this case, pain relief after paravertebral injection of 0.25% bupivacaine at the site of an excised L2 ganglion may be explained by the spread of bupivacaine to adjacent aortic plexus. Allodynia and hyperpathia associated with dissection in the common iliac artery are relieved by sympathetic block, suggesting that damage to the arterial wall may initiate abnormal reflex activity and sensory changes.

Recognition of algodystrophy is important to avoid further vascular surgery which will only exacerbate the symptoms. The permanent and complete relief of symptoms of algodystrophy by surgery or repeat chemical sympathectomy, when the condition is long established, is both impractical and impossible. The beneficial effect of β-blockers has been reported.

▶ These two articles were selected because of the curious terms in their titles. Algodystrophy covers a disparate group of painful clinical conditions, such as causalgia, reflex sympathetic dystrophy, and Sudek's atrophy. *Atrophie blanche* is a dermatologic term. From the point of view of vascular surgeons it is important to know that this is associated with atheromatous embolization, which in turn is associated with digital infarcts and erythematous flares in the skin in the presence of normal distal pulses. For dermatologists, a quotation from the article should be of some value: "The clinical or pathologic diagnosis, livedoid vasculitis, may serve as a valuable harbinger of systemic disease, notably abdominal aortic pathology."

Peripheral Embolic Phenomena From Proximal Arterial Disease
Neil R. McLean, Brian H. Irvine, and Matthew H. Calvert
J. R. Coll. Surg. Edinb. 29:205–209, July 1984 7–73

Findings in 52 consecutive patients seen in 3 years with clinical features of small peripheral emboli from proximal arterial disease were reviewed. All were nondiabetics with patent proximal major vessels. All had evidence of a proximal, potentially embolic lesion and peripheral focal ischemic lesions. Myeloproliferative and collagen disorders were absent. The 36 males and 16 females had a mean age of 60 years. Affected vessels supplied the lower limb in 72% of cases; the superficial femoral artery was most frequently involved. Two thirds of patients had a local painful but nongangrenous lesion. Only 4 patients had major tissue loss. Arterial stenosis was present in 28 patients. Ten patients had embolism just before or at the time of occlusion of a major artery. Eight patients had an aneurysm, and 4 had an ulcerated plaque. Four embolic events occurred during reconstructive arterial operations.

The embolic source was managed by reconstructive operations in 69% of cases. Antiplatelet agents were also used in many patients before operation. Thirteen patients were treated with antiplatelet drugs alone. About half the patients had spontaneous healing of the distal ischemic lesion after control of the source of emboli. Twelve patients had chemical sympathectomy with 6% aqueous phenol, but the effects of this procedure were not formally assessed.

Less severe peripheral ischemic lesions from embolism will heal, and distal amputation can be performed without reconstruction if further embolism is prevented. Antiplatelet drugs may prevent further embolism from stenotic lesions. Embolism from aneurysms often threatens limb viability. Intraoperative embolism can be avoided by making certain that the main vessels beyond the point of manipulation are first clamped.

▶ It is becoming increasingly apparent that artery to artery embolization is much more important in the genesis of peripheral artery occlusions than cardiogenic embolization. This abstract emphasizes this fact but leaves out the problem of atheromatous embolization as a cause of peripheral bypass failure. This has been addressed by our group in the past.

Thrombogenicity of Dacron Arterial Grafts and Its Modification by Platelet Inhibitory Drugs
R. C. Kester (Leeds, England)
Ann. R. Coll. Surg. Engl. 66:241–246, July 1984 7–74

When blood flows through Dacron arterial grafts, many platelets adhere to the luminal surface of the grafts. Studies of disturbed platelet function in an artificial circulation, by scanning electron microscopy of the luminal surfaces of grafts, of platelet and fibrinogen kinetics, and of clinical outcomes in narrow-bore grafts found Dacron to be highly thrombogenic.

Degree of thrombogenicity varies among types of commercially available Dacron prostheses. The thrombogenic response was studied in an artificial circulation and in patients with aortobifemoral grafts. Administration of a platelet-inhibiting regimen based on a combination of aspirin (ASA) and dipyridamole (DPM) modified the thrombogenic response to Dacron, as was reflected in the improved patency rate of Dacron grafts that occurred. Results of clinical trials suggest that 330 mg of ASA plus 75 mg of DPM given 3 times a day is a more effective antiplatelet regimen in the short term than is administration of 300 mg of ASA once a day combined with 75 mg of DPM 3 times a day. The magnitude of the thrombogenic response to Dacron probably varies both during the life-span of a graft from the day of implantation and from patient to patient. Future research will probably focus on modification of the thrombogenic surface of Dacron and on achieving effective antithrombotic measures.

▶ Attention is called to this study chiefly because within it is a prospective randomized trial of femoropopliteal Dacron bypass grafting, a study that probably could not have been carried out in North America. Sixty-five patients were studied: thirty-eight grafts in a placebo group, and thirty-five in the test group. At 3 months, 6 in the placebo group and 2 in the test group had closed; by 12 months 9 in the placebo group had closed compared to 2 in the test group. Of 27 above-knee grafts in the placebo group, 10 occluded compared to 2 out of 18 in the test group. The original paper is commended to the attention of vascular surgeons interested in prosthetic grafting.

Catheterization of Prosthetic Vascular Grafts: Acceptable Technique

Douglas C. Smith (Loma Linda Univ.)

AJR 143:1117–1118, November 1984 7–75

Percutaneous catheterization of prosthetic vascular grafts for angiography has been considered to be dangerous, despite reports of excellent results. Potential hazards are said to include graft disruption, pseudoaneurysm formation, infection, thrombosis, and uncontrollable bleeding. The author has performed more than 100 transgraft catheterizations with no complications. Aortoiliofemoral, visceral, and carotid studies were included. Mani has had more than 700 cases with a single complication unrelated to the procedure itself. The chief problem is the tight fit of the catheter at the puncture site, which can make catheter manipulation and withdrawal difficult. "Overdilation" of the puncture site can eliminate resistance there. Only 1 case of graft pseudointima disruption from catheterization has been reported.

When the native transfemoral arterial route is unavailable, catheterization of a patent graft is an alternative to axillary catheterization. The graft usually is readily punctured and a catheter easily passed through its straight course. Peripheral neurologic complications are not a concern, as they are with axillary catheterization. Catheter angiography via a graft is definitely preferable to translumbar puncture in patients with severe hypertension or borderline clotting factor values. Selective catheter placement in any aortic branch is better done via the transgraft approach. Catheterization of a patent prosthetic graft is the method of choice in most instances in which native transfemoral arterial access is unavailable.

▶ The facts contained in this abstract need to be brought to the attention of our radiologist colleagues.

Ruptured Anastomotic Pseudoaneurysm After Prosthetic Vascular Graft Bypass Procedures

Haim Gutman, Avigdor Zelikovski, and Raphael Reiss

Isr. J. Med. Sci. 20:613–617, July 1984 7–76

Anastomotic pseudoaneurysms are a late complication of prosthetic implantation, seen in 2% to 3% of all procedures. A large majority have occurred in the groin. Four cases of ruptured pseudoaneurysm, diagnosed 1½ to 12 months after initial operation, were encountered, representing 1.3% of all vascular grafts done in a 2-year period.

Man, 70, with severe lymphedema of the left leg after orchiectomy and irradiation for seminoma, was operated on for ischemia of the left foot and received an ileofemoral Gortex bypass. A pneumatic device was used to treat lymphedema 1 year later. A pulsating, tender mass was present in the left groin several months thereafter. Ultrasonography showed a pseudoaneurysm measuring 3 × 3 cm at the point at which the graft was inserted in the common femoral artery. A new extra-anatomical bypass was made from the iliac artery distal to the bifurcation, and the femoral artery was ligated. The pseudoaneurysm was excised and the wound laid open. Vagotomy and pyloroplasty were necessary for two bleeding duodenal ulcers in the postoperative period. The groin wound eventually closed by granulation. Histologic study confirmed the diagnosis and showed the presence of gram-negative bacteria.

Anastomotic pseudoaneurysms are an increasingly frequent complication of prosthetic vascular bypass operations. Urgent treatment with an extra-anatomical new bypass is indicated, with resection of the possibly infected area, allowing secondary wound healing. Any pseudoaneurysm should be treated as an emergency. Occurrence of this complication might be reduced by using end-to-end anastomoses, braided Dacron sutures, knitted Dacron grafts, and antibiotic prophylaxis.

▶ One does not usually think of the problem of pseudoaneurysm eventuating in rupture. Clearly, these aneurysms follow the course of all other aneurysms and progress to enlargement and rupture if they are allowed to pursue their own natural history.

Advantage of Revascularization of the Hypogastric Artery in Chronic Vascular Disorders of the Lower Limbs: Personal Experience in 200 Cases

M. Batt, R. Hassen-Khodja, and P. Le Bas (Nice, France)

J. Chir. (Paris) 121:443–449, June–July 1984 7–77

The authors present results in 162 patients, 38 of whom received bilateral revascularizations. In 81 cases (40%) the hypogastric revascularization was performed in the course of treating an aortoiliac aneurysm, in 65 cases (32%) after an aortobi-iliac restoration for obliterating lesions, and in 54 cases (28%) after a unilateral iliac restoration.

The lesions were classified into 4 types. In type 1 (42 cases), the hypogastric artery played a supply role through its afferent collaterals: the gluteal, iliolumbar, internal pudendal, and contralateral hypogastric vessels. In type 2 (80 cases), it played a distribution role through its efferent collaterals: the gluteal, ischiatic, and obturator arteries, In type 3 (38 cases) the hypogastric unit played a supply and distribution role through its afferent and efferent collaterals. Type 4 (40 cases) corresponded to a total thrombosis of the principal arterial axis where the hypogastric only played an indirect role.

In certain cases of aortoiliofemoral obliteration, the direct revascularization of the hypogastric represents the last possible salvage technique, a true "spare tire" that permits the indirect revascularization of the lower extremities in case of failure of the restoration of the principal arterial axis.

Thromboendarterectomy was the technique of choice in 82 cases (41%) for stenosing or obliterating iliac or aortoiliac lesions. A graft was used in 103 cases (51%) and was the method chosen in aortoiliac aneurysms. Reimplantation of the hypogastric was possible in 15 cases (8%).

Revascularization of the hypogastric artery should be considered each time an aortoiliofemoral restoration is envisioned. Direct revascularization of the hypogastrics is preferred to a risky retrograde revascularization or a revascularization of the inferior mesenteric artery that seems less important in the anatomical and physiologic plan.

Is Impotence an Arterial Disorder? A Study of Arterial Risk Factors in 440 Impotent Men

R. Virag, P. Bouilly, and D. Frydman (Paris)

Lancet 1:181–184, Jan. 25, 1985 7–78

The distribution of arterial risk factors was examined in a series of 440 impotent men seen between 1977 and 1981 in whom the penile blood pressure index (PBPI), the ratio of the lowest systolic pressure in a main penile artery to arm systolic pressure, was measured. A total of 222 men participated in a more detailed investigation of the cause of impotence, which included nocturnal penile tumescence study during rapid eye movement sleep, artificial erection and cavernosography, selective bilateral internal iliac angiography, study of bulbocavernous latency, administration of the Minnesota Multiphasic Personality Inventory, and serum hormone estimations. Normoglycemic subjects had oral glucose tolerance tests.

The mean age of all men was 47 years. Age increased with the number of arterial risk factors (diabetes, smoking, hyperlipidemia, hypertension). Organic impairment of erection was present in 80% of subjects studied in detail. Evidence of an arterial lesion was obtained in 53% of these.

Smoking, diabetes, and hyperlipidemia were all significantly more frequent in the impotent group as a whole than in the general male population of comparable age. Lower PBPIs were associated with the presence of two or more arterial risk factors. Organic impotence was present in 49% of subjects without risk factors and in all those with three or four risk factors. Clinical diabetes was the only state consistently associated with a reduced PBPI.

The increase in prevalence of impotence with advancing age is related mainly to atherosclerotic changes in the penile arteries. Arterial risk factors and the PBPI should be assessed initially in any patient with impotence. Arteriosclerotic changes in the penile arteries should be sought even when impotence appears to be an isolated symptom, particularly if any arterial risk factors are present. Impotent patients should be managed in the same way as patients with more severe arteriosclerosis at other sites.

Blood Flow in Deep Abdominal and Pelvic Vessels: Ultrasonic Pulsed Doppler Analysis

Kenneth J. W. Taylor, Peter N. Burns, John P. Woodcock, and P. N. T. Wells

Radiology 154:487–493, February 1985 7–79

The use of pulsed Doppler equipment with a real-time scanner permits precise localization of the volume of tissue from which the Doppler flow signal is sampled. The normal signals in deep abdominal and pelvic arteries and veins have now been evaluated by a real-time sector scanner with pulsed Doppler flowmeter. Signals obtained by using a 3- or 5-MHz transducer were analyzed with an integral fast Fourier transform processor. Recordings were made in 20 females admitted for diagnostic laparoscopy and in 10 volunteers.

A specific Doppler "signature" was evident for each vessel examined. The proximal, middle, and distal aortic signals showed a clear window below the systolic time-velocity pulse, implying that most cells are moving at the same velocity. This plug flow profile is typical of large arteries. A decrease in flow at the end of diastole and reversal of direction at the bifurcation reflected blood rebounding up the aorta as the velocity wave was reflected from the high impedance of the peripheral vascular bed of the legs. Plug flow in systole was more disorganized during diastole in the main celiac trunk. Persistent flow in diastole reflected the low distal vascular impedance of the hepatic circulation. Similar wave forms were recorded in the main and right hepatic arteries and from the liver parenchyma. More distal branches had flow velocity profiles approaching a parabolic form, with an even spread of Doppler shift frequencies and filling in of the spectral display. The gastroduodenal arterial wave form had Doppler shift frequencies corresponding with low flow velocities. The splenic wave form showed flow away from the probe, as did that of the proximal portion of the renal artery. Wave forms in the common and external iliac arteries resembled those in the aorta. Ovarian artery signals exhibited the low Doppler shift of a small vessel with low flow velocity.

This approach can be used to demonstrate the presence or absence and direction of flow in a given structure, to describe time-velocity wave forms, and to estimate absolute volume flow.

Internal Iliac Artery Revascularization in Treatment of Vasculogenic Impotence

D. Preston Flanigan, Kim R. Sobinsky, James J. Schuler, Dale Buchbinder, Philip G. Borozan, and Joseph P. Meyer (Univ. of Illinois, Chicago)

Ann. Surg. 120:271–274, March 1985 7–80

Internal iliac artery revascularization was evaluated as an adjunct to aortofemoral bypass in 5 impotent men in whom preoperative tests suggested vasculogenic impotence. All had abnormal penile-brachial arterial pressure indices; the mean was 0.42. The patients, however, were selected on the basis of indications for lower limb revascularization. Two patients had ejaculatory function but were impotent, and another was capable of intermittent partial erections. Mean age was 57 years. Three patients were diabetic, 4 were hypertensive, and 3 had stable coronary artery disease.

The iliac part of the procedure is done first to avoid a proximate aortic bifurcation graft. A careful nerve-sparing dissection is carried out. An open endarterectomy is performed, with patch angioplasty as an alternative, before a standard end-to-side aortic bifurcation graft procedure.

All 5 patients had regained penile erectile function 3 months after operation. Four had demonstrated adequate function for sexual intercourse. The patient who had patch angioplasty of the internal iliac artery developed retrograde ejaculation after operation but remained sexually active. The mean postoperative penile-brachial arterial pressure index was 0.80. Two patients died of myocardial infarction; the 3 survivors remained potent 3 months to 2 years after operation.

Revascularization of the internal iliac artery can correct vasculogenic impotence due to iliac occlusive disease in patients undergoing lower limb revascularization by aortofemoral bypass. All 5 patients in this series regained sexual function after operation, but it is not certain that internal iliac revascularization was responsible. The procedure is safe and it prolongs the primary operation only minimally. It seems to be warranted in patients with suspected vasculogenic impotence from severe iliac occlusive disease who require aortofemoral bypass to relieve lower limb ischemia.

► As aortic surgery has become increasingly successful, surgeons have properly turned to improving the overall results of the surgical procedure. To this end, the prevention of sexual dysfunction caused by the aortic intervention is laudatory. The internal iliac artery has remained relatively uninteresting to vascular surgeons despite its importance in allowing erection and normal sexual functioning. Hopefully, surgeons doing vascular reconstruction will pay more attention to the internal iliac artery and to prevention of damage to periaortic and iliac sympathetic nerves. With that in mind, it is disappointing to note that the pulsed Doppler analysis of blood flow within abdominal vessels is difficult to obtain from the internal iliac arteries.

The Significance of Hydronephrosis After Aortofemoral Reconstruction

Peter Schubart, George Fortner, Dana Cummings, Doug Reed, Brian L. Thiele, Dennis F. Bandyk, and Hubert M. Radke (Univ. of Washington)

Arch. Surg. 120:377–381, March 1985 7–81

Hydronephrosis from ureteral obstruction (Fig 7–17) is a rarely reported complication of aortic bypass grafting, but it was observed in several patients who had developed serious graft complications. Serial real-time ultrasound studies were performed on 96 patients who underwent aortic reconstruction at several centers, excluding patients with single-limb grafts and those with preexisting hydronephrosis. Nineteen patients were found to have postreconstructive hydronephrosis. Forty-eight patients who had undergone aortofemoral bypass without evidence of hydronephrosis were

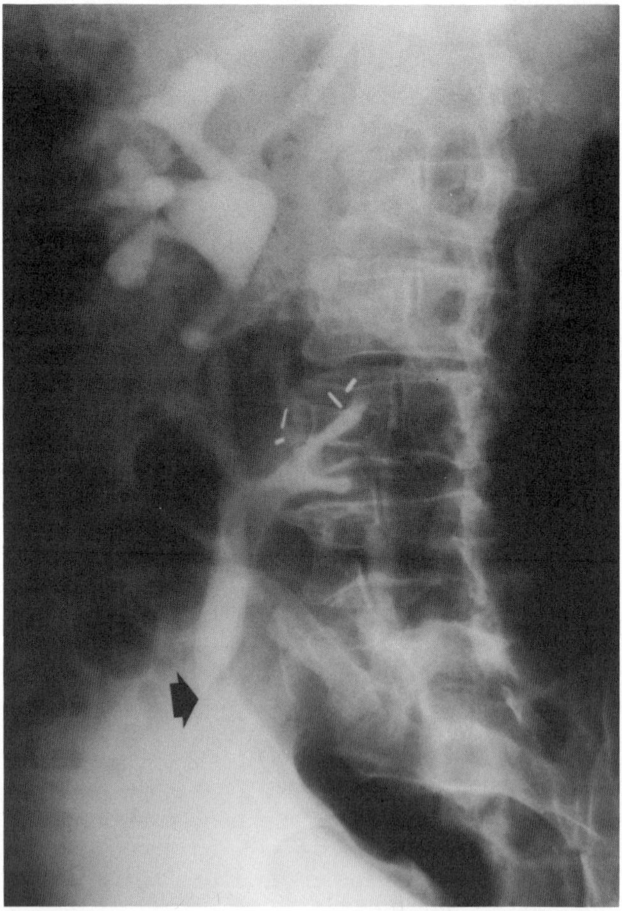

Fig 7–17.—Hydronephrosis of right kidney. Oblique intravenous pyelogram demonstrates characteristic tapering obstruction of ureter at pelvic brim *(arrow)*. (Courtesy of Schubart, P., et al.: Arch. Surg. 120:377–381, March 1985; copyright 1985, American Medical Association.)

also evaluated. Mean follow-up was 53 months. The patients with hydronephrosis were followed for an average of 6½ years after aortic grafting.

Hydronephrosis was diagnosed an average of 46 months after initial operation. Three patients had symptoms, but in 84% of cases hydronephrosis was an incidental finding. The course was generally benign, but 1 patient developed renal compromise, and 4 others had iatrogenic ureteral injury and required repair and ureteral drainage. One of these patients later died of sepsis and fistulization that were at least partly attributable to the ureteral injury. Twelve of the 19 patients with hydronephrosis had a total of 31 episodes of anastomotic pseudoaneurysm. Five patients required graft revision. Nine patients had 16 episodes of graft infection necessitating graft removal, and 2 others developed three aortoenteric fistulas. Ten patients had 32 episodes of graft thrombosis. Six patients required major amputations of nine lower extremities.

Hydronephrosis after aortic reconstruction is often asymptomatic and is probably underdiagnosed. It may develop several years after operation. The disorder is at least a marker of present or impending graft problems. All patients with overt graft infection should have intravenous ureteropyelography before reoperation, and placement of ureteral stents should be considered before graft removal. Hydronephrosis should be sought in patients who develop graft thrombosis or an anastomotic aneurysm. Ultrasonography appears to be a useful means of following patients after aortofemoral reconstruction.

Urologic Complications After Vascular Graft Surgery Within the Pelvic Area

G. Kleinhans, D. Leusmann, and D. Rühland (Univ. of Münster)
Chirurg 56:95–99, February 1985 7–82

After vascular graft operation within the pelvic area, urologic complications occur in about 10% of the patients. Of 310 cases reviewed, it was found that 4 patients suffered from ureteral lesions and 21 patients had ureteral obstructions.

Possible causes for ureteral obstructions are positioning of the ureter between vessel and prosthesis, hematoma, lymphoma, anastomotic aneurysm, prosthesis infection, and retroperitoneal fibrosis as well as trophical lesions of the ureter wall. Some authors believe that a compression is produced when the prosthesis is ventral to the anastomosed ureter; others, when it is dorsal to it. However, most authors refuse to perform a ureter resection since a water-tight anastomosis cannot be guaranteed. A primary nephrectomy for risk patients, providing the contralateral kidney is intact, is recommended by some authors. Anastomotic aneurysm is one of the most frequent late complications (3%–6%) and observed up to 12 years postoperatively. During aneurysm resection when dissecting the periaortic, the peri-iliac tissue can cause retroperitoneal hematomas and lymph drainage in the retroperitoneal space, which can lead to congestion. An infection

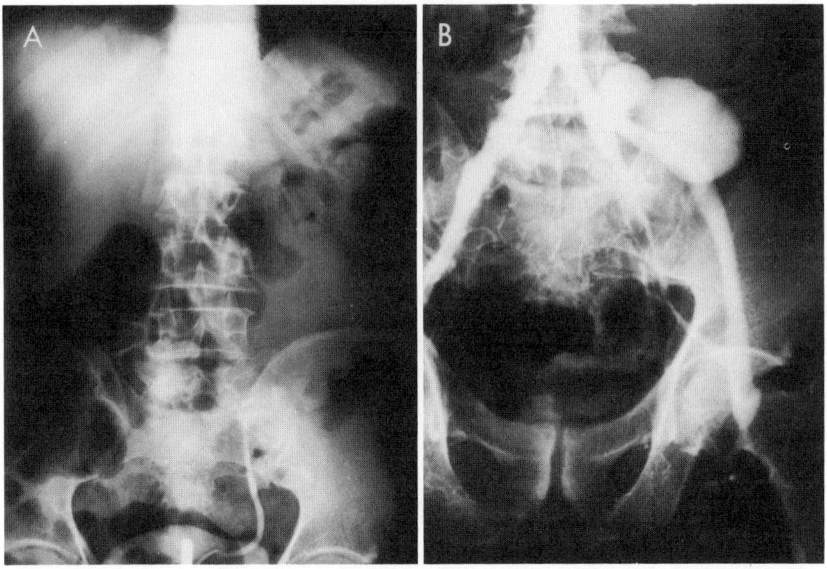

Fig 7–18.—**A**, retrograde filling; contrast medium stop. **B**, angiography; anastomosis aneurysm. (Courtesy of Kleinhans, G., et al.: Chirurg 56:95–99, February 1985; Berlin–Heidelberg–New York; Springer.)

rate of 0.3%–3% can be expected. However, after reconstruction with plastic prostheses, the rate increases. Surgical reintervention for infected aorto-femoral prosthesis is often combined with an especially high risk of ureteral lesions because of difficult retroperitoneal infected coalescences. Subtotal lesions and total ureteral separation are treated with splints; however, in a previously injured kidney, nephrectomy is indicated. Ureteral necrosis is the consequence of a trophical disturbance of the ureters, and treatment may be conservative using splints or a surgical intervention that may be less risky. Use of a ureteral splint could prevent surgical intervention in many cases.

Man, 64, because of a left subtotal iliac obstruction had an iliac femoral Teflon Bypass. Two months postoperatively the patient had colic-like pain in the left flank. The intravenous pyelogram showed severe congestion in the left space. The retrograde filling (Fig 7–18A) produced a contrast medium stop in the area of the vessel crossing. The ureteral splint was used. After 4 weeks with good position and function of the splint, the patient had pain in the left lower abdomen. Angiography (Fig 7–18B) showed an anastomotic aneurysm and revision of the prosthesis. The patient died on the first postoperative day of a fulminant lung embolism.

The authors suggest the following procedures: *(1)* Before each vascular graft intervention in the aorto-femoral area, either an infusion urogram should be made available or an angiographic diagnosis established so that the kidney vessels are shown and the pyelographic phase can be recorded. *(2)* Application of prophylactic preoperative splinting is not recommended in case of a large aneurysm, previously injured kidney, and single kidney. *(3)* Intraoperatively the ureter should lie ventral to the prosthesis. *(4)* Three and 12 months postoperatively an infusion urogram should be taken in case corresponding symptoms did not make it necessary earlier. *(5)* For compression of the ureter between vessel and prosthesis, the resection of the prosthesis and reanastomosis should take place behind the ureter. *(6)* More and more conservative treatment with ureteral splints is indicated. *(7)* Also, obstruction through the retroperitoneal fibrosis should first be treated with splints and possibly also with cortisone.

Regular follow-up examinations are absolutely necessary in order to recognize and treat postoperative lesions. The authors observed no obstruction of the ureter between the vessel and the prosthesis. In these cases, resection of the prosthesis and reanastomosis dorsal to the ureter is recommended.

▶ The importance of ureteral obstruction after aortofemoral or aortoiliac surgery is stressed by these two abstracts. In the remote past, such hydronephrosis was thought to be associated with aortic graft infection. But clearly that cause has been superceded by perigraft fibrosis and ureteral entrapment. One would like to know the nature of grafts that cause this; e.g., is perigraft fibrosis more frequent after external velour grafting? Or, is the external velour a protective element?

Detection of Abdominal Aortic Graft Infection: Comparison of CT and Indium-Labeled White Blood Cell Scans

Alexander S. Mark, Shirley M. McCarthy, Albert A. Moss, and David Price
(Univ. of California at San Francisco)

AJR 144:315–318, February 1985 7–83

The clinical diagnosis of aortic graft infection may be difficult. Both computed tomography (CT) and scanning with indium-labeled white blood cells have been reported to be helpful in identifying and assessing aortic graft infection. Eight patients clinically suspected of having aortic graft infection because of groin infection, sepsis, or both, underwent both these studies. Computed tomography was performed in conjunction with intravenous, oral, and rectal contrast administration. Scanning was done with autologous leukocytes labeled with ^{111}In complexed to oxine (8-hydroxyquinoline) sulfate. Both whole body scans and spot scintigrams of the anterior part of the abdomen and pelvis were obtained.

Five patients had surgically proved aortic graft infection extending into the retroperitoneum. Three of these had groin infections, and 2 had sepsis only. Computed tomography correctly diagnosed aortic graft infection in all 5 by showing a perigraft fluid collection, gas in the graft bed, or both. Extension of infection into the retroperitoneum was diagnosed correctly in the 3 patients with groin infection. The indium-labeled white blood cell study showed increased groin uptake in the patients with groin infection, but extension to the retroperitoneum in only 1. A repeat scan study in a patient given antibiotic therapy appeared normal. Both CT and the indium-labeled white blood cell study showed normal grafts in the 3 patients without graft infection.

Computed tomography is best able to demonstrate the precise extent of aortic graft infection through its ability to show perigraft fluid and air. Scintigraphy with indium-labeled white blood cells is less effective in demonstrating retroperitoneal extension of groin infections. This study may be misleading in patients receiving antibiotics. Computed tomography is the preferred initial imaging procedure if aortic graft infection is clinically suspected.

▶ Computed tomography is emerging as the best diagnostic method in suspected aortic graft infection.

Delayed Aortic Prosthetic Reconstruction After Removal of an Infected Graft

Linda M. Reilly, William K. Ehrenfeld, and Ronald J. Stoney (Univ. of California, San Francisco)

Am. J. Surg. 148:234–239, August 1984 7–84

Despite successful treatment of aortofemoral graft infection using extra-anatomical bypass, there is significant associated morbidity often secondary to the long-term inadequacies of the revascularization methods required to avoid infected tissue beds. Failure of extra-anatomical bypass results in multiple operations and amputation may be necessary. The incidence of multiple operations and the rate of extremity loss potentially could be reduced by delayed aortic prosthetic reconstruction, but there is concern about the risk of new prosthesis reinfection and the hazards of "redo" aortic reconstruction. The authors report the results of delayed aortic reconstruction using either an in-line aortic graft or supraceliac aortofemoral bypass performed at a mean interval of 14.5 months (range, 2 to 35 months) after removal of an infected graft in 7 patients. The procedure was performed for recurrent axillofemoral graft thrombosis in 4 patients, recurrent axillofemoral graft infection in 1 patient, progressive claudication in 1 patient, and persistent severe symptoms of leg ischemia in 1 patient.

Delayed aortic prosthetic reconstruction was performed successfully with no perioperative deaths in all 7 patients, and 6 of the 7 patients were well at a mean follow-up of 57 months (range, 1 month to 8 years). All grafts have remained patent, and no patient has required amputation for complications associated with the graft. One patient who had advanced tissue necrosis before reconstruction required amputation immediately after operation. No reimplanted graft became infected which suggested that a reimplantation interval of 6 to 12 months may be safe.

The results indicate that delayed aortic prosthetic reconstruction may be regarded as a safe and effective treatment option for patients who develop extremity-threatening recurrent ischemia or recurrent extra-anatomical graft infection after treatment of aortic vascular graft infection.

Descending Thoracic Aortobifemoral Bypass for Occluded Abdominal Aorta: Retroperitoneal Route Without an Abdominal Incision

D. E. Bowes, B. A. Keagy, C. H. Benoit, and W. F. Pharr (Danville, Pa.)

J. Cardiovasc. Surg. 26:41–45, Jan.–Feb. 1985 7–85

The need for distal bypass is complicated by the presence of infrarenal aortic occlusion, an occluded aortic bifurcation graft, and suprarenal aortic atherosclerosis. The technique of descending thoraco-aortofemoral bypass has been modified by drawing a bifurcated graft through a posterior retroperitoneal tunnel from the left lower part of the chest to the left side of the groin, avoiding an abdominal incision (Fig 7–19). A suprapubic preperitoneal tunnel is made posterior to the rectus muscle for passage of the right limb of the bifurcation graft to the right femoral artery. The graft is brought through either a retroperitoneal tunnel (Fig 7–20) or the abdominal wall muscles (Fig 7–21). The graft limbs also can be coursed retroperito-

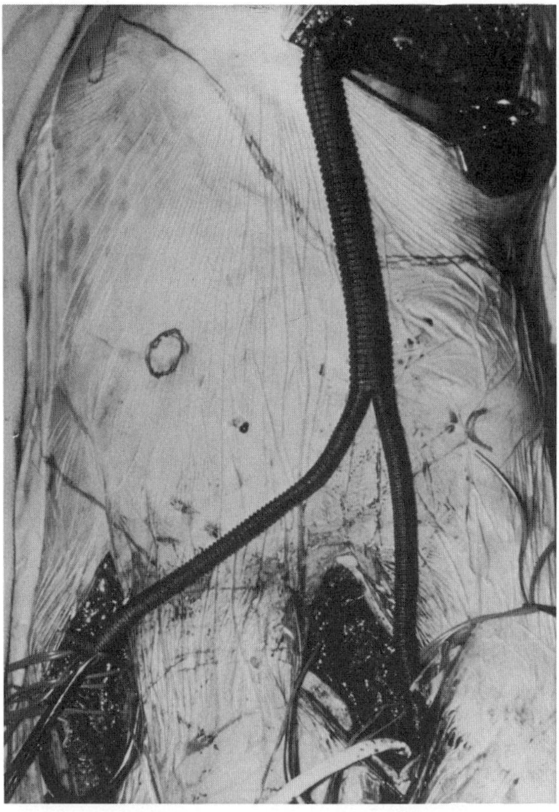

Fig 7–19.—Position of patient on operating table with left anterolateral thoracotomy incision, vertical incisions in both sides of the groin, and the preclotted standard 40-cm Dacron aortic bifurcation graft held over the course it will take. The sites of the umbilicus, subcostal margins, and inguinal ligaments have been marked with a skin pencil. (Courtesy of Bowes, D.E., et al.: J. Cardiovasc. Surg. 26:41–45, Jan.–Feb. 1985.)

neally to the external iliac arteries if acceptable for distal anastomosis.

Of 142 bifurcation grafts inserted for aortoiliac occlusive disease over a 6-year period, 12 patients underwent this procedure. Six patients had occluded aortic bifurcation grafts, 4 had juxtarenal aortic occlusion, and 2 had had multiple laparotomies. Ten patients recovered without complications, and satisfactory blood flow continued during a follow-up period lasting for 1–6 years. One early postoperative death resulted from cardiac arrhythmia in a patient with a thrombosed left main coronary artery. Another patient died of renal failure, pulmonary edema, and ischemic colitis 3 months after operation.

This operation is relatively easy technically and can be performed rapidly. The retroperitoneal tunnel approach is a useful alternative when reoperating on a patient with an occluded bifurcation graft or juxtarenal aortic disease. Patients with coronary risk factors now are screened preoperatively by dipyridamole myocardial scanning and cine coronary arteriography.

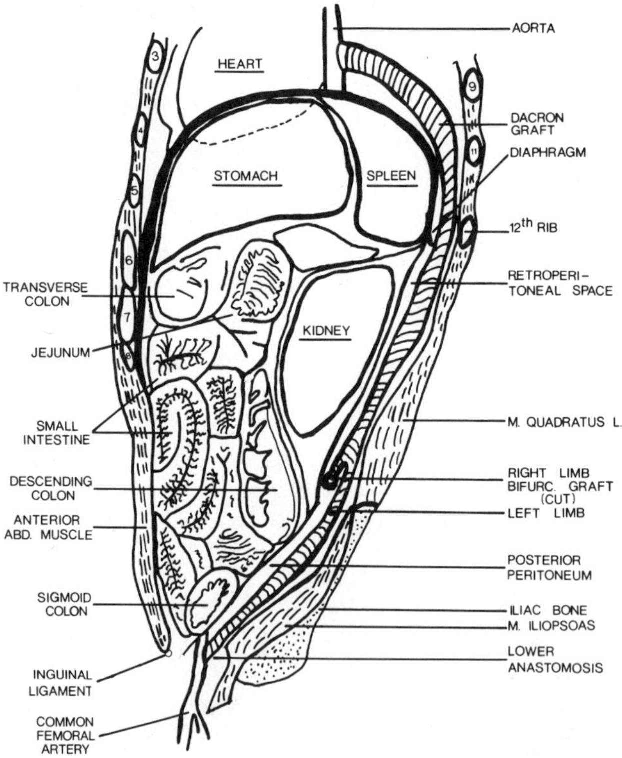

Fig 7–20.—Left half of the abdomen, sagittal view, showing Dacron graft anastomosed to the thoracic aorta at the level of the dome of the diaphragm opposite the 9th vertebra and entering the retroperitoneal space at the 12th rib. The graft passes anterior to the quadratus lumborum muscle posterior to the spleen, left kidney, and descending colon and emerges in the groin under the inguinal ligament on the anterior surface of the ileopsoas muscle. (Courtesy of Bowes, D.E., et al.: J. Cardiovasc. Surg. 26:41–45, Jan.–Feb. 1985.)

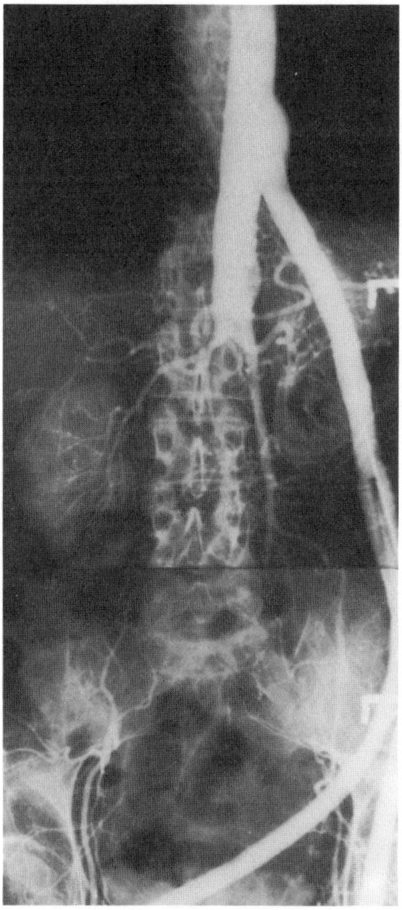

Fig 7–21.—Postoperative aortogram illustrating the second alternate retroperitoneal route for the descending thoracic aortobifemoral bypass: the graft passes more laterally and exits through the abdominal muscle near the left anterosuperior iliac spinous process. The limbs of the graft course through subcutaneous tunnels, crossing the inguinal ligaments to reach each femoral artery. (Courtesy of Bowes, D.E.: J. Cardiovasc. Surg. 26:41–45, Jan.–Feb. 1985.)

▶ The preceding two articles call attention to the fact that treatment of aortic graft infection must be a three-stage procedure; that is, removal of the infected graft, temporary revascularization (usually by an extra-anatomical route), and, finally, intracavitary reconstruction of the aorta. The two methods cited are complementary rather than competitive and should be in the armamentarium of every practicing surgeon.

Femorodistal Ischemia

Pain-Free Physical Training in Intermittent Claudication

Christine E. Boyd, Patrick J. Bird, Charles D. Teates, Harry A. Wellons, Mary Ann MacDougall, and Larry A. Wolfe (Univ. of Virginia)

J. Sports Med. 24:112–122, June 1984 7–86

Physical training is a promising noninvasive approach to claudication resulting from peripheral vascular disease. The possible therapeutic value of training by low-level endurance exercise was examined in 8 patients (6 males) with a history of vascular intermittent claudication and a mean age of 58 years. Four were diabetics and 4 smoked. Endurance exercise on a treadmill, running track, bicycle ergometer, or some combination was individually prescribed for three 25- to 40-minute sessions weekly over 12 weeks. Training intensity was set just below the threshold of pain. Muscle blood flow was estimated by the radioxenon method.

All exercise test variables increased significantly during the 12-week training period, whether estimated at the onset of pain or at the end of testing. Walking distance to onset of pain increased 138% and exercise time by 103%. Energy expenditure to the onset of pain increased 160%. Pulse volume amplitude in the lower extremities increased significantly after training. Muscle blood flow rose significantly when a subject who did not attend regularly was excluded. Body weight did not change significantly, but percent fat decreased 10% with training. Resting blood pressure and heart rate were not significantly changed after training, and exercise hemodynamics were also unchanged.

Claudication stress responses were significantly improved after individually prescribed endurance exercise training, done at a pain-free level, in these patients with vascular claudication. The exact mechanism responsible is unknown, but direct tissue analysis might be of interest. Both diabetic and nondiabetic patients responded.

▶ There has been a great deal of emphasis upon exercise training in vascular clinics in Europe but too little in rehabilitation clinics in this country. There is no doubt that a supervised exercise program produces better increases in walking distance than any of the available vasoactive drugs.

Foot Angiography in Diabetic Patients With Gangrene

Sven-Ola Hietala and Folke Lithner (Univ. Hosp. of Umeå, Sweden)

Acta Med. Scand. (Suppl.) 687:61–67, 1984 7–87

Previously, angiography of the foot was limited because it was a relatively painful procedure compared with other forms of angiography. However, the advent of less toxic and nonionic contrast material of low osmolality has allowed virtually painless and motionless angiography. A nonionic contrast medium (Amipaque) was used in 9 diabetic patients with soft tissue and skeletal lesions of the foot to categorize these lesions as ischemic or nonischemic.

No patient experienced pain on injection of contrast material, and only 2 noted a slight sensation of warmth. The digital arteries were well filled with contrast material, allowing a detailed study of the pedal arterial system both in dorsoplantar and lateral projections (Fig 7–22). Magnification and subtraction techniques allowed enhanced visualization of details and a more precise determination of the relationships between arterial lesions and osseous and gangrenous complications of diabetes.

It has been stated that osseous resorption occurs only in the presence of an adequate blood supply. Thus it appeared that 5 of the patients had resorptive skeletal changes and could be considered as having nonischemic

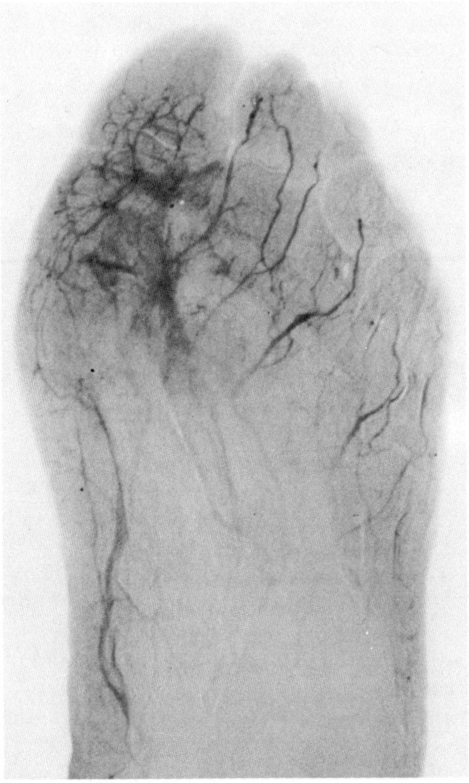

Fig 7–22.—Gangrene is seen on dorsum of left foot. Magnification angiography of foot in frontal projections shows insufficient filling of digital arteries (digits 2–5) but slightly increased vascularity to dorsomedial aspect of foot and first toe. [Courtesy of Hietala, S.-O., and Lithner, F.: Acta Med. Scand. (Suppl.) 687:61–67, 1984.]

disease, whereas 4 had no skeletal lesions and would have been categorized as having ischemic disease. Various degrees of occlusive disease were observed in the digital arteries in all patients. In most instances the venous phase was opacified, usually late in the series, indicating a slow flow rate. There was considerable variation in the collateral circulation. Two hyperemic patients exhibited a rich capillary network and increased accumulation of contrast medium at the site of osseous destructions. Correlation of the angiographic findings with the clinical course in 1 patient categorized as nonischemic indicated the need for a major amputation.

Although no definite conclusions can be drawn from the angiographic findings with regard to soft tissue and skeletal lesions in the diabetic foot because of the limited number of patients in this series, the study demonstrates that a high-quality foot angiogram can be obtained by using nonionic contrast medium and magnification and subtraction techniques.

▶ This study and careful observations obtained in the operating room after bypass grafting indicate that diabetic patients have no different pattern of arterial occlusions than nondiabetic patients. Certainly the concept of gangrene due to distal arterial occlusive disease without proximal obstruction is untenable.

Adaptation of Canine Saphenous Veins to Grafting: Correlation of Contractility and Contractile Protein Content

Charles L. Seidel, Robert M. Lewis, Rebecca Bowers, Richard D. Bukoski, Han-Seob Kim, Julius C. Allen, and Craig Hartley (Houston)

Circ. Res. 55:102–109, July 1984 7–88

Saphenous veins are widely used to replace stenotic coronary arteries. However, the contractile and biochemical functions of grafted veins are unknown. Canine saphenous veins were removed and then returned to their original location (venous autograft) or were used to replace a femoral segment (arterial graft) to characterize the contractile properties of grafted veins. This was to determine whether observed changes in contractile characteristics are associated with quantitative changes in actin, myosin, and collagen, and to determine which of the observed contractile or biochemical changes resulted from surgical procedure and which resulted from placement in the arterial circulation. Graft patency was assessed at 1, 4, or 8 weeks after grafting. Patent grafts (36 of 40) were then removed and compared with the contralateral saphenous vein.

Both venous autografts and arterial grafts had increased contractile sensitivity to norepinephrine but not to potassium chloride. The venous autograft showed a reversible reduction in myosin content and in the maximum contractile response (force/cross-sectional area) to potassium chloride and norepinephrine. At no time did the venous autografts show a significant change in circumference or wall cross-sectional area. In contast, the arterial grafts had a significantly increased circumference and wall cross-sectional area and a significantly increased wall thickness. The total protein content of venous autografts was unchanged, whereas the protein content per unit length in arterial grafts was significantly increased and correlated with graft duration. Unlike venous autografts, arterial grafts showed a significant reduction in maximum contractile response despite increased net production of actin and myosin. Normalization of maximum force to cross-sectional area or heavy-chain myosin content did not return maximum contractile response values to normal.

The results suggest that, except for elevated sensitivity to norepinephrine, the saphenous vein is able to recover from the effects of surgery within 8 weeks. However, when the vein is placed in the arterial circulation, recovery is delayed and a hypertrophic response is begun, which includes diminished contractile function. This attenuation of contractile function may result from structural reorganization of contractile filaments and muscle cells within the vessel wall, as well as alterations in the chemomechanical transduction process.

Optimal Techniques for Harvesting and Preparation of Reversed Autogenous Vein Grafts for Use as Arterial Substitutes: A Review

O. T. Adcock, Jr., Gayle L. D. Adcock, Jock R. Wheeler, Roger T. Gregory, Stanley O. Snyder, Jr., and Robert G. Gayle (Eastern Virginia Med. School)
Surgery 96:886–894, November 1984 7–89

Despite being the preferred material for reconstruction, reversed autogenous vein is not an ideal arterial substitute. The most significant problem is the structural alterations in the implanted vein that predispose to graft failure. Most of these failures occur within the first few months after graft implantation and are thought to be due, in part, to endothelial damage incurred during harvesting and preparation of the reversed vein grafts. The authors have focused on the technical aspects of vein graft harvesting associated with alterations in endothelial morphology including dissection technique, types of irrigation and storage solutions used, temperature of these solutions, distention pressures, and pharmacologic agents.

An optimal technique for reversed vein graft harvesting and preparation includes *(1)* marking of the skin overlying the vein before operation with the patient standing, to facilitate identification of the tract of the vein in the operating suite; *(2)* infiltration of papaverine solution (0.12 mg/ml) subcutaneously along the tract of the vein before skin incision; *(3)* perivenous injection and adventitial irrigation with papaverine solution after exposure and at intervals during dissection of the vein to reduce smooth muscle spasm that causes endothelial "buckling" and sloughing that result in endothelial injury; *(4)* use of a precise, atraumatic dissection technique with minimal handling of tissue; *(5)* ligation of tributaries 2 to 3 mm from the vein wall; *(6)* irrigation and gradual distention of the graft with a solution of heparinized autologous whole blood containing papaverine, at body temperature, to a pressure of 100 mm Hg; *(7)* storage, while distended, in cold (4 C), heparinized, autologous blood containing papaverine; and *(8)* reimplantation by atraumatic technique.

The use of such techniques has resulted in decreased endothelial damage by morphological criteria. However, it is doubtful that reversed vein grafts prepared even with optimal techniques will have endothelial preservation superior to that with in situ grafts. These techniques should produce improved endothelial preservation and better long- and short-term patency rates when compared with techniques in widespread use at present.

Relationship Between Vasa Vasorum and Blood Flow to Vein Bypass Endothelial Morphology

John D. Corson, Robert P. Leather, Alex Balko, Vijay Naraynsingh, Allastair M. Karmody, and Dhiraj M. Shah (Albany, N.Y., VA Med. Center)
Arch. Surg. 120:386–388, March 1985 7–90

The method used for vein preparation before arterial bypass grafting is relevant to its future performance, especially when small veins are utilized. A canine model was used to assess the role of the vasa vasorum in preserving venous endothelial integrity. In 8 dogs part of an exposed length of external jugular vein was freed from all vasa vasorum by sharp dissection, and both ends of the vein were clamped 1 hour before fluorescein was injected into the ipsilateral forelimb vein. Fourteen in situ external jugular vein-to-carotid artery bypasses were created in 7 dogs. After arterialization of the bypasses, the vasa vasorum along the complete length of one vein were interrupted by sharp dissection. The bypasses were sampled at intervals up to 3 weeks after implantation.

The in vivo studies showed that, even in the absence of intraluminal blood flow, the vasa vasorum maintained endothelial integrity. The endothelium was quite sensitive to loss of the vasa vasorum, which was associated with the presence of fibrin and platelet aggregates on the largely denuded endothelial layer. In the vein bypass study, arterialization of the vein maintained endothelial integrity despite division of the vasa vasorum.

Blood flow through the vasa vasorum can supply nutrients to the entire vein wall, including the endothelium. Continuous arterial flow is important in vein bypasses. When an in situ vein is used as a bypass conduit, the vasa vasorum supply to the vein should be preserved and arterial flow established as rapidly as possible to avoid ischemic injury to the vein wall and to preserve the endothelium. Ideally the vein should be arterialized before being mobilized, and side branches with arteriovenous fistulas should be left intact. The lower distal part of the vein is most at risk of ischemic injury and should be dissected en bloc with its surrounding fat and accompanying vasa vasorum; loupe magnification is helpful.

▶ Studies such as these show damage to the veins caused by the harvesting technique. Perhaps such studies will raise the cumulative patency rate from its present level of 80%–85% at 1 year to a much more acceptable level. There is no question but that the first 90 days after bypass grafting is the critical time for any distal reconstructive arterial procedure. Corson et al. show that the vasa vasorum maintained endothelian integrity and that the endothelium is quite sensitive to loss of the vasa. All of this may affect 90-day patency.

The Relation of Risk Factors to the Development of Atherosclerosis in Saphenous-Vein Bypass Grafts and the Progression of Disease in the Native Circulation: A Study 10 Years After Aortocoronary Bypass Surgery

Lucien Campeau, Marc Enjalbert, Jacques Lespérance, Martial G. Bourassa, Peter Kwiterovich, Jr., Sholom Wacholder, and Allan Sniderman (McGill Univ., Montreal)

N. Engl. J. Med. 311:1329–1332, Nov. 22, 1984 7–91

Little is known about the long-term effects of aortocoronary bypass surgery on graft-patency rates and progression of atherosclerosis. The authors examined 82 patients 10 years after aortocoronary saphenous-vein bypass surgery in an attempt to relate the development of atherosclerosis in the grafts and progression of disease in the native circulation to the major risk factors for coronary artery disease. All patients underwent sequential coronary angiographic examinations. Blood pressure, fasting blood sugar level, cigarette smoking, and plasma lipids were assessed.

Of 132 grafts that were patent 1 year after surgery, only 50 (37.5%)

were unchanged at 10 years; 43 (33%) showed atherosclerotic lesions, and 39 (29.5%) were completely occluded. Among 85 arteries without grafts, 25 of 53 coronary arteries with previous stenosis showed disease progression whereas 15 of 32 arteries that were previously normal showed new obstruction. Atherosclerotic lesions did not develop in 15 patients, whereas in 67 patients they developed in the grafts, native circulation, or both. There was no significant difference between the 2 groups in the incidence of hypertension, diabetes, age, or smoking. Univariate analysis showed that very low-density lipoproteins and low-density lipoproteins (LDLs) were higher and high-density lipoproteins (HDL) were lower in those with new lesions than in those without. Both plasma cholesterol and triglyceride levels were significantly higher at time of surgery and at the 10-year examination in those with new lesions. Multivariate analysis showed that among the lipoprotein indexes, levels of HDL cholesterol and plasma LDL apoprotein B best distinguished the 2 groups. Seventy-nine percent of patients without new lesions had normal lipoprotein phenotypes, whereas 92% of patients with new lesions had abnormal phenotypes.

The data show that atherosclerosis in grafts and progression of coronary artery disease in the native circulation are both very common 10 years after aortocoronary bypass surgery and that the course of such disease may be related to the plasma lipoprotein levels. Plasma levels of LDL apoprotein B and HDL cholesterol are the principal factors that predict the presence or absence of atherosclerosis; this may be a clue to prevention of coronary artery disease.

Atherosclerosis in Vascular Grafts for Peripheral Vascular Disease: Autogenous Vein Grafts

K. W. Walton, G. Slaney, and F. Ashton (Univ. of Birmingham)
Atherosclerosis 54:49–64, January 1985 7–92

Patients with peripheral arterial disease warranting vascular bypass are susceptible to atherosclerosis in general, but it remains uncertain whether true atheromatosis develops in autologous vein grafts and, if it does, whether it contributes to late graft failures. Twenty-nine lower extremity vein grafts in place from a few days to more than 12 years were examined by conventional and immunohistologic techniques. The patients were 23 men and 3 women aged 39–73 years. Control samples of contralateral "normal" saphenous vein were taken from 2 patients with unilateral vein grafts and from 8 age-matched subjects without significant peripheral arterial disease. In a majority of study patients the grafts were replaced because of impaired patency.

Changes seen within 3 months of graft placement included increased thickness of the graft wall, mostly due to marked intimal proliferation. Superficial fibrinous deposits were seen at this stage and in grafts present for 5–18 months. The latter were removed for thrombotic occlusion and showed little or no evidence of lipid infiltration of the occluded segment.

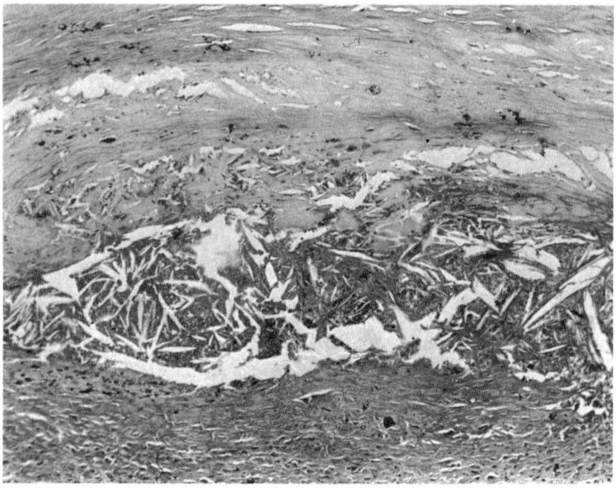

Fig 7–23.—Section from cold-ethanol-fixed vein graft removed after 11 years in position with "atheroma-like" pool in depth of graft. This contains "cholesterol clefts" and is surrounded by dense fibrosis. Alcianophilic material (blue-green) seen in original in and around lipid pool. Corresponding frozen section from adjacent block of tissue showed anisotropic crystals (cholesterol ester) in midst of lipid in this "atheroma." Alcian blue-chlorantine fast red; original magnification ×125. (Courtesy of Walton, K.W., et al.: Atherosclerosis 54:49–64, January 1985.)

Lipid deposit was seen in grafts of longer duration, especially in those in place for 4–12 years and those from patients who had marked hyperlipidemia and other risk factors for atherosclerosis. Extracellular lipid corresponded with the distribution of specific fluorescence for apolipoprotein B-containing lipoproteins (Fig 7–23). Fibrinogen-related antigens were also deposited in thickened grafts. Some graft complications were stenosis or occlusion, ulceration, calcification, and aneurysm formation. Some grafts removed after 5 years had plaquelike areas of fibrosis on the intimal surface, strongly resembling organized thrombi.

A process indistinguishable from "true" atherosclerosis appears to take place in vein grafts present for some time in the lower extremities of patients with peripheral arterial disease. Changes were consistently found in grafts in place for 2 years or longer. The lesions appeared to have arisen as largely extracellular deposits of fibrinogen-related antigens and apolipoprotein B-containing lipoproteins in areas of active mesenchymal proliferation. Lipid deposit also occurred on the surface of collagen fibers in organizing thrombi in grafts present for a longer time.

Venous Grafting in Femoropopliteal Obstructions: A 16-Year Experience

Piergiorgio Settembrini, Piero Zannini, Massimo Pisacreta, Rocco Antonio Maruotti, and Giuseppe Pezzuoli (Univ. of Milan)

Int. Surg. 69:271–275, July–Sept. 1984 7–93

A total of 172 femoropopliteal saphenous vein bypass procedures were done in 151 patients seen in a 15-year period with chronic obstructive

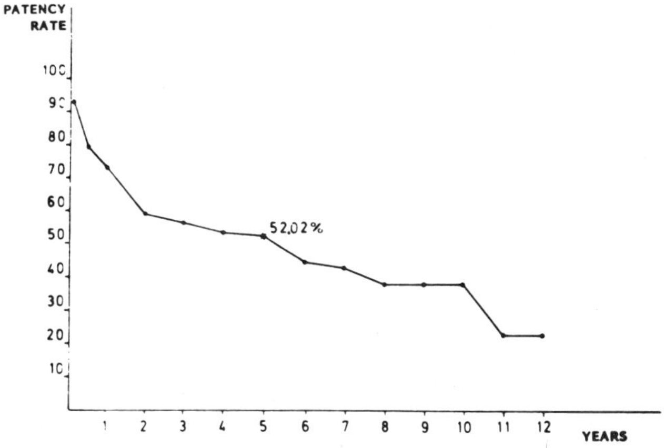

Fig 7–24.—Patency curve. After 10 years, curve becomes less reliable due to small number of bypasses at risk. (Courtesy of Settembrini, P., et al.: Int. Surg. 69:271–275, July–Aug. 1984.)

arterial disease. The 141 men and 10 women had a mean age of 62 years. Eighty-one patients had rest pain, trophic lesions, or both at the time of operation. The distal anastomosis was above the knee in 57 patients and below the knee in 115. Nine patients were lost to follow-up which extended for 6 months to 12 years.

Operative mortality was 1.3%; both deaths were due to heart failure. Later mortality was similar to that in the general population of the same age. Early rupture of the vein occurred in 2 patients. Five femoral false aneurysms developed. Patency rates over time are shown in Figure 7–24. Seventy-eight bypasses were occluded, 12 in the immediate postoperative period and 32 in the first year of follow-up. Major amputations were necessary in 23 patients, most within 1 year of operation.

Good results were obtained by femoropopliteal saphenous vein bypass grafting in this series, even in a majority of patients with trophic lesions or rest pain. Direct arterial reconstruction is the only effective approach if a limb will otherwise have to be amputated. Survival is not improved, but the operation improves the quality of life. Autogenous vein grafts are the most reliable and the most suitable for delicate anastomoses.

▶ The preceding three abstracts show, once again, that atherosclerosis occurs in saphenous vein bypass grafts and that such atherosclerotic lesions are partly related to operative trauma and partly due to lipoprotein abnormalities intrinsic to the patient population.

Inhibition of Platelet Deposition on Polytetrafluoroethylene Grafts by Antiplatelet Agents

Neal D. Kon, Kimberley J. Hansen, Matt B. Martin, J. Wayne Meredith, Jesse H. Meredith, and A. Robert Cordell

Surgery 96:870–873, November 1984 7–94

The poor patency rates of polytetrafluoroethylene (PTFE) grafts for femoral artery replacement have been caused by the formation of neointimal fibrous hyperplasia that results from excessive proliferation of subendothelial smooth muscle cells in response to mitogenic factors released by platelets. Agents that inhibit platelet aggregation have been known to retard this process.

The effects of ibuprofen, dipyridamole, and prostacyclin on the deposition of platelets on PTFE grafts were studied on 21 mongrel dogs. Autologous platelets labeled with ^{51}CR were reinjected into the dogs 15 minutes before crossclamping. Four dogs (8 grafts) received ibuprofen (12.5 mg/kg), and 5 dogs (10 grafts) received dipyridamole (2.5 mg/kg), each given by a single intravenous injection. Five dogs (10 grafts) received prostacyclin (50 ng kg^{-1} $minute^{-1}$ by continuous intravenous infusion; 7 dogs (14 grafts) that served as controls received saline as a single intravenous injection. A 5.5-cm PTFE graft with an internal diameter of 4 mm was anastomosed to the femoral arteries. Arterial flow was maintained at 65 ml/minute and monitored continuously. Grafts were removed 2 hours after implantation, and radioactivity was determined in 4 segments of each graft (proximal, midproximal, middistal, and distal with inclusion of both anastomoses) with a γ-counter.

Platelet deposition in control dogs averaged 10,033.9/10 minutes. The decrease from control values was fourfold in the prostacyclin-treated dogs, averaging 2,513.7/10 minutes, and twofold in the ibuprofen-treated dogs, averaging 5,453.4/10 minutes. No significant difference was noted in the group treated with dipyridamole (average, 11,213.7/10 minutes). In all 4 groups a greater concentration of platelets appeared on the anastomotic segments than on the middle portions of the PTFE grafts.

The study indicates that deposition of platelets on PTFE grafts is inhibited to a greater extent by prostacyclin than by ibuprofen and not at all by dipyridamole. Prostacyclin is an endogenous substance secreted by the vascular endothelial cell, and it prevents aggregation of platelets and promotes platelet deaggregation. Its use is limited by its instability at biologic pH and its intravenous route of administration. Ibuprofen is a nonsteroidal anti-inflammatory agent that acts as a reversible inhibitor of cyclooxygenase and promotes endogenous production of prostacyclin; it can be administered both orally and intravenously. This study also shows the advantage of using direct measurement of platelet deposition which allows rapid evaluation of different drug effects on graft patency as opposed to more time-consuming studies.

Platelet Function is Altered by Autogenous Vein Grafts in the Early Postoperative Months

Anthony H. Gershlick, Y. Denise Syndercombe Court, Andrew J. Murday, Terence Lewis, and Peter G. Mills (London)

Cardiovasc. Res. 18:119–125, February 1984 7–95

Indirect evidence implicates platelets in the intimal hyperplasia observed after autogenous vein graft placement. In vitro demonstration of a platelet-derived growth factor supports a role for platelets in the development of smooth muscle cell hyperplasia. A new model was developed in the lop-eared rabbit to examine the effects of autogenous vein graft on platelet function. The reversed external jugular vein was grafted to the ipsilateral carotid artery, and the platelet activation index (PAI), reflecting platelet responsiveness to adenosine diphosphate, was estimated at varying postoperative intervals.

No significant changes in the PAI were associated with anesthesia or surgical exposure in control studies. Platelet activation increased significantly 1 week after grafting, and the effect persisted at 1 and 2 months. After 4 months the PAI was not significantly different from preoperative values. A significant increase in PAI was observed in distal carotid artery samples 1 week and 1 month postoperatively when both proximal and distal samples were obtained.

Platelets activated by an autogenous vein graft may be involved in the occurrence of intimal hyperplasia in the graft wall, but platelet modification by drug treatment may be necessary only in the early months after graft placement. Further work is needed to detect any platelet deposition associated with the activation. This model should be useful in assessing the effects of antiplatelet drugs on the development of intimal hyperplasia in autogenous vein grafts.

Effect of Ticlopidine on Saphenous Vein Bypass Patency Rates: A Double-Blind Study

M. Chevigné, J.-L. David, P. Rigo, and R. Limet (Univ. of Liege, Belgium)

Ann. Thorac. Surg. 37:371–378, May 1984 7–96

In a 3-month-long, double-blind study, 75 patients undergoing aortocoronary bypass graft procedures received ticlopidine, 250 mg twice daily, and 75 were given placebo. Graft patency was assessed by repeat angiography in 38 patients and by resting and stress myocardial scintigraphy in 93; combined angiography and scintigraphy was used in 36.

Compared with placebo, ticlopidine significantly increased bleeding times ($P < .001$) and significantly diminished platelet aggregation ($P < .001$). Excluding 7 patients with discordant biologic results and poor compliance, the rate of graft occlusion was significantly lower in those who responded to ticlopidine than in those given placebo (7.1% and 21.8%, respectively; $P < .02$). However, several months after discontinuation of therapy the rate of occlusion was similar in both groups. Blood flow in the occluded graft appeared lower in patients receiving ticlopidine than in the placebo group. The overall graft attrition rate was 10.1% in patients treated with ticlopidine compared with 20.3% in the placebo group ($P < .1$). Graft permeability was more frequent among patients responding to ticlopidine ($P < .05$); however, no differences were observed between groups after discontinuation of therapy. Hematologic side effects were minor; patients receiving ticlopidine had a slightly elevated platelet count on day 10 and a slight reduction in the leukocyte count on day 45.

Ticlopidine appears to be an effective drug for protecting graft patency, provided that its biologic effects are present. Because its protective effect disappears when the drug is discontinued, it would seem advisable to prescribe ticlopidine for at least 1 year after operation.

Activation of Platelets by Autogenous Vein Grafts Is Not Prevented by Acetylsalicylic Acid and Dipyridamole

Anthony H. Gershlick, Y. Denise Syndercombe-Court, Andrew J. Murday, C. Terence Lewis, and Peter G. Mills (London Hosp.)

Cardiovasc. Res. 18:391–396, July 1984 7–97

Previous reports have shown that experimental autogenous vein grafts activate platelets for up to 4 months after operation. The effect of acetylsalicylic acid (ASA) in combination with dipyridamole on the activation of platelets was studied in a rabbit vein graft model consisting of reversed external jugular vein grafted into the ipsilateral carotid artery. Dipyridamole was started 48 hours before operation and ASA was started the morning after operation.

In the first part of the study 13 animals were followed up to 8 months and were treated with a middle dose of ASA, 10 mg kg^{-1} 24 $hours^{-1}$, plus dipyridamole, 8 mg kg^{-1} 24 $hours^{-1}$. In the second part, animals were followed up for 1 month and received either a low dose of ASA, 0.5 mg kg^{-1} 24 $hours^{-1}$, plus dipyridamole, 8 mg kg^{-1} 24 $hours^{-1}$, (8 animals) or a high dose of ASA, 40 mg kg^{-1} 24 $hours^{-1}$, plus dipyridamole, 8 mg kg^{-1} 24 $hours^{-1}$, (10) or dipyridamole alone, 2 mg kg^{-1} 6 $hours^{-1}$, (7). Platelet activation was measured by aggregometry. The platelet activation index (PAI), which is the slope of the linear portion of the dose response curve, was used to quantitate platelet aggregation in response to adenosine diphosphate.

Platelets were activated by the vein graft for up to 4 months after operation despite treatment with a middle dose of ASA plus dipyridamole. However, after this time, the PAI was not significantly different from the preoperative value. Similarly, treatment with low or high doses of ASA plus dipyridamole or dipyridamole alone did not prevent the vein graft-induced activation of platelets. Full inhibition of arachidonic acid metabolism was demonstrated in the group that received high doses of ASA plus dipyridamole.

The results suggest that the interaction between the vessel wall and platelets is not inhibited by ASA plus dipyridamole and that factors other than arachidonic acid metabolites are involved. Other reports have suggested that the initial adhesion, spread, and aggregation of platelets in the presence of high doses of collagen and thrombin is not dependent on arachidonic acid metabolism. Deendothelialization of vein grafts that occurs in the early postoperative period will expose high concentrations of collagen and cause local generation of thrombin. Despite the presence of an "effective" inhibitory dose of ASA, platelet activation by vein grafts is probably the result of exposure of subendothelial collagen. Platelet-derived growth factor may also be released in the presence of ASA.

It is concluded that the combination of ASA and dipyridamole is unlikely to prevent the development of intimal hyperplasia in the graft wall that results from activation of platelets. However, this combination of drugs may be useful in preventing early occlusion of coronary artery bypass grafts caused by formation of thrombus in the first 3 months after operation. This effect likely results from the inhibition of platelet aggregates (through the effect on the arachidonic acid pathway) which prevents the formation of thrombus.

▶ These abstracts teach that activation of platelets is produced by both polytetrafluoroethylene (PTFE) grafts and autogenous vein grafts during the early postoperative period. They do not present convincing evidence that pseudointimal hyperplasia is produced by such platelet activation and, in fact, two of these abstracts conclude that aspirin and dipyridamole do not improve the overall patency of vein or PTFE bypass grafts. In light of these conclusions, it is difficult to accept the findings of the ticlopidine study. Clearly, not all of the answers are in on this subject and, in fact, the causes of subintimal fibrous hyperplasia must be elucidated in the future.

Effect of Aspirin and Dipyridamole on the Patency of Lower Extremity Bypass Grafts

T. R. Kohler, J. L. Kaufman, G. Kacoyanis, A. Clowes, M. C. Donaldson, E. Kelly, J. Skillman, N. P. Couch, A. D. Whittemore, J. A. Mannick, and E. W. Salzman (Boston)

Surgery 96:462–466, September 1984 7–98

Recent clinical studies have shown that aspirin and dipyridamole improve graft patency rates in patients with infrainguinal polytetrafluoroethylene (PTFE) grafts and aortocoronary grafts. The authors undertook a prospective, double-blind study to determine whether these drugs administered postoperatively to patients with PTFE or vein infrainguinal bypass grafts would improve graft patency during the first 24-month period. One hundred patients received either 325 mg of aspirin and 75 mg of dipyridamole or placebo tablets 3 times a day, orally, beginning on the first postoperative day. Graft patency was assessed at intervals by review of symptoms, palpation of the graft, measurement of Doppler ankle-arm pressure ratios, and, if indicated, angiography, for 24 months. Patency rates were compared by computing standard life tables and comparing cumulative patency rates.

One hundred two grafts in the 100 patients were included in the study. A cumulative patency rate of 62% at 24 months was not significantly different for the treatment (57%) vs. control (67%) group. Two-year cumulative patency rates were not significantly different between diabetics and nondiabetics, between distal and proximal popliteal anastomoses, and between vein grafts and PTFE grafts.

Fibrous intimal hyperplasia, the main cause of vascular graft failures between 3 and 24 months, begins with platelet deposit on sites of endothelial denudation at operation and progresses by proliferation of smooth muscle in response to mitogens released by platelets. Low-dosage aspirin retards this process by irreversibly acetylating platelet cyclo-oxygenase and blocking the production of thromboxane A_2. Higher dosages of aspirin may block the generation of prostacyclin, a potent inhibitor of platelet aggregation. The mechanism of the antiplatelet action of dipyridamole is not well understood. However, studies have shown that it enhances the platelet-inhibiting effect of circulating prostacyclin brought about by aspirin.

Aspirin and dipyridamole given postoperatively in the dosages used in this study do not improve the overall patency rates of vein or PTFE infrainguinal bypass grafts. The relatively high dosage of aspirin used in this study may have adversely affected graft patency by inhibiting vascular prostacyclin production. Further studies with low-dosage aspirin (0.45 mg/kg daily) are needed to clarify this issue.

▶ It is clear that the results of this study are at variance with conclusions derived from the coronary bypass study abstracted earlier in this volume.

Comparative Study of Leg Wound Skin Closure in Coronary Artery Bypass Graft Operations

G. D. Angelini, E. G. Butchart, S. H. Armistead, and I. M. Breckenridge (Cardiff, Wales)

Thorax 39:942–945, December 1984 7–99

Autogenous saphenous vein is most often used in coronary bypass grafting. Removal of the entire long saphenous vein for multiple grafts requires a long leg incision, and little attention has been given to management of this wound. A prospective study of four methods of skin closure was carried out in 113 patients undergoing coronary bypass grafting. The groups were comparable in age, sex, body weight, and length of the leg incision. A continuous nylon vertical mattress suture was used in 27 patients, a continuous subcuticular Dexon suture in 29, metal skin staples (Autosuture) in 27, and adhesive sutureless skin closure (Op-site) in 30. All incisions were closed by the same surgeon after protamine was given after cardiopulmonary bypass.

Wound discharge was least in those closed with subcuticular Dexon suture at day 5. Inflammation was less with both subcuticular Dexon and Op-site than with nylon mattress sutures or metal staples. Overall incidence of established wound infection was 4.5%. No infections occurred in the subcuticular Dexon group. The cosmetic results on day 45 were better in the subcuticular Dexon group than in the mattress suture and staple groups and as good as in the Op-site sutureless skin closure group. The Op-site method was the most rapid; the Dexon method took the most time.

Continuous subcuticular Dexon suture closure was the best means of managing the leg wound after saphenous vein removal for coronary bypass grafting in this study. The method can be recommended for general use in all cases. Cost and speed of insertion were not optimal, but these factors are relatively unimportant compared with the advantages of the method.

▶ Since saphenous vein is the graft material of choice, this study of skin closure will aid in decreasing morbidity of autogenous vein bypass grafting. This study has fortunately confirmed prejudices of our group, which has used the continuous subcuticular Dexon suture closure for all wounds for more than 10 years.

Intraoperative Assessment of In Situ Saphenous Vein Bypass Grafts With Continuous-Wave Doppler Probe

Timothy D. Spencer, Mitchell H. Goldman, John W. Hyslop, H. M. Lee, and Robert W. Barnes

Surgery 96:874–877, November 1984 7–100

Intraoperative evaluation of in situ saphenous vein bypass grafts by using angiography is less than perfect in identifying retained competent posterior valvular leaflets and arteriovenous fistulas. Twenty-five such grafts were evaluated during operation by using a 5 mHz bidirectional continuous-wave Doppler probe for localization of persistent competent valves and arteriovenous fistulas.

After the saphenous vein bypass was anastomosed, the Doppler evaluation was begun at the common femoral artery and continued over the entire length of the graft including the distal anastomosis and recipient artery. The probe was held to closely approximate a 60-degree angle with the artery or graft throughout the evaluation, particularly over the distal aspect of the graft as it traversed the superficial to deep tissue planes to join the recipient artery. If there was no evidence of a retained valve or fistula, the probe was placed over the proximal graft and the distal graft was occluded with finger pressure (no flow should be detected). Completion angiography was then performed.

When recordings of the intraoperative evaluation were studied, it was found that the Doppler was able to distinguish a retained valve from an arteriovenous fistula on clinical grounds but not by waveform analysis. The Doppler produced a high-pitched sound over the problem area, and when the probe was passed over the soft tissues on either side of the graft, the high-pitched signals were heard away from the graft when a fistula was present. A retained valve was suspected if, when the vein was circumferentially dissected by the probe, a fistula was not identified.

At least one arteriovenous fistula per case and 5 retained posterior valvular leaflets were identified with the Doppler before completion of angiography. The waveforms of both retained valves and arteriovenous fistulas showed an increase in peak systolic frequency as well as diastolic frequency. As the lesion became more hemodynamically significant, turbulent flow was evidenced by poor wave configuration.

Intraoperative assessment of in situ saphenous vein bypass grafts with the continuous-wave Doppler can identify retained valves that might be missed by angiography. It can reduce the number of angiograms needed to demonstrate a technically perfect graft, thus saving operative time and load of contrast agent.

The authors recommend this technique when an in situ saphenous vein bypass graft is performed. However, problems may occur when a high-flow distal arteriovenous fistula is present because the Doppler cannot be used to evaluate the graft proximal to the fistula until it is ligated. After ligation, the flow will be reduced so that less hemodynamically significant fistulas or valves are identified. Another problem, although rare, can occur when no arteriovenous fistula or retained valve is found at the area of high-pitched signal; exploration is usually performed and a preexisting stenosis, presumably caused by phlebitis, is usually found.

▶ The in situ technique is an important addition to the vascular surgery armamentarium, and this intraoperative assessment with continuous-wave Doppler is a way of simplifying the operation.

In Situ Vein Bypass to Distal Tibial and Limited Outflow Tracts for Limb Salvage

John D. Corson, Allastair M. Karmody, Dhiraj M. Shah, Vijay Naraynsingh, Howard L. Young, and Robert P. Leather

Surgery 96:756–763, October 1984 7–101

The in situ saphenous vein bypass has been utilized, with the valve incision technique, for long bypasses to vessels in the lower leg and foot and for bypasses to discontinuous tibial arteries. Of 492 complete in situ saphenous vein bypasses done in 1976–1983, 307 were carried to infrapopliteal vessels, and 96 of these bypasses in 92 patients had distal anastomoses to either a tibial artery that was discontinuous from the plantar arch, in 13 cases, or a vessel within 10 cm of the ankle joint or in the foot, in 83 instances. The average age of patients was 68 years. More than half the patients were diabetic, and nearly 80% of operations were done for gangrene or nonhealing ulcers. All bypasses were done by the valve incision technique.

Four of the 13 bypasses to discontinuous vessels have occluded. One diabetic patient required a below-knee amputation because of infection of a transmetatarsal amputation despite a functioning bypass. Eight of the bypasses with distal anastomoses in the ankle region or foot failed within the first month and 5 others subsequently. The cumulative patency rate at 3 years was 70%. Use of a vein less than 3.5 mm in diameter at the distal anastomosis did not prejudice the results. The patency rate at 3 years was similar to that for shorter tibial bypasses. Four limbs in the distal bypass group required major amputation after bypass failure. Several patients healed after transmetatarsal or digital amputations with a functioning bypass. The overall average follow-up has been 12.7 months.

The in situ vein bypass permits limb salvage using more distal bypasses with smaller veins in the lower extremity. The length of bypass itself does not influence the long-term patency rate. Discontinuous tibial vessels can be successfully used as an outflow tract for limb salvage. Use of the valve incision technique increases the operability rate where limb loss is threatened.

Revascularization of Popliteal and Below-Knee Arteries With Polytetrafluoroethylene

J. T. Christenson, A. Broomé, L. Norgren, and B. Eklöf

Surgery 97:141–149, February 1985 7–102

The expanded polytetrafluoroethylene (PTFE), or Goretex, graft is the most commonly used synthetic graft when an alternative to saphenous vein is needed. The authors used Goretex grafts 281 times in revascularizing popliteal and calf arteries between 1976 and 1980. The series included 153 above-knee and 74 below-knee femoropopliteal bypass grafts and 54 femorotibial-peroneal bypass grafts. Severe ischemia was the chief indication for reconstruction. Patients received dextran after operation, and 95% received antibiotics prophylactically. Minimum follow-up was 1 year after operation.

There were no operative deaths. Graft infection occurred in fewer than 5% of cases. Cumulative 6-year limb salvage rates in cases of severe ischemia were 87% and 59%, respectively, in the above-knee and below-knee femoropopliteal bypass groups and 57% in the femorotibial-peroneal bypass group. Graft patency rates were somewhat higher when operation was performed for disabling claudication than when severe ischemia was the indication in the above-knee femoropopliteal bypass group. Cumulative graft patency rates at 6 years were 43% in the below-knee femoropopliteal bypass group and 39% in the femorotibial-peroneal bypass group. Early and late graft thrombosis were more frequent in more distal anastomosis placements.

Satisfactory results have been obtained 6 years after Goretex grafting in the lower extremity. This material is an adequate alternative to the saphenous vein, even for below-knee reconstructions to revascularize the distal popliteal artery and the crural arteries. Disease in the outflow tract is probably the most critical factor limiting the function of vascular grafts.

Polytetrafluoroethylene Grafts as the First-Choice Arterial Substitute in Femoropopliteal Revascularization

William J. Quinones-Baldrich, Vicente Martin-Paredero, J. Dennis Baker, Ronald W. Busuttil, Herbert I. Machleder, and Wesley S. Moore (Univ. of California, Los Angeles)

Arch. Surg. 119:1238–1243, November 1984 7–103

Although excellent results have been reported by using polytetrafluoroethylene (PTFE) grafts in the femoropopliteal position, the results in more distal revascularizations have been poor, thus underscoring the importance of preserving the saphenous vein for coronary or distal revascularizations, or both.

Sixty-three femoropopliteal bypass operations were studied in 55 patients in whom PTFE grafts were used as the first-choice of arterial substitute, regardless of the availability of the saphenous vein, to determine whether reduced extremity morbidity and late patency justify this approach to preserve the saphenous vein for other, more critical tibial bypass surgery.

Forty-three grafts (68%) were placed for limb salvage, and 20 grafts (32%) were placed for disabling claudication. Diabetes mellitus was present in 23 cases (42%). Patients were followed for 9 to 53 months (mean, 23 months). All patients had preoperative aortographic study with visualization of runoff. Forty-seven grafts had distal anastomosis above the knee, and 16 had anastomosis below the knee. The procedure was the first attempt at revascularization in 55 cases.

Operative mortality was 1.8%. There were no deep wound or graft infections. Significant morbidity was seen in 3 patients (5.4%), including severe edema of the extremity in 2 patients that appeared after revascularization of an acutely ischemic extremity.

Overall patency rate at 30 months was 76.7%. Cumulative patency rate at 30 months for patients with claudication was 89.3%, and there were no amputations. Cumulative patency rate at 30 months for limb salvage procedures was 70.1%, with a limb salvage rate of 81.2%. Despite no significant difference between the 30-month patency rate for limb salvage with above-the-knee distal anastomosis (72.2%) and for popliteal anastomosis placed below the knee (63.1%), it was noted that the difference was further reduced when salvage between the two groups was compared. Thus, the patency rate in the group with below-the-knee distal anastomosis may be as dependent on the location of the anastomosis as on coexisting factors in patients who require a more distal reconstruction. The 30-month cumulative patency rate for 35 femoropopliteal bypasses with good runoff was 84.6%, compared to 63.7% in 28 procedures with poor runoff.

Although the difference between the 30-month cumulative patency rate for insulin-dependent diabetic patients (66.1%) and that of nondiabetic patients (80.8%) was not statistically significant, it was highly suggestive. There was no difference in patency rate between diabetic patients (83.4%) and nondiabetic patients (84.1%) when both had good runoff; however, diabetic patients with poor runoff fared worse (58.2%) than nondiabetic patients with poor runoff (69.2%).

Because the 30-month patency rates and limb salvage patency rates are comparable with those in other series in which autogenous saphenous veins were used, particularly in the series reported by Bergan et al., it is concluded that PTFE grafts may be considered the first choice of arterial substitute for femoropopliteal reconstruction. Morbidity is low with no graft infections noted. The avoidance of multiple skin incisions and dissection necessary to harvest the saphenous vein decreases the incidence of postoperative edema, eliminates the possibility of saphenous nerve injury, and contributes to a shorter operative time.

However, until longer follow-up studies are available, reversed autogenous saphenous vein should probably be considered the graft of first choice in patients less than age 60 years with no significant coronary artery disease who are undergoing femoropopliteal revascularization.

▶ Most vascular surgeons would agree with the last line of one of the abstracts:

"The expanded PTFE graft seems to be a good alternative when autologous vein is not available."

But informed vascular surgeons would never say that this is the first-choice material. The UCLA Study, in fact, had a mean follow-up period of less than 2 years, and 75% of the grafts were from the femoral to the above-knee popliteal artery. That is certainly one of the most favorable types of grafts in the lower extremity. Objective hemodynamic measures were not employed in evaluation of patency in this study. Therefore, we must conclude that, whenever possible, autogenous veins should be used to revascularize the lower extremity.

Early Aneurysmal Degeneration of Human Umbilical Vein Bypass Grafts
G. T. Layer, R. B. King, and C. W. Jamieson
Br. J. Surg. 71:709–710, September 1984 7–104

Development of aneurysms within functioning arterial prostheses made of human umbilical vein (HUV) supposedly is a late and rare defect, although few patent grafts have been followed for more than 3 years. Three cases of early formation of aneurysms in modified HUV grafts in the femorodistal segment are described. One is the first in which multiple true aneurysms are reported.

Man, 62, presented with rest pain in the right leg and foot. He had undergone left iliofemoral endarterectomy and profundoplasty 3 years previously. A HUV graft was inserted in the lateral aspect of the right lower extremity extending from the common femoral to the anterior tibial artery. Severe rest pain developed in the left foot 1 month later, requiring a similar HUV bypass procedure. The left prosthesis failed 10 months later, was unsuccessfully thrombectomized, and became infected, requiring its removal. A false anastomotic aneurysm was found in the left groin, and a left above-knee amputation followed. One year after insertion the right-sided HUV graft was observed to be dilating. Angiography performed 27 months after operation confirmed the clinical impression of multiple aneurysms of the graft (Fig 7–25). Ulceration of the skin seemed imminent and there appeared to be a serious risk of embolism to his solitary patent distal vessel. The abnormal graft was excised and bridged with another HUV graft without complication.

Examination of the excised graft revealed three saccular dilatations of the biograft, with the largest measuring 3×2.5 cm. Section of the swellings showed absence of the vein segment, with the Dacron mesh being the only lining of the

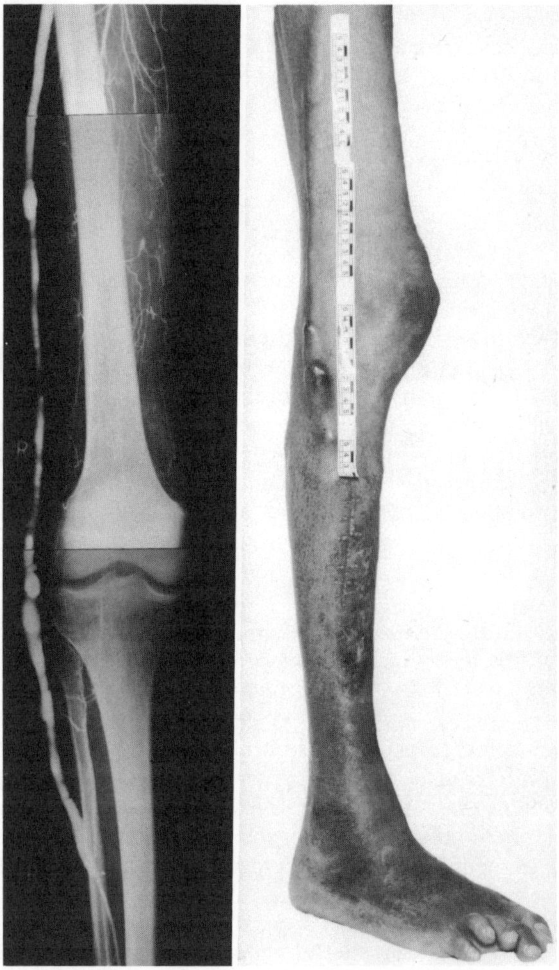

Fig 7–25.—Angiogram and photograph of right leg. There are multiple aneurysms of subcutaneous graft. (Courtesy of Layer, G.T., et al.: Br. J. Surg. 71:709–710, September 1984.)

inner vessel segment; an organized thrombus was attached to it. Grossly normal zones showed good preservation of both the biologic and synthetic portions. Section of the aneurysm showed destruction of the biologic component, with organized thrombus and rupture of the mesh; adjoining areas exhibited early dissection. Graft culturing revealed no evidence of infection.

The cause of aneurysmal degeneration of the HUV graft remains to be determined. Thinning of the umbilical vein as a result of poor preservation or trauma may lead to dilatation and subsequent rupture of the Dacron mesh. In the patient described here inadequate tanning of the graft by glutaraldehyde was considered to be the cause of early degeneration. Arteriographic follow-up of biografts may be an appropriate study in patients with a good life expectancy.

Occlusion of Femoropopliteal Bypasses (Biografts)
A. H. Boontje (Univ. of Groningen)
J. Cardiovasc. Surg. 25:385–389, Sept.–Oct. 1984 7–105

Acceptable results have been obtained from use of the Biograft, or modified human umbilical cord vein, in femoropopliteal bypass operations, but graft failures are fairly frequent. Review was made of 225 Biografts inserted as femoropopliteal bypasses for atherosclerotic occlusive disease between 1978 and 1983. Disabling claudication was the indication for 175 procedures and limb-threatening ischemia for the other 50. Fifty-seven failures resulted from occlusion of the Biograft. The 5-year patency rates were 82% for above-knee and 47% for below-knee reconstructions. Forty-five percent of below-knee procedures failed, compared with 14% of above-knee operations. In only 9 cases was claudication converted to limb-threatening ischemia by graft occlusion. Five patients operated on for limb salvage had only claudication after graft failure. The chief cause of failure was progressive atherosclerotic disease, especially of the outflow tract. Kinking of the graft was responsible in 7 patients with a below-knee distal anastomosis. Five of these were among the 11 failures seen within a month of operation.

Forty-nine failures were managed operatively. Iliofemoral endarterectomy was possible in 6 cases of inflow tract obstruction. Failures of above-knee grafts were managed by inserting a jump Biograft and performing thrombectomy. Biograft-related failures were managed by simple thrombectomy if kinking was responsible. The overall initial success rate was 77%. A few patients required further reoperations. Five with persistent failure had amputation of the leg; none of these patients had the initial operation for claudication only.

Progressive atherosclerosis is the chief cause of Biograft failure in femoropopliteal bypasses. Most Biograft-related failures have been due to kinking; none resulted from changes in the Biograft itself. An aggressive approach to Biograft failures seems to be worthwhile. An occluded Biograft need not be replaced by a new one. Intraoperative angiography should follow thrombectomy to demonstrate any anastomotic stenosis or outflow problem.

Umbilical Vein Bypass in Patients With Severe Lower Limb Ischemia: A Report of 121 Consecutive Cases
L. I. Andersen, O. M. Nielsen, and H. J. Buchardt Hansen (Copenhagen)
Surgery 97:294–298, March 1985 7–106

The umbilical vein graft was used in 121 consecutive femoropopliteal and femorodistal reconstructions since 1977 in patients with severe lower extremity ischemia where no suitable saphenous vein was available. Nine patients had grafts placed bilaterally. There were 75 men with a median age of 60 years and 37 women with a median age of 61 years in the series. Reconstructive operation had been done on nearly half the patients. Sur-

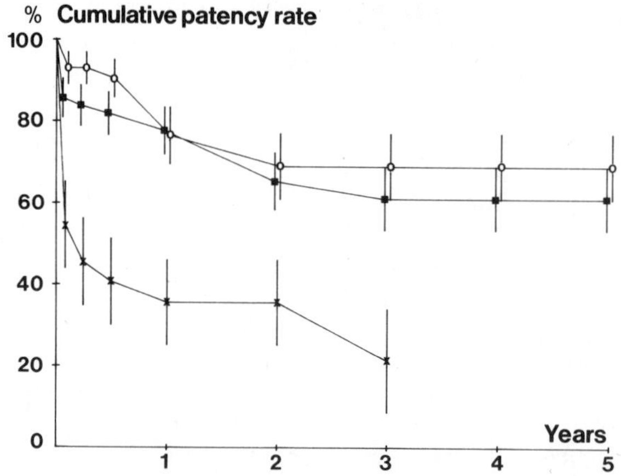

Fig 7–26.—Cumulative patency rates for the grafts with distal anastomosis to the popliteal artery above the knee *(squares)*, the popliteal artery below the knee *(circles)*, and to one of the crural arteries *(x)*. Vertical bars depict SD. (Courtesy of Andersen, L.I., et al.: Surgery 97:294–298, March 1985.)

gical procedure was done for extremity salvage in 78% of the patients and for disabling claudication in 22%. All grafts were placed in anatomical position with end-to-side anastomoses. An additional arterial reconstruction was necessary proximal to the bypass to ensure inflow in 40% of the procedures.

The patency rate for all femoropopliteal and femorodistal reconstructions was 70% after 1 year and 57% after 5 years. Mean follow-up was 2 years. Grafts with distal anastomosis to a crural artery had a relatively low patency rate (Fig 7–26). More graft failures tended to occur with decreasing runoff but not to a significant degree. Two deep infections occurred; 1 caused late graft failure. One false aneurysm at the proximal anastomotic site was excised. Several early failures may have been due to inadequate runoff. Most late failures were related to progressive arteriosclerotic disease in the distal arterial tree.

These results justify using the human umbilical vein for lower extremity graft procedures if a suitable saphenous vein is not available. The distal anastomosis should be below the popliteal artery only where the extremity is threatened. Runoff cannot be used to predict graft patency. The polytetrafluoroethylene grafts appear to fail more often than umbilical vein grafts. Patient variation makes comparison with saphenous vein grafting difficult.

Thromboxane Production in Umbilical Vein Grafts

Pia Saldeen, Carlos O. Esquivel, Claes-Göran Björck, David Bergqvist, and Tom Saldeen
Thromb. Res. 33:259–267, 1984 7–107

Thrombosis is a common cause of failure of small vascular prostheses. Platelet survival is reduced in the first year after vascular grafting, suggesting platelet consumption on the graft surface and possibly resultant thrombosis. Disordered prostacyclin-thromboxane metabolism in the neointima may be responsible. The in vitro production of 6-keto-prostaglandin $F_1\alpha$ ($PGF_1\alpha$) and thromboxane B_2, stable hydrolysis products of prostacyclin and thromboxane A_2, respectively, was examined in vascular grafts placed in the sheep carotid artery. Twelve glutaraldehyde-tanned human umbilical vein grafts, half treated with heparin and alcohol and the rest with heparin solution alone, were placed for 90 days. The grafts perfused at physiologic blood flow. Other grafts were removed 10 days after placement.

Production of prostaglandin metabolites was similar in parent grafts with and without small thrombi and occluded grafts. Grafts removed at 90 days showed high production of thromboxane B_2, compared with native carotid artery and jugular vein. As much thromboxane B_2 was present in the anastomosis as in the midgraft region. Production of 6-keto-$PGF_1\alpha$ was not significantly different from that in native vessels, although lower production was evident in the midgraft region. Grafts placed for 10 days showed a less marked elevation of thromboxane B_2 production.

The reduced ratio of 6-keto-$PGF_1\alpha$ to thromboxane B_2 observed in these grafts suggests low resistance to platelet adhesion and aggregation. This may contribute to the thrombogenicity of vascular grafts and may be involved in the pathogenesis of neointimal fibrous hyperplasia. The thromboxane synthesis inhibitor UK 37,248 (Dazoxiben) prevents production of thromboxane B_2 in the vessel wall but leaves 6-keto-PGF production unchanged. Another thromboxane inhibitor, ibuprofen, reduces the thrombogenicity of polytetrafluoroethylene grafts.

▶ The above four abstracts present the state of the art with regard to umbilical vein bypass grafting and, in particular, the paper from the *British Journal of Surgery* emphasizes the late development of true aneurysms in the human umbilical vein graft. In retrospect, when one recalls that thin-walled knitted Dacron grafts have been seen to become aneurysmal, it would be too much to expect that a nylon mesh would contain an aneurysm that forms in a collagen tube.

Patency of Femoropopliteal and Femorotibial Grafts After Outflow Revascularization (Jump Grafts) to Bypass Distal Disease

George Andros, Robert W. Harris, Leopoldo B. Dulawa, Robert W. Oblath, and Sergio X. Salles-Cunha (St. Joseph Med. Center, Burbank, Calif.)

Surgery 96:878–885, November 1984 7–108

Secondary vascular reconstructions have extended the patency of hemodynamically failed arterial grafts and have salvaged extremities at risk of amputation because of impending graft occlusion. Repair of failing femorodistal bypass grafts with secondary distal "jump" grafts was performed 34 times in 33 patients. Salvage of an extremity was the only indication for operation for all distal jump grafts and for 85% of initial femorodistal bypass grafts. Angiograms performed before initial femorodistal bypass or secondary jump grafting were classified according to the number of infrapopliteal vessels that were patent or segmentally patent.

Bypass grafts from the greater saphenous, lesser saphenous, and cephalic and basilic veins were used in 28 of 33 initial femorodistal grafts (85%) and in 29 of 34 secondary jump grafts (85%). Twenty-nine (87%) of the initial grafts originated from the common or superficial femoral arteries and 16 (48%) extended to the infrapopliteal level. Thirty jump grafts originated from the initial femorodistal bypass grafts and 19 terminated in foot or ankle arteries. Average follow-up was 34 months.

Poor runoff, even at the time of initial bypass grafting, was common among patients who eventually required a distal jump graft. Only 4 extremities were still viable 5 years after the initial femorodistal bypass grafting. The need for a distal jump graft occurred mainly during the first year after the initial bypass. The 12 jump grafts performed in the first 2 months after the initial graft were associated with high rates (9%) of graft thrombosis and amputation. Early loss of viability of initial grafts probably resulted from technical and judgment errors (2 cases) or underestimation of distal occlusive disease (10). Progression of distal disease in 11 cases produced late failure after 1 year of implantation of the initial graft.

The 1-year patency rate of the initial femorodistal grafts was 63%of which only 32% were viable and were not at risk of amputation. Distal jump grafts produced a 49% improvement in limb viability (from 32% to 81%), and an increase of 11% in the initial graft patency rate (from 63% to 74%) at 1 year. The 50% survival rate was 3 years after the jump graft and 7 years after the initial operation. Survival rate 1 year after amputation was 50%.

The study shows that jump grafts improve the patency rate of previously inserted femoropopliteal and infrapopliteal grafts and definitely contribute to salvage of the extremity despite the presence of extensive arterial occlusive disease. Although there was only a 50% survival of patients 3 years after distal jump grafting, this operation is warranted in graft failures that will otherwise result in amputation. The triad of a good pulse (usually the popliteal) in a previously inserted graft, loss of foot pulses, and recurrence of ischemic signs and symptoms is diagnostic of distal occlusive disease and identifies a possible candidate for a jump graft.

Successful Long-Term Limb Salvage Using Cephalic Vein Bypass Grafts

Robert W. Harris, George Andros, Leopoldo B. Dulawa, Robert W. Oblath, Sergio X. Salles-Cunha, and Roseanne Apyan (Burbank, Calif.)

Ann. Surg. 200:785–792, December 1984 7–109

Patients with ischemia of an extremity but absent or inadequate saphenous veins remain a problem in vascular surgery. At Saint Joseph Medical Center 70 cephalic vein bypass grafts were placed in the lower extremities of 67 patients between 1972 and 1983. The 51 men and 16 women were aged 41 to 90 years. Twenty-five patients (37%) were known diabetics and 47 (70%) smoked cigarettes. Fifty-eight operations (83%) were done for limb salvage; the others were done because of disabling claudication. previous bypass surgery with a saphenous vein had been done in 32 (46%) of cases. Twenty-one (30%) of patients had had saphenous stripping; 17 (24%) had an inadequate saphenous vein. In 6 instances other graft materials were used with the cephalic vein. Most grafts originated from the common, profunda, or superficial femoral artery.

Follow-up averaged 31 months. Two graft occlusions occurred in hospital, and there were 14 late cephalic vein graft occlusions. Eight of these extremities required further vascular surgery for salvage. Patency rates for cephalic vein bypasses were 85% at 1 year and 68% at 5 years. Popliteal artery grafts did better than tibial grafts. Inflow or outflow procedures were necessary in 13 extremities with patent cephalic vein grafts. The

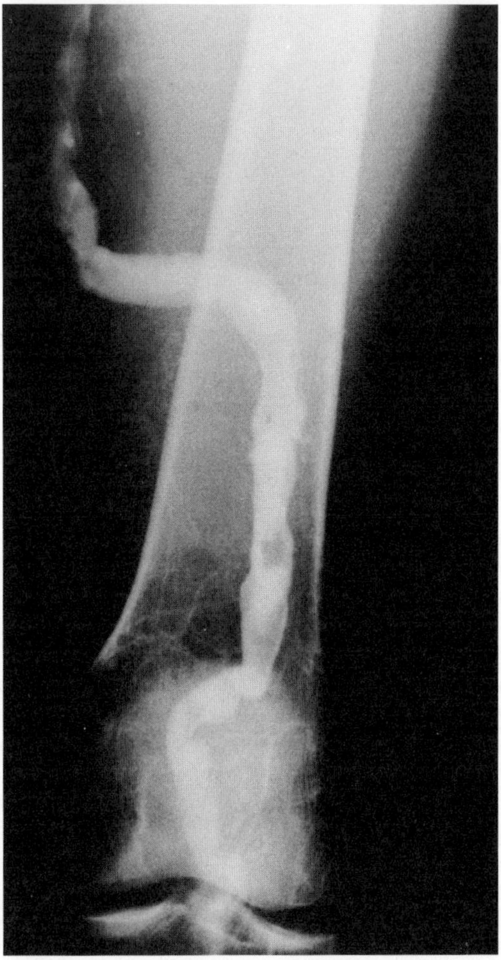

Fig 7–27.—Dilatation of cephalic vein bypass graft which was still patent and viable 43 months later. (Courtesy of Harris, R.W., et al.: Ann. Surg. 200:785–792, December 1984.)

ultimate salvage rate of extremities from all procedures was 93% at 1 year and 85% after 4 years. Six amputations were necessary, all in patients operated on for salvage. There was no hospital mortality.

The same sequelae observed with saphenous vein bypass grafts have been seen with cephalic vein grafts (Fig 7–27), but no graft rupture, embolization, or failure due to dilatation has been encountered. The high patency rate of cephalic vein bypass grafts makes the technical difficulties worthwhile in patients with severe ischemia of an extremity. These grafts are used when a suitable saphenous vein is not available. The authors believe that all reasonable attempts at using autogenous tissue should be made before resorting to prosthetic graft materials.

▶ Andros and his group have championed the use of upper extremity veins as bypass grafts whenever lower extremity veins were unavailable. His long-term follow-up shows few serious dilations of the thin-walled veins, as is shown in the second abstract chosen here. He has paid attention to hemodynamic failure of distal bypass grafts by extending the revascularization to a more distal location. The revascularization of these severely ischemic limbs requires attention to such nuances of observation and to the need for repetitive operations.

Pseudoaneurysm Secondary to a Protruding Screw as a Result of Normal Growth and Remodeling Following Supracondylar Osteotomy: A Case Report

David P. Falconer (Louisville, Ky.) and Uriel Adar (Albert Einstein College of Medicine)

J. Bone Joint Surg. (Am.) 66-A:1126–1128, September 1984 7–110

The potential for growth must be considered when internal fixation is used in children. A child is described in whom the relative migration of an implanted plate caused by skeletal growth resulted in vascular compromise of the lower extremity.

Girl, 6, with bilateral knee flexion contractures underwent bilateral closing-wedge supracondylar femoral osteotomy in which fixation was achieved with a two-hole plate and screws. Six years later the patient complained of transient episodes in which the lower extremity turned blue. Films of the right femur revealed proximal relative migration of the plate and screws that resulted from the femoral growth, with the distal screw penetrating beyond the medial section of the cortex at the junction of the middle and distal thirds of the femur. Femoral arteriography showed formation of a pseudoaneurysm in association with a protruding screw in the distal portion of Hunter's canal. At surgery a pseudoaneurysm was identified and the protruding screw point was found lying in the center of the aneurysmal sac. Resection and end-to-end anastomosis was performed. The patient returned to baseline functional level.

In a growing child orthopedic implants may not remain where they were originally placed. The broad distal metaphyseal region is remodeled into diaphyseal cortex of uniform diameter as part of normal femoral growth. Screws previously contained within the metaphysis may become prominent, with resultant risk to adjacent soft tissue structures. It has been suggested that a pseudoaneurysm is usually the result of erosion of an arterial wall that pulsates against a protruding screw rather than of penetration by a drill or bone fragment. Removal of screws that project beyond the medial part of the cortex has been recommended to avoid this complication.

Thrombosis of the Popliteal Artery Due to Osteochondroma of the Upper End of the Tibia. A Case Report

Y. Boscher, F. Lescalie, P. Moreau, B. Enon, J. M. Chevalier, and J. Pillet (Angers)

J. Chir. (Paris) 121:327–330, May 1984 7–111

Isolated or multiple osteochondromas represent a group of benign tumors, generally well tolerated, with only rare complications. Although unusual, vascular sequelae have occasionally been reported with particular predilection for the lower end of the femur. The present case involves thrombosis of the popliteal artery due to an exostosis of the upper end of the tibia.

A man aged 41 years sought consultation for progressively incapacitating left leg pain of about 1 year's duration that was most troublesome at the end of the day. For the last 4–5 months, a growing cramplike pain in the left calf was reported even after short walks. Left popliteal and distal pulses were not palpable. An arteriogram showed thrombosis of the left popliteal artery 3 cm proximal to the level of the articular cartilage with periarticular revascularization. Surgical procedure revealed an exostosis of the posterior side of the tibia at the level of the popliteal artery that compressed the artery and caused the thrombosis. Excision of the exostosis and resection of the thrombosed arterial segment was followed by interposition of a saphenous graft. Postoperative course was unremarkable, the pain disappeared, and all distal pulses of the left leg were palpable.

This lesion should be considered in the differential diagnosis in young adults with lower extremity ischemia. Follow-up should be by Doppler after arteriography to serve as a reference.

▶ These abstracts were selected because vascular surgeons must know about these phenomena. In fact, one abstract describes a common location of osteochondromas, and experience shows that these can produce false aneurysms of the popliteal artery, with or without secondary thrombosis. Such a lesion should not be a surprise to the educated vascular surgeon.

Pathogenesis of the So-called Cystic Adventitial Degeneration of Peripheral Blood Vessels

Hans Jörg Leu, John Largiadèr, and Bernhard Odermatt (Univ. of Zurich)

Virchows Arch. (Pathol. Anat.) 404:289–300, October 1984 7–112

Ruppell et al. suggested that the cysts in cystic adventitial degeneration of peripheral vessels may correspond with ganglia of adjacent joints. This has been corroborated in a study of 11 cases by light and in 3 by electron microscopic examination. The 7 men and 4 women had respective mean ages of 39 and 49 years. Eight cases involving arteries were associated with intermittent claudication and ischemic symptoms in healthy, mostly young subjects. Three cases of venous involvement were found incidentally on biopsies. The popliteal artery was involved in 7 subjects.

The findings are shown in Figures 7–28 and 7–29. The cystic changes were within the adventitial layer. Changes of primary dysplasia of the media were not seen. There were no accumulations of myocytes with increased numbers of cytoplasmic organelles. No necrosis of cells or nuclei was observed. The cysts often were multiple or multichambered. Their lumina were filled by mucinous, alcian blue-positive fluid. The nature of the lining cells was not clarified by immunohistochemical study. No factor VIII was detected, and tests for keratin were negative. In 3 cases a pedicle was found connecting the cysts and an adjacent joint, and in 1 of these the pedicle was followed to its junction with the knee joint capsule.

So-called cystic adventitial degeneration is not a primary dysplasia of

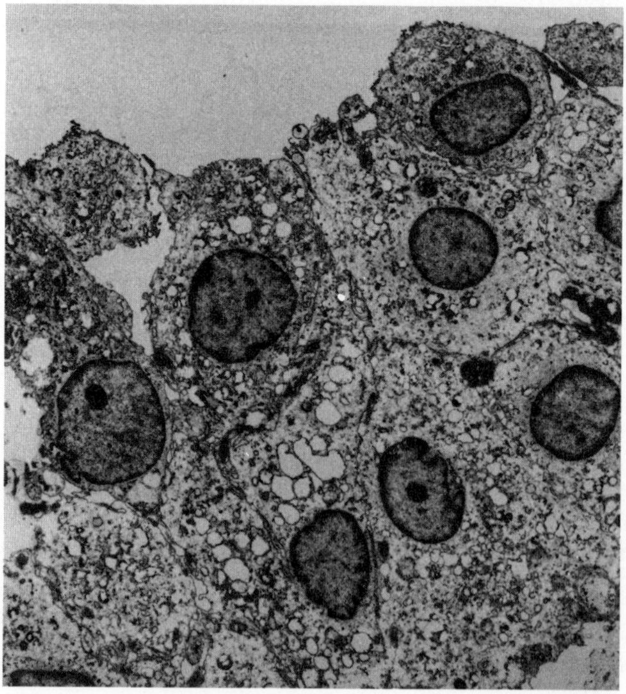

Fig 7–28.—Several cell layers lining adventitial cyst. Large, round nuclei with marginated chromatin, numerous vacuoles, and inclusion of mucinous fluid. Phosphate-buffered glutaraldehyde; original magnification ×3600. (Courtesy of Leu, H.J., et al.: Virchows Arch. [Pathol. Anat.] 404:289–300, October 1984; Berlin–Heidelberg–New York: Springer.)

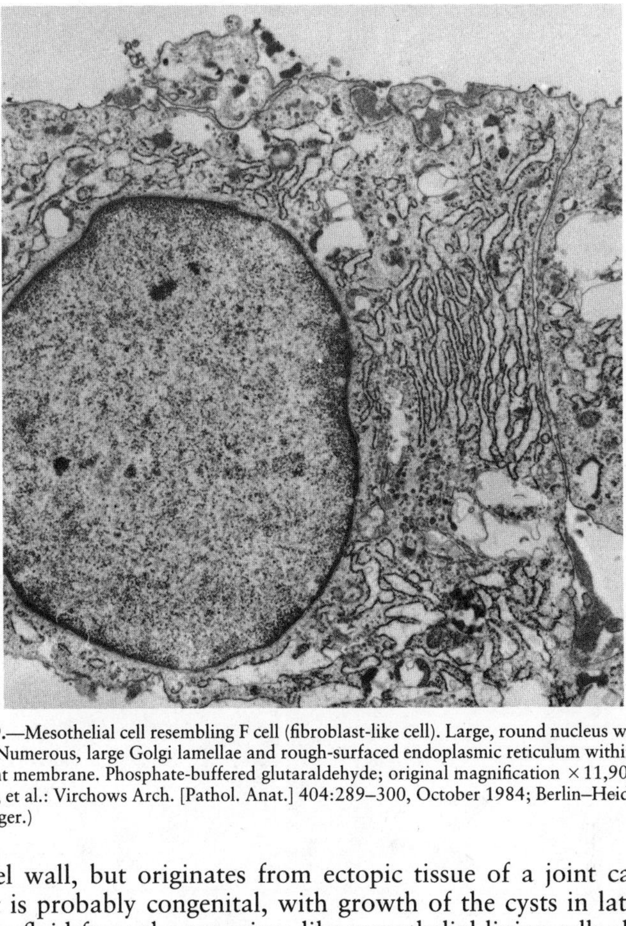

Fig 7–29.—Mesothelial cell resembling F cell (fibroblast-like cell). Large, round nucleus with dispersed chromatin. Numerous, large Golgi lamellae and rough-surfaced endoplasmic reticulum within cytoplasm. No basement membrane. Phosphate-buffered glutaraldehyde; original magnification ×11,900. (Courtesy of Leu, H.J., et al.: Virchows Arch. [Pathol. Anat.] 404:289–300, October 1984; Berlin–Heidelberg–New York: Springer.)

the vessel wall, but originates from ectopic tissue of a joint capsule or bursa. It is probably congenital, with growth of the cysts in later life as muciform fluid from the synovium-like mesothelial lining cells slowly accumulates. The amount of fluid in the cysts may vary and cause intermittent ischemic symptoms by compressing the arterial lumen. A pedicle, if present, must be ligated at the level of the joint capsule to prevent recurrence.

The Autogenous Vein Graft as Popliteal Artery Substitute: Long-Term Follow-up of Cystic Adventitial Degeneration

Tor Hierton and Anders Hemmingsson (Uppsala, Sweden)

Acta Chir. Scand. 150:377–383, 1984 7–113

A small proportion of popliteal artery occlusions are due to an adventital cystic disorder. Young men are chiefly affected. At University Hospital 3 active men aged 24 to 32 years had a reversed saphenous vein graft inserted after resection of the affected arterial segment and were followed for 27 to 30 years. All had intermittent claudication and were found to have popliteal stenosis or occlusion ranging in length from 2 to 10 cm. The vein graft was anastomosed end to end to the popliteal artery. Cystic formation with mucoid change was found in the resected segments. In 1 patient there was necrosis of the compressed media.

Postoperative recovery was uneventful, and the patients regained unlimited walking capacity. The functional results have remained excellent for up to 30 years. Postoperative angiography showed the vein grafts to be patent, but some anastomotic narrowing was present and it progressed moderately over time (Fig 7–30). The transplants themselves widened, but no kinking was seen (Fig 7–31).

The cause of this rare disorder is unknown, but pathogenically the structure and cystic formation of the diseased segment resemble that of a ganglion within the adventitia. Autogenos saphenous vein grafts have done quite well over 3 decades of follow-up. These 3 patients had no signs of relapse of the femoropopliteal disease. Continued arteriographic follow-up of asymptomatic patients is necessary, because aneurysmal changes may not be detected by currently used noninvasive methods for checking the status of the peripheral circulation.

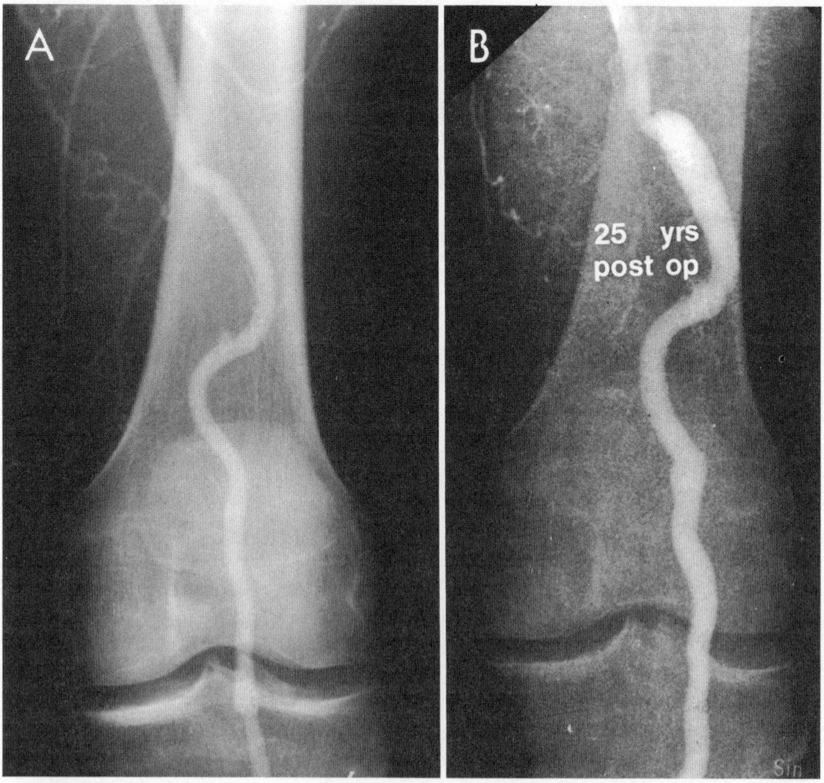

Fig 7–30.—**A**, angiography 3 weeks after operation. Transplant is somewhat long with a curved course. There is slight narrowing of proximal anastomosis. **B**, angiography 25 years after operation, same patient. Transplant is still open with unchanged slight narrowing of proximal anastomosis. Moderate widening of transplant has developed. (Courtesy of Hierton, T., and Hemmingsson, A.: Acta Chir. Scand. 150:377–383, 1984.)

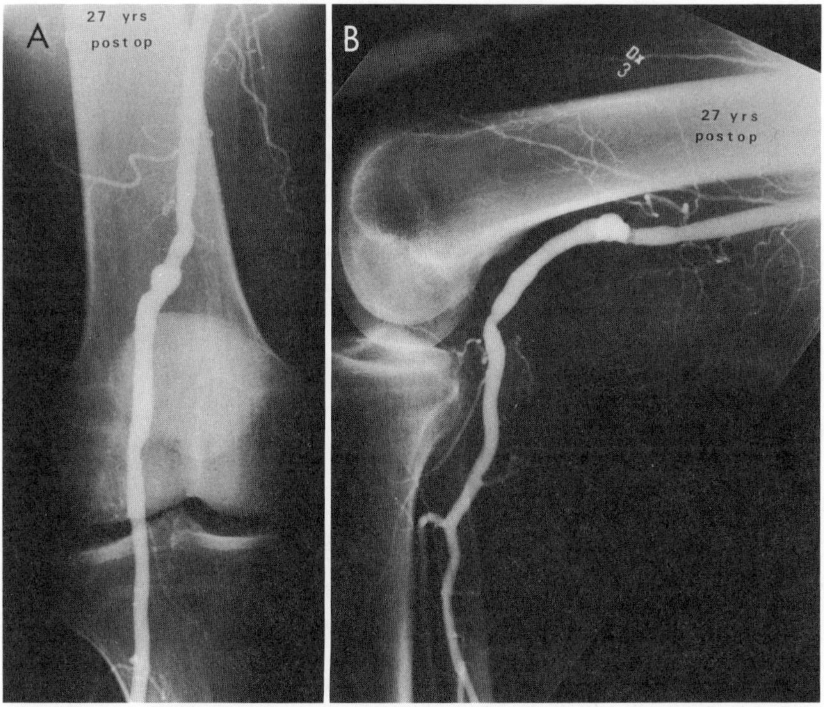

Fig 7–31.—**A**, angiogram 27 years after operation (another patient) shows transplant is still open and no evident narrowing of anastomoses is seen. Some widening of transplant has developed. Although transplant is somewhat too long, no kinking appears at flexion of knee (**B**). (Courtesy of Hierton, T., and Hemmingsson, A.: Acta Chir. Scand. 150:377–383, 1984.)

▶ Tor Hierton is to be commended for the careful documentation of his reconstructions for cystic adventitial disease and for persistence in following these patients. His observations teach us that, as many as 30 years after autogenous vein grafting, the veins stand up under arterial pressure and do not become aneurysmal. This paper is a landmark presentation that caps a very distinguished surgical career.

In a review of worldwide experience with cystic adventitial disease, it was predicted that ultimately the etiology of this condition would be found. It is appropriate that this was accomplished in a cooperative study involving a surgical clinic and an institute for pathology (Flannigan, P. D., et al.: *Ann. Surg.* 189:165, 1979). Vascular surgeons must know about this condition, its pathogenesis and treatment, and whether or not the artery is anatomically occluded.

Lower Extremity Amputation for Peripheral Vascular Disease: A Low-Risk Operation

T. J. Bunt, Lawrence L. Manship, Raymond P. H. Bynoe, and James L. Haynes (Univ. of South Carolina)

Am. Surg. 50:581–584, November 1984 7–114

A review of a representative series from the literature of above-knee amputation for end stage peripheral vascular disease revealed average mortalities of 15% to 30% (table). Review of 253 consecutive major amputations of the lower extremity for peripheral vascular insufficiency performed in the elderly (median age, 68 years) showed that adherence to a protocol of aggressive medical management with timely operation allows a mortality appropriate to the age and general debility of this population. All operations were performed by junior surgical residents under direct supervision of the vascular surgical attending staff or the chief resident on the vascular service.

Patients undergoing elective operation had any deficits corrected before the procedure. Hydration was begun at least 12 hours before anesthesia, patients with a hematocrit of less than 32 gm/dl were given transfusions before operation, and diabetics underwent stabilization of serum glucose concentrations and were managed by the Izzo method intraoperatively. Two-dose perioperative cephalosporine prophylaxis was given. Patients with pedal gangrene, progressive cellulitis, or signs of systemic toxicity underwent intensive care for preoperative medical stabilization before amputation. Broad-spectrum antibiotics and vigorous hydration were started, with Swan-Ganz catheter and radial artery pressure monitoring. Prophylactic digitalis and low-dose dopamine were given for cardiotonic support, and intravenous nitroprusside or nitroglycerin drips were given for hypertension. Physiologic amputation of the lower extremity in a Dry Ice boot was undertaken, and formal amputation was delayed until maximal cardiopulmonary function was obtained, usually 48 to 72 hours. No patient underwent emergency amputation. With electrocautery dissection, above-knee amputations were performed with standard two-layer closure of a fish-mouth incision; below-knee amputations used a long posterior flap, with the fibula resected ¾ in. shorter than the tibia, which was beveled in its anterior third. Operative mortalities were 0.9% for 113 below-knee

Representative Mortalities of Above-Knee Amputations

Author	Year	Number of Patients	Mortality (%)
Mandelberg	1946	128	33
Dale	1962	385	20
Lempke	1963	200	12
Otteman	1965	370	42
McClure	1966	457	23
Gorman	1967	72	18
Warren	1968	372	28
Eidemiller	1968	436	19.7
Rosenberg	1970	342	28
Wray	1972	256	8
Silverstein	1973	320	35
Berardi	1978	101	13.9
Huston	1980	100	15
Pollock	1980	32	12
Rush	1981	146	16
Bunt	1984	140	2.8

(Courtesy of Bunt, T.J., et al.: Am. Surg. 50:581–584, November 1984.)

and 2.8% for 140 above-knee amputations. Deaths were due to pulmonary embolus in 2 patients, extension of a preoperative myocardial infarction in 1, and pneumonitis in 1.

Acceptance of higher operative mortalities for lower extremity amputations for peripheral vascular insufficiency is unwarranted. Aggressive preoperative medical and surgical management under the direction of an involved vascular surgeon is a prerequisite to extremity amputation. Sepsis can be controlled by physiologic amputation and broad-spectrum antibiotics. The risk of pulmonary embolism may be decreased by perioperative anticoagulation. Myocardial infarction can be prevented by vigorous rehydration and restoration of optimal myocardial performance with digitalis, dopamine, and Swan-Ganz-determination of cardiac output. Avoidance of intraoperative blood loss is another preventive measure.

▶ This modern study refutes previous observations of high mortality following lower extremity amputation. Clearly, there is a need for this information so that we in vascular surgery can regard the amputation event as a beginning of rehabilitation rather than the end of a series of failed operations.

Streptokinase Therapy: Complications of Intra-arterial Use

Erich K. Lang (Louisiana State Univ.)

Radiology 154:75–77, January 1985 7–115

Complications from low-dose, intra-arterial streptokinase therapy have been noted quite frequently, and the author has encountered a disturbing number of renal complications following streptokinase therapy. Low-dose, intra-arterial treatment was given to 86 patients, 71 men and 5 women aged 38–77 years, with thrombotic or thromboembolic arterial occlusion. The primary artery was injected in 37 cases, and an occluded prosthetic bypass graft or native artery in the leg was injected in 35 cases. Limb amputation had been recommended in 18 patients. Streptokinase was perfused at a rate of 5,000 units per hour via a 5 F catheter. Heparin was added to maintain the partial thromboplastin time at 1½–2 times normal. Cryoprecipitate was administered where indicated. Fractional heparin therapy was continued for 5 days after successful thrombolysis or until surgery was performed.

Complete thrombolysis and restitution of flow in distal runoff vessels were achieved in 27 of 35 patients; bleeding from the catheter entry site occurred in one fifth of these cases. One patient had distal embolism. Significant myoglobinuria occurred in 10 patients. Three of 17 patients without ischemic necrosis or compartment syndrome had trace myoglobinuria. In 5 of 13 patients with compartment syndrome but without ischemic necrosis, massive myoglobinuria developed on the same day as thrombolysis. One of these patients later experienced acute tubular necrosis, as did 2 of 5 patients with both ischemic necrosis and compartment syndrome. Ischemic necrosis did not appear to compromise the efficacy of streptokinase therapy.

Compromise of perfusion may result in myoglobinuria after low-dose streptokinase therapy is given for thrombolysis in an extremity unless the muscle is properly decompressed by fasciotomy and by fibulectomy, if necessary. Acute tubular necrosis can also result. Any attempt to salvage irreversibly damaged tissue by re-establishing the circulation entails an unacceptable risk of renal complications and can threaten the patient's life.

▶ The swing of the pendulum with regard to streptokinase therapy has begun. In the future we will see less treatment with lytic agents.

Gender and Preatherosclerotic Lesions: Effects on Prevalence in Human Abdominal Aortas

Garth E. Austin (Emory Univ.) and Thomas J. Moss (UCLA School of Medicine)

Arch. Pathol. Lab. Med. 108:811–813, October 1984 7–116

Atherosclerosis may be more severe in men than in women because women have fewer or less extensive precursor lesions, or because the lesions progress at a more rapid rate in men. The prevalence of fatty streaks and fibromusculoelastic lesions was estimated in autopsy specimens of aortas from 39 male and 37 female patients, aged 9–30 years, none of whom had lipid-metabolic disorders. Respective mean ages were 20.5 and 20.9 years.

Fatty streaks were seen in the aortic segments from 27 male and 25 female patients, not a significant difference. The proportions of aortic surfaces involved did not differ significantly between sexes. Early fibromusculoelastic lesions were seen in 26 male and 20 female patients, also not a significant difference; and late fibromusculoelastic lesions were comparably frequent in the 2 groups. No substantial age differences were observed in this population.

Preatherosclerotic lesions in the upper abdominal aorta were similarly frequent in younger male and female patients in this autopsy study (most of these preatherosclerotic lesions apparently are present by about age 15 years). More rapid progression of lesions may explain the more severe atherosclerosis seen in men. Hormonal or other factors that protect women may act mainly by retarding the progression of precursor lesions.

▶ This observation of similar incidence in boys and girls of fibrofatty streaks in the aorta has not been reported before and is an important finding.

Atherosclerosis in the Young: A Virulent Disease

Robert A. McCready, Anne E. Vincent, Richard W. Schwartz, Gordon L. Hyde, Sally S. Mattingly, and Ward O. Griffen, Jr. (Univ. of Kentucky)

Surgery 96:863–869, November 1984 7–117

Data on 47 patients aged 40 years and younger who required peripheral vascular or coronary bypass operations for atherosclerotic occlusive disease in 1968–1983 were reviewed. Twenty-five patients, 14 men and 11 women, aged 24–40 years, required peripheral vascular procedures. All had strong family histories of atherosclerosis, and heavy smoking was prominent. Seven of 8 women followed for an average of 6 years after operation for lower extremity disease were asymptomatic. Thirteen men were operated on for limb salvage and 1 for renovascular hypertension. The men required 45 further procedures, including 15 amputations. Most graft failures were due to recurrent disease at the distal anastomoses or progressive outflow disease.

Twenty-two patients, 21 men and 1 woman, aged 27–40 years, required coronary bypass grafting. All but 1 were smokers. Nineteen had had a total of 26 infarctions, and 13 patients had angina. There was 1 postoperative death. Five patients had infarctions during follow-up. Five patients required a second coronary bypass procedure during an average follow-up of 4 years. Only two thirds of patients were asymptomatic when last evaluated. All 3 evaluable patients continued to smoke.

Young patients with atherosclerotic occlusive disease of either the peripheral vascular system or the coronary arteries appear to have a virulent disease. Patients requiring revascularization have a high rate of recurrent or progressive disease. Males with lower limb ischemia have frequently required amputation. Premature atherosclerosis in these patients seems to be strongly associated with cigarette smoking, and patients who continue to smoke after operation have a particularly poor prognosis.

Lower Limb Ischemia in Young Adults: Prognostic Implications

Peter C. Pairolero, John W. Joyce, Clay R. Skinner, Larry H. Hollier, and Kenneth J. Cherry, Jr. (Mayo Clinic and Mayo Foundation)

J. Vasc. Surg. 1:459–464, May 1984 7–118

Lower limb ischemia in young adults is rare and commonly associated with premature atherosclerosis obliterans or thromboangiitis obliterans. The authors report their experience in a 28-year period with lower limb ischemia in 50 patients, 41 men and 6 women, younger than age 36 years.

Claudication was the presenting symptom in 30 patients (60%) and distal ulceration in 20 (40%). Mean age was 28.3 years (range: 20–35 years). Premature atherosclerosis obliterans was diagnosed in 24 patients (48%), thromboangiitis obliterans in 12 (24%), and the other 14 patients had a variety of uncommon etiologies. All patients with premature atherosclerosis obliterans had at least one risk factor; 95% of patients smoked at least one pack of cigarettes per day; 70% had two or more risk factors, such as diabetes mellitus, hyperlipidemia, hypertension, positive family history, or use of contraceptives. Arteriography showed localized atherosclerosis in 10 patients and diffuse atherosclerosis in 14 patients. All patients with localized disease presented with claudication, all improved with reconstruction arterial surgery, none came to amputation, only 10% developed coronary artery disease, and only 10% died of myocardial infarction. Ten (71%) patients with diffuse atherosclerosis presented with lower extremity ulceration, only 31% were successfully revascularized whereas 54% ultimately required amputation, 69% developed coronary artery disease, and 31% died of myocardial infarction. Smoking was the dominant risk factor among patients with thromboangiitis obliterans. Arterial reconstruction was not possible in all 12 patients with thromboangiitis obliterans because of severe tibioperoneal occlusive disease; all underwent lumbar sympathectomy. Seventy-three percent of patients had lower limb amputation. All 14 patients with uncommon etiologies presented with claudication with risk factors present in 9. Arterial reconstruction was done in 8 patients, embolectomy in 4, and popliteal muscle release in 1, resulting in long-term relief of claudication in 12 patients. In summary, 22 patients with claudication underwent arterial reconstruction; 3 had sympathectomy. Arterial reconstruction was possible in only 3 patients with ulceration; 17 had sympathectomy. No operative deaths or early amputations occurred. At follow-up, averaging 13.5 years, 24 patients with claudication were improved, 3 were unchanged, 1 developed ulceration, 1 required late amputation, and 1 was lost to follow-up. Four patients with ulceration were improved, 1 was unchanged, 14 required late amputation, and 1 was lost to follow-up. Ten patients, all with atherosclerosis obliterans, developed coronary artery disease; 5 died of myocardial infarction. No patient developed cerebrovascular disease.

The authors conclude that reconstructive arterial surgery for claudication can be performed with a low risk and a strong likelihood of long-term improvement. Most patients presenting with ulceration, however, will ultimately require amputation. Because of the difference in prognosis between patients with localized and diffuse atherosclerosis, arterial reconstruction should be considered in patients with localized disease who present with claudication and in patients with diffuse atherosclerosis presenting with impending tissue loss. Identification of patients with uncommon etiologies is important since arterial reconstruction results mostly in long-term improvement. Patients with atherosclerosis obliterans are at risk for coronary artery disease and death from myocardial infarction.

▶ The strong smoking history in these two series suggests there is a need for further investigation of the smoking effect on the arteries in young adults. We all encounter these patients in our practice and yet there is no answer to their problems.

Placebo-Controlled Double-Blind Trial of Ketanserin in Treatment of Intermittent Claudication

Jean De Cree, Hedwig Geukens, Jos Leempoels, and Herman Verhaegen (Merksem, Belgium)

Lancet 2:775–779, Oct. 6, 1984 7–119

Serotonin (5-HT) is a potent vasoconstricting and platelet aggregating agent that enhances vasoconstriction and platelet aggregation induced by other agents, e.g., norepinephrine, angiotensin, and prostaglandins. Ketanserin, a specific 5-HT antagonist at 5-HT_2 receptors, antagonizes vasoconstriction and platelet aggregation induced by 5-HT and also increases red blood cell deformability. The effect of ketanserin (20–40 mg 3 times a day) was assessed in a 3-month, double-blind, placebo-controlled study of 20 patients with intermittent stage II claudication. Blood pressure ratios (thigh/arm) were measured by Doppler velocimetry and by plethysmography.

During ketanserin therapy, the blood pressure ratio between the thigh and arm, the reactive hyperemia profile as determined by electrocardiographically triggered venous occlusion plethysmography, blood filterability, and claudication distance on a treadmill progressively and significantly improved, whereas no such changes were observed in the placebo group. The mean arterial pressure also fell significantly in patients receiving ketanserin compared with the placebo group. Mean claudication distance on the treadmill increased by 140%, and 4 of the 11 patients receiving ketanserin were able to continue walking beyond the time limit of the exercise test. No significant changes were noted in any of the parameters evaluated in the nonclaudicant leg in either the ketanserin or placebo groups. When blood pressure ratios were compared, plethysmography showed a definite upward shift at thigh level in favor of ketanserin-treated patients, suggesting improvement in the collateral circulation. Side effects occurred in only a few patients and were minor.

The results suggest that 5-HT may be involved in the pathogenesis of peripheral arterial obstructive disease. Additional studies are needed to define the therapeutic role of ketanserin in affected patients.

▶ Evaluation of claudication must be done by hemodynamic measurements before and after exercise. It is unlikely that resting ankle pressure will evaluate drug effect, such as by ketanserin. If ankle pressure does not drop after exercise we would accept the drug treatment as effective. Otherwise, drug trials provide more benefits to pharmaceutical firms than to the patients.

Incidence of Positive Inguinal Lymph Node Cultures During Peripheral Revascularization

T. J. Bunt and Jerry D. Mohr (Univ. of South Carolina)
Am. Surg. 50:522–523, October 1984 7–120

Infection of a synthetic vascular graft is a catastrophic complication in peripheral vascular surgery. Most infections occur in the early postoperative period, usually at the inguinal incision. Some workers have found an increased infection rate if active infection is present distally, whereas others suggest that graft contamination at the inguinal site may result from transected lymphatics or lymph nodes proximal to a site of infection.

Superficial inguinal nodes were harvested during 45 consecutive elective peripheral revascularizations, most of them femoropopliteal or femorotibial bypasses. All patients received two doses of cephalothin perioperatively. The skin was prepared with povidone-iodine. Distal infections were present in 15 of the 45 extremities; they were open ulcers or gangrenous toes.

Eight of 30 inguinal nodes from normal legs had 1+ cultures for *Staphylococcus epidermidis*. No wound or graft infections occurred in these patients. Two of 15 nodes from limbs with known distal infection had similarly positive cultures. These patients had no graft or wound infection. Two other patients had a cephalothin-resistant isolate in node cultures, identical with the isolate from the distal infection. Methicillin-resistant *Staphylococcus* was present in 1 and *Actinobacter* in the other. Both these patients had graft infections by the same organism.

Contamination of synthetic vascular grafts by bacteria in inguinal lymph appears to be a possibility. Ideally, operation would be deferred until the infective source was eliminated, but infection is usually a result of arterial insufficiency and will not be corrected without revascularization. Culture-directed antibiotic coverage might be indicated in this circumstance or broader-spectrum therapy be given for a longer period.

Perigraft Seromas Complicating Arterial Grafts

Robert M. Blumenberg, Michael L. Gelfand, and W. Andrew Dale

Surgery 97:194–204, February 1985 7–121

A perigraft collection of clear, sterile fluid confined within a fibrous pseudomembrane is a distinct clinicopathologic entity. Four cases of perigraft seroma involving both Dacron and polytetrafluoroethylene (PTFE) grafts were encountered, and 275 previously unreported cases were reviewed. The latter were provided by 165 surgeons who were among 320 who responded to a questionnaire.

About half the cases involved axillofemoral and bifemoral grafts. Knitted Dacron was involved in 55% of cases and PTFE in 34%. Six autogenous vein grafts were reported to be affected. Perigraft swelling was seen within 1 month after operation in one fourth of cases. The middle and distal thirds of the grafts were most often involved. Only 1 of 45 patients who had cultures had positive results. Operative removal of the pseudocyst without graft excision carried an infection rate of 12%. The effects of instilling tetracycline and other nontoxic substances were unpredictable. Removal and replacement of the graft provided a cure in 92% of instances. Replacement with a prosthesis of different material seemed to be preferable. Observation alone was associated with cyst resolution in two thirds of 22 cases. Histologic study of the surgical specimens showed no secretory cells in the inner lining, which consisted of fibrous tissue. Inflammatory cells were not abundant.

Perigraft seroma complicating an arterial graft should be removed with the original graft, which should be replaced by a graft of different material, rerouted through a new anatomical route if feasible. Observation or multiple aspirations may be tried in poor-risk patients. Avoidance of wetting of PTFE grafts, and nontraumatic tunneling may be helpful. Areas of cyst excision should be drained with soft, sump-type drains and antibiotic prophylaxis given. Prosthetic angulation should be avoided, especially near anastomoses.

Vascular Graft Infection: Analysis of 62 Graft Infections in 2,411 Consecutive Implanted Synthetic Vascular Grafts

J. E. Lorentzen, O. M. Nielsen, H. Arendrup, H. H. Kimose, S. Bille, J. Andersen, C. H. Jensen, F. Jacobsen, and O. C. Røder

Surgery 98:81–86, July 1985 7–122

Sixty-two graft infections occurred among 2,411 consecutive arterial reconstructive procedures done in Denmark in a 4-year period, using synthetic prosthetic materials, for an incidence of 2.6%. Incidence rates were similar in cases of occlusive atherosclerotic disease and abdominal aortic aneurysm. Graft infections occurred only when the groin had been incised. More peripheral reconstructions seemed to be associated more often with graft infection. Predisposing factors were identified in 50 patients; the most frequent were poor surgical technique producing wound complications, reoperation, and long-lasting bowel paralysis. About half the infections occurred within 1 month of operation. The infection appeared in the femoral wound in three fourths of cases. Gram-positive cocci were isolated in 70% of cases.

Treatment ranged from local wound care and systemic antibiotic therapy to graft excision with immediate revascularization. Conservative measures failed in several bifurcation graft cases. Graft excision consistently ended the infection. Mortality from graft infection was 26%, and the amputation rate was 31%. Two patients had chronic infections with fistulas to the prosthesis. The cure rate was 40%. An average of 1.4 operations was done.

An incidence of graft infection of about 2% is acceptable in most vascular surgery centers. More emphasis on nontraumatic surgical technique is needed, particularly in making groin incisions. A rational prophylactic antibiotic regimen is essential, as are improved antiseptic precautions. The authors presently use cephalosporin and ampicillin in combination for prophylaxis.

▶ Synthetic graft complications continue to be a challenge to vascular surgeons. Perigraft seroma is an entity that must not be confused with an infected graft.

Should inguinal nodes be cultured in all bypass procedures?

A study similar to culture of the contents of the abdominal aortic aneurysm should be done to establish the role of infected nodes in the pathogenesis of infected grafts.

The Optimal Contrast Material for Digital Subtraction Angiography of the Renal Arteries: Ionic or Nonionic?

Kerry K. Ford, Glenn E. Newman, and N. Reed Dunnick (Duke Univ.)
Invest. Radiol. (Suppl.) 19:S244–S246, Sept.–Oct. 1984 7–123

Digital intravenous subtraction angiography (DISA) is now the screening procedure of choice for renal artery stenosis at many centers. Nonionic contrast materials are better tolerated by patients, and they are less toxic than conventional ionic materials. Their role in DISA was examined in a double-blind comparison of the nonionic contrast material iopamidol with the conventional ionic medium meglumine sodium diatrizoate in 84 patients undergoing renal artery DISA. Patients older than age 18 years received iopamidol, 370 mg of iodine per ml, iopamidol, 300 mg of iodine per ml, or diatrizoate, 370 of iodine per ml, via the antecubital fossa or a superior or inferior vena cava catheter. A 40-ml volume of contrast was used. Only 4 of the 84 patients received central contrast injections.

None of the groups had significant changes in pulse, blood pressure, or serum creatinine concentration. No significant electrocardiographic abnormalities were seen in the 59 patients monitored. One diatrizoate-treated patient with extravasation had pain. Image qualities were comparable in all groups on average, but substantially more patients in the iopamidol 370 group had excellent images. All 10 adverse reactions were minor; nausea, vomiting, or both, was most frequent. All but 1 of these reactions occurred in diatrizoate-treated patients.

The nonionic contrast material iopamidol can produce better images than diatrizoate in renal DISA, with less patient discomfort and fewer adverse reactions. Nonionic contrast material may be superior to conventional ionic material in DISA. The better image qualty obtained with iopamidol in this study was not attributable to decreased patient motion.

Outpatient Arteriography: Its Safety and Cost Effectiveness

Donald A. Wolfel, Bruce P. Lovett, Arthur I. Ortenburger, Lawrence S. Johnson, and David L. Sommerville (Presbyterian Hosp., Albuquerque, N.M.)
Radiology 153:363–364, November 1984 7–124

Invasive arteriography has long been deemed an in-hospital procedure because of the fear of potential complications that might be dealt with inadequately in an outpatient environment and the fear of medicolegal consequences. In an 11-year period 2,029 outpatient arteriograms were performed at this 500-bed community hospital with active vascular and cardiovascular services.

Each patient is interviewed personally or by telephone before the procedure is scheduled. To avoid dehydration, oral fluids are encouraged the morning of an early-morning procedure, and a light breakfast with emphasis on fluids is encouraged for late-morning or early-afternoon procedures.

Angiography is performed only by experienced angiographers. Catheters range in size from 5 F to 8 F. After stable hemostasis is achieved at the puncture site, outpatients are observed for approximately 3 hours. At discharge patients are instructed to remain quiet at home for the remainder of the day and to resume normal, nonstrenuous activities the next day.

A total of 5,893 arteriograms were performed from July 1972 through June 1983; 2,029 were done as outpatient and 3,864 as inpatient procedures. Multiple areas of the body were studied as part of the same outpatient procedure, i.e., aortic arch, brachiocephalic vessels, abdominal aorta, and femoral runoff arteries. There were 39 major complications (0.66%); 33 occurred in inpatients (0.85%) and 6 occurred in outpatients (0.30%). Total dollar savings for all outpatient arteriograms was estimated at more than $702,000. No malpractice litigation arose as a result of outpatient arteriography.

The authors encourage the use of conventional arteriography on an outpatient basis because it can be done safely and economically, and it provides images that are generally of higher quality than those obtained with digital subtraction angiography, which is emerging as a less costly and less invasive vascular procedure. Furthermore, the patient's understanding of the procedure and rapport with the angiographer is better in outpatients.

Renal Dysfunction After Arteriography

Robert A. Mason, Leonard A. Arbeit, and Fabio Giron (SUNY at Stony Brook)
JAMA 253:1001–1004, Feb. 15, 1985 7–125

Acute renal failure has complicated diagnostic angiography in a small proportion of cases, but the incidence of subclinical renal dysfunction precipitated by contrast angiography is uncertain. The effects of hyperosmotic contrast medium were assessed in a prospective study of males undergoing 120 angiographic procedures. Average age was 62 years. Most studies involved the abdominal aorta and runoff. Diabetes was present in 28% of patients and hypertension in 38%. Baseline creatine clearance was less than 60 ml per minute in 26%.

Creatinine clearance was reduced by 25% or more after 31% of procedures. Reductions were similar in patients with baseline serum creatinine concentrations of 1.5 mg/dl or above and those with lower values, and depressed creatinine clearance did not increase the risk of renal dysfunction after angiography. Diabetics had a more depressed renal function at baseline, but the group did not have a higher rate of dysfunction after angiography. Hypertension and a higher dose of contrast also were not associated with an increased risk of renal dysfunction after angiography. Multiple contrast injections into the abdominal aorta, however, were associated with an increased risk. Only 4 patients had overt oliguric renal failure after angiography. Each had a baseline creatinine clearance of less than 50 ml per minute. One patient died of sepsis, and another continued to have renal dysfunction. All 9 patients with subclinical dysfunction who were followed had baseline creatinine clearance values within 1 week.

Up to a third of patients may have a 25% or greater fall in creatinine clearance after arterial angiography. A combination of the hemodynamic effects of hyperosmolar contrast material and direct toxic effects may be responsible. Renal function should be assessed before angiography and patients at risk of oliguric renal failure monitored after the study. A well-hydrated patient is at lower risk of renal dysfunction. Contrast injections should be minimized, especially in azotemic patients undergoing abdominal aortic studies.

▶ As 31% of patients studied by Mason et al. sustained a significant reduction in creatinine clearance after arteriography, this should alert surgeons not to use outpatient arteriography indiscriminately. Outpatient arteriography is cost effective, but it should not be used in those patients who are at risk of developing renal failure.

Unfortunately, the cost of nonionic contrast media makes it prohibitive for routine use. Otherwise, it is relatively pain-free, which should make it an ideal contrast material.

Epidural Electric Stimulation in Severe Limb Ischemia: Pain Relief, Increased Blood Flow, and a Possible Limb-Saving Effect

Lars E. Augustinsson, Carl A. Carlsson, Jan Holm, and Lennart Jivegård (Univ. of Göteborg)

Ann. Surg. 202:104–110, July 1985 7–126

A way to relieve pain and improve blood flow is needed for elderly patients with severe atherosclerosis in whom vascular surgery has failed or is not feasible. Epidural spinal electric stimulation (ESES) was evaluated in 34 patients seen since 1978 with severe limb ischemia and rest pain in whom arterial surgery was technically impossible. The 21 men and 13 women had an average age of 64 years. Twenty-six patients had atherosclerosis, 5 in association with diabetes. Seven patients had severe vasospastic disorders, and 1 had Buerger's disease. Most patients had ischemic ulcers, and some had partial gangrene at the time ESES was begun. Operation had previously failed in many patients. The electrode was placed epidurally with fluoroscopic control and a Touhy needle, and the radio receiver was placed in a subcutaneous pouch above a costal arch and connected to the electrode via a subcutaneous extension. Patients were taught to use the radio transmitter at a voltage producing comfortable paresthesias in the affected limb.

Most patients used the stimulator for 2-hour periods at 2-hour intervals during the day; some used it continuously. All but 6% of patients had a reduction in pain during stimulation. Vasospastic patients had the most improvement. Morphine use was no longer necessary in most instances. Skin ulcers healed in many patients. Ten arteriosclerotic or diabetic patients had amputations during follow-up. Digital blood pressures increased with stimulation. There was one infectious complication. Repositioning of the electrode or lead exchange was necessary in 6 patients.

Epidural electric stimulation is a promising means of relieving symptoms of severe limb ischemia where a reconstructive operation is not feasible. Pain relief is the main benefit, but favorable effects on wound healing are also evident. The procedure may avoid the need for amputation in some cases. The mechanisms involved in the beneficial effects of ESES remain to be clarified.

▶ This article should be of interest to "inoperable surgeons."

Restenosis Following Transluminal Angioplasty in Experimental Atherosclerosis

David P. Faxon, Timothy A. Sanborn, Vance J. Weber, Christian Haudenschild, Susan B. Gottsman, Wanda A. McGovern, and Thomas J. Ryan (Boston)

Arteriosclerosis 4:189–195, May–June 1984 7–127

Considerable attention has been given to the use of percutaneous transluminal angioplasty in the treatment of obstructive atherosclerotic lesions. However, restenosis often occurs, thus limiting the long-term effectiveness of this approach. To study the process by which angioplasty may induce restenosis, a model of atherosclerosis was developed in 16 New Zealand rabbits. Balloon deendothelialization and administration of a diet containing 2% cholesterol were used for 6 weeks to induce atherosclerosis in 1 or both iliac vessels.

Angiography performed after the 6-week period showed a narrowing of the luminal diameter by 0.7–1.8 mm. In 9 iliac vessels, transluminal angioplasty was successful, increasing the luminal diameter by a mean of 0.9 mm ($P < .01$). After an additional 4 weeks of using a high-cholesterol diet, all animals were again studied by angiography; significant progression of disease was seen in only 6 of 14 control vessels, but in all 9 dilated vessels. Compared with the diameter at initial angiography, the control vessels were not changed significantly, whereas the dilated vessels decreased in size by an average of 1.6 mm ($P < .01$). Histopathologic examination of the dilated segment at 4 weeks revealed a pattern of fibrocellular tissue suggestive of the original neointimal tears, with the spaces filled by abundant loose connective tissue that was lipid-rich and edematous; a new fibrocellular cap was seen creating a further occlusive process. Other patterns included a multilaminated neointimal process with layers of loose connective tissue and lipid alternating with more dense fibrocellular tissue. Varying degrees of thrombus formation were noted in 5 animals. All but 1 of these thrombi occurred in totally occluded vessels, whereas thrombus was seen in only 1 of the 14 control vessels ($P < .01$).

Thus, restenosis can occur after transluminal angioplasty and may occur more frequently than in the natural progression of disease in a rabbit model of atherosclerosis. This process appears to be related to intraluminal thrombosis and acceleration of atherosclerosis. Studies to evaluate the effectiveness of antiplatelet drug treatment in the prevention of restenosis would seem warranted.

Outcome of a Failed Percutaneous Transluminal Dilation

P. G. Kalman and K. W. Johnston (Univ. of Toronto)
Surg. Gynecol. Obstet. 161:43–46, July 1985 7–128

Percutaneous transluminal dilation (TLD) has been successfully used to treat patients with peripheral arterial occlusive disease, but the consequences of failure are uncertain. A total of 631 dilations performed between 1978 and 1983 were reviewed. Of the 223 failures, 198 were followed for at least 6 months. The patients who did well after TLD and those in whom the procedure failed were generally comparable, but there were relatively more femoropopliteal and fewer aortoiliac cases in the failure group. Failure occurred shortly after the procedure or during follow-up in 175 cases. Twenty-three failures occurred when the balloon catheter could not be passed through the stenosis.

No change in clinical grade occurred in 85% of failed cases. Improvement occurred in 5.5% of cases, and 9.5% of patients were worse. The average ankle-brachial systolic pressure ratios were 0.53 before and 0.54 after TLD. Dilation was repeated in 18% of cases, whereas 29% of patients underwent arterial reconstruction. The results of repeat TLD were not different from the overall results. All 12 amputations were in patients who had TLD for advanced ischemia and were considered to result from the ischemia.

Percutaneous transluminal dilation is a relatively safe procedure that can be considered as an alternative to operation in selected cases of peripheral arterial disease. No limb losses were attributed directly to the procedure in this series. The early results of operation after failed TLD are similar to those obtained in patients who have not previously undergone dilation.

Percutaneous Transluminal Angioplasty of the Arteries of the Lower Limbs: A 5-Year Follow-Up

A. Gallino, F. Mahler, P. Probst, and B. Nachbur (Univ. of Bern, Switzerland)
Circulation 70:619–623, October 1984 7–129

Data were reviewed concerning 482 percutaneous transluminal angioplasties (PTAs) of the lower limbs performed on 411 patients between 1977 and 1983. Initially, 134 iliac PTAs and 251 femoral PTAs were successful, the early patency rates being 95% and 87%, respectively. The patency rates at 1 year were 86% for iliac PTA and 61% for femoral PTA, and the corresponding rates at 5 years were 83% and 58%, respectively.

As percentages of initially successful, rather than of attempted, procedures, 5-year patency rates were 87% for iliac PTA and 67% for femoral PTA. The impression of clinical improvement was confirmed by a significant reduction in the mean arm-ankle pressure difference from 48 mm Hg before to 17 mm Hg 2 years after iliac PTA ($P < .01$), and from 73 mm Hg before to 28 mm Hg 2 years after femoropopliteal PTA ($P < .01$). Of the 140 patients who underwent femoral PTA, 61% initially had claudication and 39% had pain at rest or gangrene. Two years later, 69% were without symptoms, 23% had claudication, and only 8% had pain at rest or gangrene. Most occlusions occurred within the first year after PTA. Stenoses or occlusions of less than 3 cm had an associated favorable long-term patency rate of 74%. In contrast, patients with femoropopliteal occlusions who had pain at rest, diabetes, occlusions of more than 3 cm in size, or poor distal runoff had an increased rate of reocclusion. Complications, occurring in 8% of all patients, included local hemorrhage, dissection, embolism, and spasm requiring surgical intervention. After redilatation was performed in 52 patients, the 2-year patency rate was similar to that seen after primary PTA. There were no deaths directly attributable to PTA. The use of PTA in the lower limbs may be regarded as a valid complementary procedure to vascular surgery in patients with occlusive disease of the peripheral arteries.

▶ How good is percutaneous transluminal angioplasty for arterial occlusive disease? It appears that failure of such procedures when done by experienced operators does not worsen the condition in the vast majority of patients.

In successful percutaneous transluminal angioplasty, 5-year follow-up yields a respectable patency rate, especially in the iliac artery. Perhaps a more liberal use of antiplatelet drugs may prevent restenosis, as demonstrated in the animal study.

On the Nervous Control of Collateral Arterial Tone in the Human Lower Limb With Large-Artery Obstruction During Postural Change

Kim Agerskov (Copenhagen)

Dan. Med. Bull. 31:316–329, August 1984 7–130

The effects of postural changes and muscular exercise in the upright position on resistance in collateral arteries in patients with chronic occlusive arterial disease of the legs are uncertain. These effects were examined in patients who represented difficult management problems for vascular surgery. Catheters were placed in the brachial artery, the common femoral artery and vein, and the popliteal artery and vein. Blood flow in the common femoral artery was measured by the indicator dilution technique.

In 15 limbs with superficial femoral artery occlusion and in 6 with superficial femoral or external iliac stenosis, a reduction in flow caused an equal drop in pressure gradient over the collaterals where only a few collateral vessels were present in association with stenosis. With occlusion and many collaterals, however, head-up tilt did not alter the pressure gradient over the collateral arteries. Studies of acute central sympathetic blockade with carbocaine suggested that central sympathetic outflow contributes to the tone in collateral arteries under supine resting conditions. Studies with phentolamine indicated that collateral tone is largely influenced by changes in neurogenically mediated α-receptor stimulation. β-Receptor blockade with propranolol led to augmented collateral tone in the supine position. Heel-raising exercise blocked the augmented neurogenically mediated constriction of the collaterals in the upright position in patients with superficial femoral occlusion.

Collateral vessels in the thigh that bypass a large-artery occlusion constrict when the erect position is assumed. Collateral tone is determined chiefly by centrally elicited sympathetic α-adrenergic activity. Redistribution of blood flow makes it unlikely that lumbar sympathectomy will improve perfusion in ischemic vascular beds in the foot. Collateral resistance is reduced but not abolished during muscular exercise. Further studies are needed to determine the effect of β-receptor blockade on the exercise-induced fall in collateral arterial resistance.

Local Regulation of Subcutaneous Forefoot Blood Flow During Orthostatic Changes in Normal Subjects, in Sympathetically Denervated Patients, and in Patients With Occlusive Arterial Disease

Jens H. Eickhoff and Ole Henriksen (Copenhagen)

Cardiovasc. Res. 19:219–227, April 1985 7–131

Orthostatic changes in local blood flow in the forefoot were examined by the radioxenon washout method in 21 normal subjects, in 39 patients with atherosclerotic changes in the lower limbs, and in 6 sympathetically denervated legs in 5 patients. One of the patients in the last group had Shy Drager syndrome; the rest had had lumbar sympathectomy.

Blood flow was decreased 36% in normal limbs when the foot was lowered 40 cm below the heart. Flow remained unchanged on elevation to 20 cm, and decreased only 10% on further elevation to 40 cm, corresponding to a 15% decrease in vascular resistance. Blood flow decreased only 6% in the sympathetically denervated limbs. Autoregulation was preserved. Blood flow decreased 19% in extremities with intermittent claudication from atherosclerosis. Vascular resistance was not, however, significantly different from normal when the added increase in arterial pressure was taken into account. Autoregulation was preserved in these extremities. In limbs with pain on resting, blood flow rose 28% on lowering. Vascular resistance increased 21% when the added rise in arterial pressure was taken into account. Blood flow fell significantly on elevation; estimated vascular resistance did not decrease significantly.

Local blood flow in the subcutaneous tissues of the lower extremity is regulated by a local vasoconstrictor response during lowering, and by autoregulation of flow during elevation. The findings provide reason to discourage exercise training in patients with rest pain or low distal blood pressures.

Effects of Increased Tissue Pressure on Regional Blood Flow in the Lower Limb of Man

Henrik Vagn Nielsen (Univ. of Copenhagen, Denmark)

Dan. Med. J. 31:425–438, December 1984 7–132

Most clinical studies relating tissue pressure to regional blood flow have used external pressure on an extremity level with the heart; in the upright position, however, blood pressure is passively increased in the dependent limb, and dynamic muscular exercise also may be a factor. Vascular adjustments to increased tissue pressure in a lower limb were examined, using the local radioxenon washout technique to assess flow separately in the superficial and subfascial compartments. Thirty-seven healthy subjects, aged 22–40 years, participated in the study. Both indirect and direct arterial pressure recordings were obtained. Dynamic muscular exercise was performed by heel-raisings.

The precapillary vessels collapsed with cessation of blood flow. When diastolic backflow in the inflow vessels was prevented by inflating a cuff, the vascular bed was distended and flow reappeared in the formerly ischemic subcutaneous and skeletal-muscle tissues. Autoregulation was evident when the arterial pressure was reduced by 30 mm Hg. External compression of the leg was associated with postcapillary collapse, indicating increased flow resistance in the subcutaneous tissues. Subfascial flow in the calf was greatly increased in exercising legs in head-up tilted subjects, chiefly because of a reduction in subfascial venous pressure, thus eliminating the arteriolar constrictor effect of the veno-arterial reflex mechanism.

It is diastolic pressure that underlies microcirculatory blood flow in severe arterial hypotension or severe vascular compression. Arterial compression may play a role in compartment syndromes. Compression of an elevated limb may be hazardous in patients with severe arterial insufficiency.

Circumferential Skin Blood Flow Measurements in the Ischemic Limb

P. T. McCollum, V. A. Spence, and W. F. Walker (Dundee, Scotland)

Br. J. Surg. 72:310–312, April 1985 7–133

Circumferential differences in skin blood flow (SBF) around the ischemic extremity could invalidate the results of the Kety method of measuring flow. Measurements of SBF were made in conjunction with Doppler ankle pressure measurements at multiple sites in the lower extremity in 47 consecutive patients referred for assessment of amputation level. All had critical ischemia. The average age was 73 years. Sixteen patients were diabetic. Skin blood flow was estimated at the posterior, medial, and lateral aspects of the lower limb by the iodoantipyrine clearance technique. A dose of 0.1 mBq of ^{125}I-4-iodoantipyrine was deposited intradermally at each site.

The mean SBF was 9.0 ml/100 gm per minute at the medial site, 8.3 ml posteriorly, and 6.5 ml laterally. The values obtained on the medial and posterior aspects of the leg were significantly higher than those at the lateral site. Patients with the most extreme ischemia and SBF values of less than 3 ml usually had greater medial than lateral SBF values, and medial values were also greater than posterior values in most instances. Values for SBF generally did not correlate well with presenting symptoms. Ankle pressures did not correlate closely with SBF values at any of the sites. Four below-knee amputations failed to heal, 1 because of skin flap ischemia. The posterior SBF in this case was less than 1 ml/100 gm per minute.

Measurements of SBF in the medial and posterior aspects of the ischemic leg are higher than in the lateral aspect of the leg. It seems wise to obtain at least three SBF measurements at different sites in the ischemic leg. The time needed is worthwhile if above-knee amputations can be reduced without increasing morbidity. A more medially based posterior flap might be useful in below-knee amputations in certain cases. Bypass grafting could conceivably prejudice the outcome of below-knee amputation by interrupting small vessels on the medial side of the knee.

▶ In calcified arteries, the use of Doppler pressure measurement will be invalid to determine the level of amputation. Blood flow measurement, as suggested by McCollum et al., is of interest. Unfortunately, the complexity of the measurement will not lend itself to a routine study. Nevertheless, the importance of a more medially based posterior flap to ensure complete healing in the performance of below-knee amputation should be kept in mind.

The effect of increased tissue pressure on orthostatic changes in blood flow has received little attention. Reports by Danish workers, especially on rest pain, are of interest. Relief of rest pain in the dependent position is due to an increase in arterial pressure rather than to dilatation of arterioles.

Multiple Arterial Lesions Associated With Von Recklinghausen's Disease: One Case

C. Debure, J. N. Fiessinger, P. Bruneval, N. P. Vuong, J. M. Cormier, and E. Housset (Paris)

Presse Med. 13:1776–1778, July 1984 7–134

Arterial lesions are believed to be rare in neurofibromatosis. However, full vascular exploration showed diffuse lesions in many arteries in one case studied.

Woman, 36, diagnosed with neurofibromatosis in 1977, was hospitalized in May 1982 for treatment of hypertension from which she had been suffering since the age of 16. Vascular involvement was suspected because of periumbilical abdominal and right femoral souffles, a dampening of the right femoral pulse, and the absence of the posterior tibial and foot pulses. Arterial pressure was 160/100 mm Hg. Aortography and arteriography of the lower extremities revealed stenosing lesions affecting the subdiaphragmatic aorta, right common iliac, right hypogastric, and left renal arteries. In the legs, only the peroneal artery on the right side and the anterior tibial artery on the left side were visible to the feet. Aneurysmal lesions were found at the juxtahilar splenic and left renal arteries and at the bifurcation of the right common iliac artery. Numerical angiography of the supra-aortic trunks with intracranial views revealed a voluminous aneurysm of the left carotid axis.

Revascularization of the renal arteries did not appear justified; nevertheless, in view of possible decompensation of the arterial hypertension, an exploratory laparotomy was performed to verify the state of the aortic wall. The arterial lesions were confirmed, and yet the aorta appeared macroscopically normal and there were no intra-abdominal neurofibromas. A splenectomy and an excision of the splenic aneurysm were performed. Histologic study of the splenic artery, macroscopically normal, revealed changes that suggested medial fibrodysplasia.

The originality in this case was the diffusion of lesions involving the intracranial carotid, subrenal aorta, renal and iliac arteries, and also, what is most original, the extremity axes. Other than a moderate hypertension, these different localizations were asymptomatic. This leads to the proposal that arteriographic exploration of the principal regions be conducted whenever vascular involvement is discovered in the course of von Recklinghausen's disease since the discovery of other localizations will influence the choice of therapy. Such was the case here, where the renal revascularization, initially proposed, was abandoned because of the potential risk to the intracranial lesion.

Surgery for Arteritis After 70 Years of Age

P. Langeron, G. Mahieu, M. H. Gohier, P. Puppinck, and Ph. Patenotre (Lomme, France)

J. Chir. (Paris) 121:437–442, June–July 1984 7–135

The authors analyzed data from 176 cases from a larger group of 385 after excluding lumbar sympathectomies and operations for ruptured aortic aneurysms. There were 21 operations at the aortoiliac level, 119 at the subinguinal level, and 36 atypical grafts.

One of the questions that can be posed for aged patients is whether an amputation is not preferable to a complex operation when the chance for success is not assured. In this series, the comparison between early and secondary death after immediate amputation and surgical restoration was convincing. The mortality was doubled after amputation. Furthermore, the mortality after secondary amputation (i.e., after failure of a salvage attempt) was far less than that following immediate amputation. These data argue persuasively in favor of conservative operation.

The results of the restorative surgical procedure were broken down according to the type of operation. Among the 21 arterial reconstructions at the aortoiliac level, good medium-range results were obtained in 80.9% of the cases, although it must be noted that this operation was reserved for patients in good general condition. At the subinguinal level, the failure rate including deaths and amputations was higher, but good results were obtained in 66.3% of the 119 cases. Atypical grafts (i.e., axillofemoral or crossed femorofemoral grafts) performed on elderly patients or patients in bad condition who could not tolerate direct aortoiliac operation, yielded a higher rate of primary or secondary mortality and of secondary amputations. However, 55.5% of the 36 patients obtained beneficial medium-term results.

The authors attribute the improvement in mortality to the use of peridural and spinal anesthesia and to use of two operating teams that resulted in the percentage of immediate amputations falling from 32.3% in 1978–1979 to 17.3% in 1981–1982. This maximum conservatism was accompanied by more frequent placement of grafts at peripheral sites.

New Aspects of Thromboangiitis Obliterans (Von Winiwarter-Buerger's Disease)

P. Berlit, C. Kessler, R. Reuther, and K.-H. Krause (Heidelberg)
Eur. Neurol. 23:394–399, Nov.–Dec. 1984 7–136

The status of thromboangiitis obliterans as a clinical entity has long been debated despite reports of several typical features, including a predilection for young men, the frequent inclusion of hand and wrist vessels in the inflammatory process, a close association with cigarette smoking, and accompanying migratory superficial thrombophlebitis. The distinctive noninflammatory form of arteriosclerosis in this condition is especially problematic, as is the cerebral form of thromboangiitis obliterans. The lack of organ involvement contrasts with most other immunovasculitides; and relapsing brain infarctions can occur that are visualizable by computed tomography while arteriography remains negative.

Apart from nonspecific inflammatory features in the blood and cerebrospinal fluid, laboratory findings can be obtained that indicate the autoimmune nature of the disease. Antielastin antibodies, IgE, and anticollagen antibody activity are detectable in serum. The authors found specific immunohistologic changes in temporal artery biopsy specimens from 3 patients, suggesting that such procedures could be diagnostically helpful in young stroke patients.

Hence the cerebral form of von Winiwarter-Buerger's disease is an entity. In addition to platelet-inhibitors, corticoid therapy is used in acute cases and azathioprine for long-term treatment. Smoking is forbidden.

Takayasu Arteritis: A Study of 32 North American Patients

Stephen Hall, W. Barr, J. T. Lie, A. W. Stanson, F. J. Kazmier, and G. G. Hunder (Mayo Clinic)
Medicine (Baltimore) 64:89–99, March 1985 7–137

Takayasu arteritis is a chronic inflammatory arteriopathic condition of unknown cause that affects large vessels, including the aorta and its main branches. The disorder typically affects young Oriental women, although it may present differently in different countries. The findings in 32 patients in North America, 23 of them Caucasian, were reviewed. Only 3 subjects were of Oriental descent. Patients older than age 50 years and those with known causes of vasculitis were excluded. Median interval from initial symptoms to diagnosis was 18 months.

Systemic features such as fever, weight loss, and malaise were frequent. Fifteen patients had symptoms of vascular insufficiency in the upper limbs, usually arm claudication. All but 2 patients had multiple vascular bruits, most often in the carotid artery and abdominal aorta. Sixteen patients had no pulse. Postural dizziness was significant in 39% of patients. Five patients had symptoms of ischemic heart disease. Aortic incompetence was noted in 3 cases. Thirteen patients were hypertensive initially as were 5 others on follow-up. Arthralgias and myalgias were frequently described. Mild anemia and moderate thrombocytosis were common findings. Angiographic abnormalities were most frequent in the left subclavian and superior mesenteric arteries and in the abdominal aorta.

All but 3 patients received steroid therapy, and systemic inflammatory symptoms improved greatly in all treated patients. The sedimentation rate was helpful in monitoring treatment. Twelve patients had surgical treatment, with mostly satisfactory results. One of 16 patients died of aortic rupture during a median follow-up period of 5 years. Another death resulted from pneumonia 8 years after diagnosis. Twenty of 27 patients evaluated were working full time with minimal disability. No patient experienced heart failure or stroke after diagnosis. Seven patients had significant functional impairment related to angina, limb claudication, or steroid therapy.

Takayasu arteritis is more frequent in North America than previously thought. It is treated with steroids and vascular reconstruction.

Adventitial Cystic Disease of the Popliteal Artery

Andrew C. Wilbur, George F. Woelfel, Joseph P. Meyer, D. Preston Flanigan, and Dimitrios G. Spigos (Univ. of Illinois)

Radiology 155:63–64, April 1985 7–138

The primary diagnostic considerations in a young adult with calf claudication are adventitial cystic disease of the popliteal artery and popliteal entrapment syndrome. The former disorder is characterized by formation of a mucin-containing cyst in the popliteal artery wall in a patient whose arteries are otherwise normal.

Man, 26, had sudden onset of mild cramping pain in the left lower leg, followed by nonprogressive intermittent calf claudication for 6 weeks before admission. Popliteal, posterior tibial, and dorsalis pedis pulses were absent in the left leg. Aortoileofemoral angiography by a right femoral approach showed a smooth crescentic obstruction of the proximal left popliteal artery (Fig 7–32). Computed tomography with brachial contrast infusion showed a cyst-like mass producing eccentric compression of the arterial lumen (Fig 7–33). Real-time sonography showed a fusiform mass with the arterial lumen narrowly patent at times. The mass contained scattered low-level echoes. A radiologic diagnosis of adventitial cystic disease of the popliteal artery was made.

Computed tomography showed eccentric luminal compression by a thin-walled mass having an enhanced rim in this case. The mass was intrinsic to the artery and expanded its outer contour. This lesion presumably represents a form of ganglion associated with the knee joint. Surgical aspiration or incisional evacuation of the cyst generally is done when the artery remains patent, or resection and grafting are carried out when it is occluded.

▶ In the treatment of vascular problems, vascular surgeons should be familiar with nonatherosclerotic causes of arterial occlusive disease. Because of changes in the immigration pattern, it is expected that Takayasu arteritis will be seen often in North America.

The diagnosis of Buerger's disease has always been questioned. Recently the role of an abnormal immunologic response was implicated as a contributing factor rather than smoking alone. Immunologic testing, such as cellular sensitivity to human type I or type III collagen, may help to understand the etiologic factor in Buerger's disease (Adam et al.: *N. Engl. J. Med.* 308:1113, 1983). Popliteal cystic disease can now be diagnosed in claudicants by a CT scan.

Finally, the busy vascular service of Dr. J. M. Cormier has called attention to a rare form of arterial lesions in von Recklinghausen's disease.

Fig 7–32.—Upper popliteal artery is obstructed by a smooth indentation along its lateral aspect. Note the crescentic or "scimitar"-like contour of the obstructing mass, its obtuse upper and lower margins, and the meniscus-shaped tapering of the arterial lumen. This was a classic appearance of popliteal adventitial cysts. (Courtesy of Wilbur, A.C., et al.: Radiology 155:63–64, April 1985.)

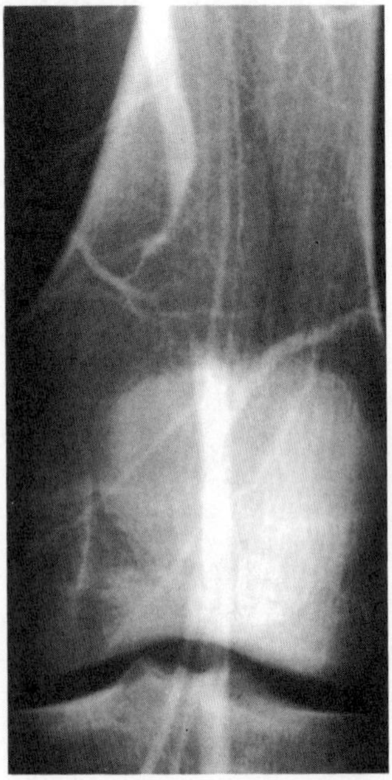

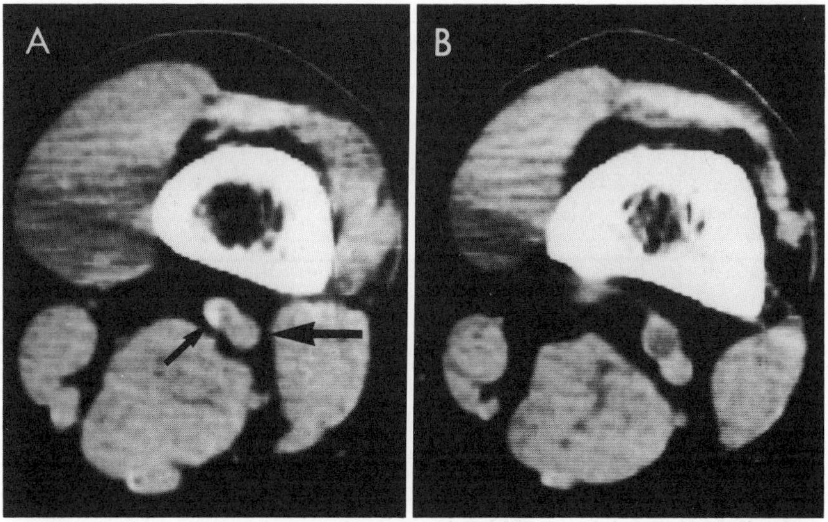

Fig 7–33.—Contrast-medium-enhanced transverse computed tomographic sections at the level of the upper (**A**) and middle (**B**) portions of the cyst. **A**, there is narrowing of the lumen by the upper margin of the cyst. *Large arrow,* popliteal vein; *small arrow,* popliteal artery. **B**, cyst expands the enhanced adventitial perimeter of the artery. (Courtesy of Wilbur, A.C., et al.: Radiology 155:63–64, April 1985.)

Arterial Thromboembolism: A 20-Year Perspective

Roy L. Tawes, Jr., Edmund J. Harris, William H. Brown, Perry M. Shoor, James J. Zimmerman, Gerald R. Sydorak, John P. Beare, Robert G. Scribner, and Thomas J. Fogarty

Arch. Surg. 120:595–599, May 1985 7–139

Review was made of 739 patients with peripheral lower limb thromboembolism who had been treated since the introduction of the Fogarty balloon catheter (1963). Embolism was responsible for potential limb loss in more than 90% of cases. Men predominated in a ratio of about 3 to 2. Mean age was 66 years. Embolic obstruction was most frequent in the femoral artery. Thirty-five patients had bilateral or saddle emboli. A total of 161 secondary operations was performed in 135 patients after embolectomy. Forty-four patients received direct treatment for a cardiac source of emboli.

Patient mortality was 12%, and the limb salvage rate was 95%. Heparin was used after embolectomy later in the series. Additional surgery did not result in major limb amputations or deaths. About 80% of deaths were due to cardiopulmonary dysfunction, mostly myocardial infarction. Wound complications were a serious problem in 56 patients. Thirty-eight patients required evacuation of a large hematoma to prevent wound dehiscence, infection, or skin necrosis.

These improved results would seem to justify an aggressive approach to peripheral arterial thromboembolism. Combined embolectomy and heparin administration is recommended as primary treatment. The results presented here are attributed to appropriate patient selection, early diagnosis, correction of underlying sources of emboli, and secondary operative procedures where necessary.

Symptoms and Therapy of Embolism of the Aortic Bifurcation
W. Bätz and R. Brückner (Univ. of Mainz)
Chirurg 56:166–169, March 1985 7–140

Acute aortic bifurcation embolism is rare among arterial occlusions of the extremities, whereas chronic obstructions of the terminal aorta are frequent. Because of specific clinical symptoms, relatively high mortality, and amputation rates after embolectomy, acute aortic embolisation deserves special attention.

Thirty-one patients underwent embolectomy for acute embolism of the aortic bifurcation. In most instances paraplegia (84%) was present. Neurologic disease had been considered in 55%. The heart was the source of embolism in 92%. Postoperative complications were mainly due to renal failure (23%) and irreversible extremity ischemia (10%) requiring amputation. In 3 patients irreversible muscle necrosis made amputation necessary as a second operation. Two patients developed a new occlusion and had successful reembolectomy following which the circulation remained open. Mortality after embolism to the bifurcation was 39%. The major cause of death was cardiac failure (58%) followed by renal failure and pulmonary embolism.

According to the literature the main source of embolism is arteriosclerotic rather than rheumatic (in this study, 68% and 24%, respectively). Ten percent of emboli locate at the bifurcation.

Isolated arterial embolism of the extremities is often characterized by ischemic muscle pain, and the history and absent pulse makes an on-the-spot diagnosis. Pain was observed in 100% of patients, and paralysis of the extremity was present in only 27%. With bifurcation embolism, the authors frequently observed signs of striking weakness to paralysis and simultaneously developing numbness. Unless suspicion of a chronic block or an incomplete embolus causing a distinct palpable pulse suggests low-grade ischemia, a noninvasive digital subtraction angiography can replace conventional angiography.

Intraoperative angiography is recommended for control and documentation of results of embolectomy and is requisite when intraoperatively an adequate blood supply cannot be assured. Because of relatively mild and uncharacteristic symptoms of bifurcation embolism, especially by incomplete occlusion, only 13% of the patients are diagnosed correctly. The interval between embolism and therapy is a deciding factor. The duration of the circulatory interruption is especially important in embolic occlusions since the collateral circulation is not developed as well as in chronic occlusion. Even after a long delay (4 weeks), successful operation is possible when adequate collateral circulation is supplying the extremity.

▶ These two papers present an overview of the past; that is, emboli largely of cardiogenic origin affect large vessels. As pointed out elsewhere in this volume, modern day embolism is characterized by particulate matter traveling from atherosclerotic ulcerations and aneurysms in one part of the arterial stream and lodging in the distal arborizations. As such, atheromatous embolization becomes an important part of clinical vascular practice. Its treatment by medical means is as important as embolectomy.

8 Congenital Arterial Abnormalities

Surgical Treatment of Cavernous Hemangioma

Eric P. Lofgren and Karl A. Lofgren (Mayo Clinic)

Surgery 97:474–480, April 1985 8–1

Congenital cavernous hemangioma of the lower limb is a form of angioplastic dysplasia involving the venous trunks and capillaries. Elastic support can provide good symptomatic control (Fig 8–1), but surgical removal of large abnormal superficial veins and ligation of incompetent perforators may be of definite value in selected cases. Chronic disability also can be reduced by excising thrombosed veins, eroding cutaneous veins, and localized hemangiomas. Conventional stripping is not adequate, however, because of the fragility of the thin-walled varicosities and their communication with deep veins through numerous large perforators. Perforators should be ligated under direct vision at the deep fascial level. Deeper anomalous veins are not excised. Any large vein should be occluded by finger pressure before being ligated. The saphenous veins are not routinely removed.

Forty-six patients underwent surgery for cavernous hemangioma during a 20-year period. Sixteen of them had two operations. A cutaneous port-wine stain was evident in two thirds of cases. Twenty patients had a hypertrophied extremity. Incompetent perforators were found in 30 cases. The greater saphenous system was involved in 11 cases and the lesser saphenous system in 10. Twenty-five of the 28 evaluable patients had excellent or good surgical results, whereas 3 had fair results. Eight patients received sclerotherapy postoperatively. Only 8 of 29 subjects were satisfied with the appearance of the leg. Most patients who were followed have continued to use elastic support.

Klippel-Trenaunay Syndrome: Clinical, Radiologic, and Hemodynamic Features and Management

P. A. Baskerville, J. S. Ackroyd, M. Lea Thomas, and N. L. Browse (St. Thomas' Hosp., London)

Br. J. Surg. 72:232–236, March 1985 8–2

Klippel and Trenaunay, in 1900, described a congenital vascular abnormality consisting of a cutaneous nevus, varicose veins, and bone and soft tissue hypertrophy involving one or more extremity. Other soft tissue, lymphatic, and bony abnormalities are often present, but there are no hemodynamically significant arteriovenous communications. Forty-nine

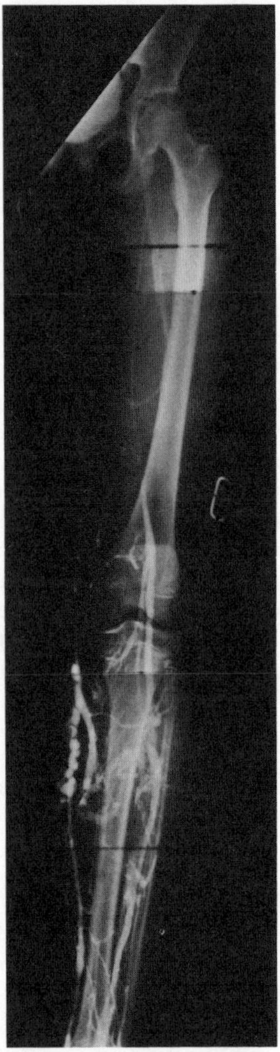

Fig 8–1.—Venogram showing presence but small size of superficial femoral vein with preferential collateral flow into the deep and saphenous systems. Surgery for the incompetent saphenous vein was not recommended, and the patient did well with an elastic support. (Courtesy of Lofgren, E.P., and Lofgren, K.A.: Surgery 97:474–480, April 1985.)

cases of Klippel-Trenaunay syndrome (KTS) seen in the past 2 decades were reviewed. Forty patients were evaluated clinically. X-ray scanography was performed in 38 cases. Foot volumetry was also performed, and calf blood flow was measured plethysmographically.

The 49 patients had 53 affected legs and three involved arms. Mean age at review was 28 years, and mean follow-up was 9½ years. All patients had visible varicosities. All but 2 had a nevus, and the same number had limb hypertrophy. Abnormality was observed at birth in 43 patients. In one fourth of cases the nevus involved more than the affected extremity. All long bones of the affected limb were lengthened. Varicosities were associated with limb pain and swelling in nearly 90% of cases. Nine patients had episodes of rectal bleeding. Seven patients had lymphedema, and 10 had cutaneous lymphatic vesicles. Congenital bony abnormalities were frequent. Only 5 patients had evidence of an inefficient calf pump on foot volumetry. Calf blood flow was significantly greater than in control limbs. Nearly one fourth of patients had venous thromboembolism. Thirty-eight patients have had 88 operations, most commonly stripping of the lateral venous trunk and other superficial varicosities.

Thromboembolism is a frequent complication of KTS. Symptoms in most patients respond to the use of compression stockings, but operation is occasionally necessary. Ligation and stripping of superficial varicosities has generally relieved local symptoms.

Congenital Arteriovenous Dysplasia: Indication for Treatment, Angiographic Documentation, and Combined Percutaneous and Surgical Treatment

R. J. A. M. van Dongen, M. G. M. H. Barwegen, J. G. Kromhout, J. G. van Baal, and J. W. P. Marsman (Academic Med. Center, Amsterdam)

Chirurg. 56:65–72, February 1985 8–3

Knowledge of embryogenesis of the vessels helps to understand the variations of angiodysplasia. There are malformations combining polydysplasias with arterial, venous, capillary, and lymphatic components. The treatment is mostly palliative, symptomatic, or cosmetic (varicose operation, extirpation of hemangiomas, lymphangiomas, and other vessel proliferations). Most therapeutic procedures are related to vessel dysplasias, especially pathologic arteriovenous short circuits. These can have a reaction on the total circulation and cause cardiac and vascular decompensation. The condition can destroy soft and osseous tissue parts in such a way as to give the appearance of a malignoma.

Treatment is indicated in all cases where the presence of active arteriovenous short circuits have caused such complications. There is no conservative treatment and no spontaneous healing. The danger in fact exists for later complications in the form of ulcers, gangrene, or nerve injury. The surgical procedure consists of: *(1)* far-reaching extirpation of the dysplastic vessels and the angiomatous tissue; *(2)* embolic obliteration of all remaining vessels of the pathologic area over all fistula feeding branches of the main artery; and *(3)* skeletization of the stem vessels over a long stretch.

Technical flawless arteriograms are decisive for the planning and performing of the surgical and percutaneous combination therapy. Detailed angiograms are especially important when the arteriovenous dysplasia is in the hand or foot area. A decision has to be made about which dysplastic vessels should be extirpated or embolized and which should be saved and thus prevent ischemia of fingers and toes. When the fistula is in the hand area or in 1 or more fingers (Fig 8–2, A) the distal section of the forearm artery of the diseased half and the corresponding hand arc with its branches are denudated. With the angiograms and the surgical findings, each case must be evaluated as to which branches should be ligated, resected, or embolized.

When the surgeon proceeds carefully and most accurately, he is able to treat an arteriovenous dysplasia of the hand or even a finger successfully (Figs 8–2, B through D). Sixty-five patients with congenital arteriovenous fistulas of various localizations were treated with the combination procedure. In 58 patients the complaints disappeared or were tolerable after combination operation. In 7 patients improvement was achieved for only a short time or not at all. Five patients with recurrent conditions after 2–4 years had to be treated with renewed percutaneous or surgical embolization. Three patients had preoperative necrosis, and small amputations could not be avoided. Two patients suffered from postoperative neurologic complications that undoubtedly were caused by ischemia. After 4–6 months the function of these nerves was completely restored. The authors find ligature of the afferent arteries and intervention of efferent veins of little value. With skeletization alone the shunt volume decreases postoperatively; it increases again after some weeks or months, and therefore the results are discouraging. As an alternative a long-stretch resection of the main artery with a prosthesis replacement or a venous transplant can be

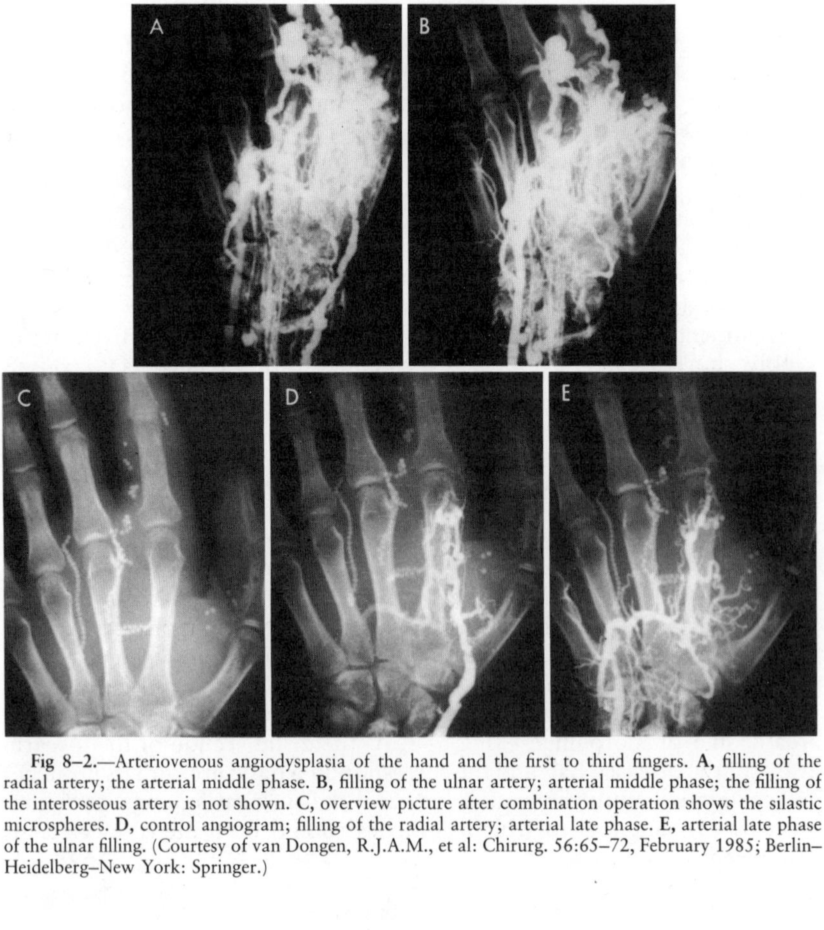

Fig 8–2.—Arteriovenous angiodysplasia of the hand and the first to third fingers. **A,** filling of the radial artery; the arterial middle phase. **B,** filling of the ulnar artery; arterial middle phase; the filling of the interosseous artery is not shown. **C,** overview picture after combination operation shows the silastic microspheres. **D,** control angiogram; filling of the radial artery; arterial late phase. **E,** arterial late phase of the ulnar filling. (Courtesy of van Dongen, R.J.A.M., et al: Chirurg. 56:65–72, February 1985; Berlin–Heidelberg–New York: Springer.)

performed. However, collaterals develop from nearby vessel areas without interference and thus therefore is of no advantage.

Percutaneous transcatheter embolization makes it possible to embolize the arteriovenous area and to turn off the total dysplastic vessel convolution. This method has the advantage of avoiding difficult, long-lasting operations often connected with blood loss. Mostly it is possible to repeat this treatment in case of any recurrence. The combination procedure offers the opportunity to remove the dysplastic vessels and tissue affected by pathologic vessels.

▶ These three articles summarize the current treatment of arteriovenous malformation. In the past, arteriography was the only radiologic investigation employed in the evaluation of this difficult problem. Now CT gives us tremendously valuable information in the third dimension. This, combined with more extensive use of venography, may allow us to identify anomalies of the arterial and venous systems which lend themselves to appropriate surgical treatment. Embolization may be helpful in certain conditions, but its value probably is most often found in reducing vascularity to prepare for surgical intervention.

Persistent Sciatic Artery: Clinical, Embryologic, and Angiographic Features

Valerie S. Mandell, Paul F. Jaques, David J. Delany, and Victor Oberheu

AJR 144:245–249, February 1985 8–4

Persistence of the sciatic or axial artery as the major arterial channel to the lower part of the leg is an uncommon but clinically significant anomaly that may be apparent as a buttock aneurysm or as ischemic or embolic disease. The authors describe the clinical and angiographic features in 16 cases of persistent sciatic artery.

Acute or chronic ischemic symptoms were present in 13 of the 16 patients. One patient with bilateral persistent sciatic arteries was symptomatic on only one side, the side of the thrombosed aneurysm, indicating that the sciatic artery may be silent until aneurysm, thrombosis, or embolus develops. An embolic source was suspected clinically in 6 patients, and 7 had sciatic artery aneurysm. Five patients had painful, tender swelling over the buttock. In 1 patient an aneurysm ruptured suddenly, resulting in death. The 3 youngest patients (aged 19, 23, and 30 years) had clinically prominent veins associated with a mass over the thigh. One patient with a history of thigh trauma may have had an acquired arteriovenous malformation involving the persistent sciatic artery. Surgical treatment may include excision of the aneurysm or bypass or simple ligation of the aneurysm.

Differentiation of persistent sciatic artery from superficial femoral artery occlusion can be clinically challenging. Fifteen of the 16 patients underwent diagnostic angiography. In every case, retrograde femoral or translumbar aortograms demonstrated the sciatic artery. However, in many cases, slow flow made it difficult to fill the vessels below the knee, despite totally

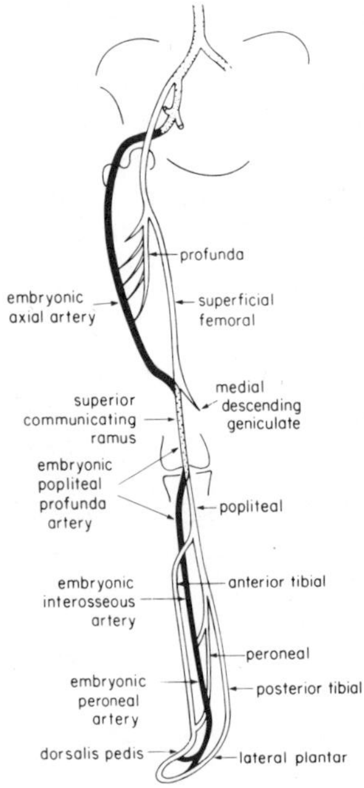

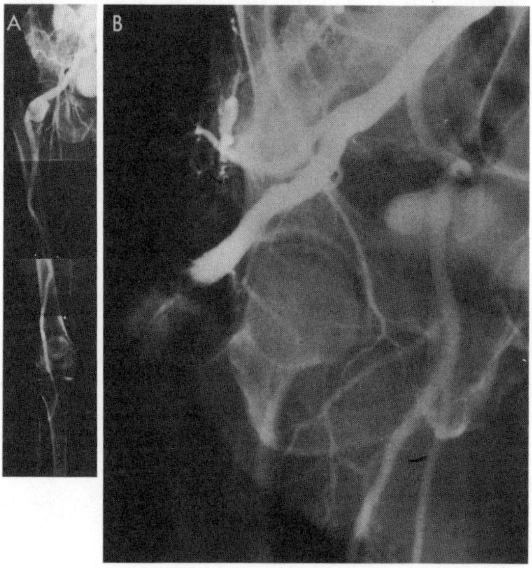

Fig 8–3 (left).—Embryonic and adult vasculature to lower extremity. Stippled and solid vessels represent embryonic flow. Solid parts eventually regress, whereas stippled segments form part of adult system. Open adult arteries are seen in relation to common embryonic segments.

Fig 8–4 (right).—**A,** ectatic artery courses lateral to common femoral artery and is superimposed on femoral head in anteroposterior projection. Aneurysm is seen, but vessel is patent, and filling of normal trifurcation occurs late in this composite run. Note forked appearance of tapered distal superficial femoral artery. **B,** oblique iliac arteriogram. Ectatic vessel originates from internal iliac artery. Saccular aneurysm of persistent sciatic artery lies posterior to femoral neck and is projected over greater trochanter on oblique views.

(Courtesy of Mandell, V.S., et al.: AJR 144:245–249, February 1985.)

patent distal runoff. In 6 cases, another injection with unusually delayed timing or a selective internal iliac artery injection was required to visualize more distal vessels. Selective injection into the common femoral or external iliac artery to the exclusion of the internal iliac artery was one cause of failure to fill the popliteal artery and its branches. An incongruity between the degree of demonstrated collateral vessels below the knee and the clinical condition or Doppler pressures at the ankle should raise suspicion about the accuracy of the angiographic runoff demonstrated.

The angiographic appearance is classic. The internal iliac artery has a larger caliber than the external iliac, is nontapering, courses laterally at the level of the femoral head, and is recognized as posterior on oblique films. The external iliac and common femoral arteries are usually normal or small. The superficial femoral artery gradually tapers as it runs into the thigh and bifurcates close to the level of the adductor canal. Near this tapering, the ectatic sciatic artery appears tortuous, most likely marking the convexity described in embryonic specimens at the anticipated sites of anastomosis with the distal superficial femoral artery (Fig 8–3). The distal vessels may be normal or show signs of atherosclerosis. In every patient the sciatic artery was ectatic, with irregular walls (Figs 8–4A and B). This ectasia with its slow flow is similar to the ectasia associated with aberrant subclavian arteries and the arteriomegalic form of atherosclerotic disease.

Sequelae of distal embolization may be observed, and the axial artery itself may be entirely thrombosed or ruptured.

Rare Variations of the Femoral Artery

Von P. Anger, K. Seidel, G. Kauffmann, and B. Urbanyi (Freiburg)

Fortschr. Geb. Rontgenstr. Nuklearmed. Ergänzungsband 141:318–326, September 1984 8–5

One of the 3 rare variations of the large arteries of the thigh that is

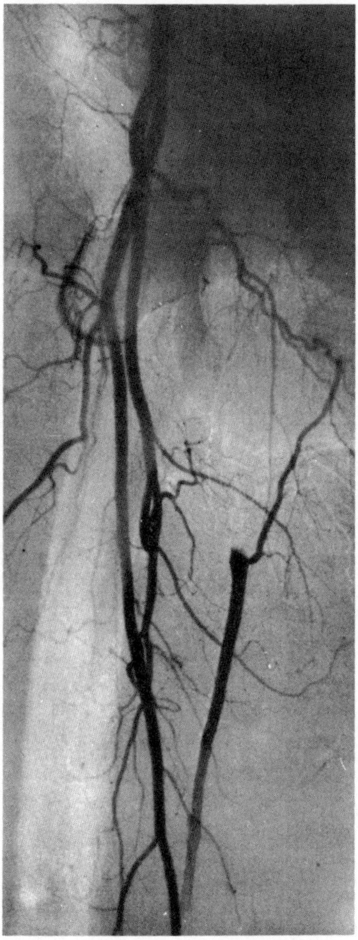

Fig 8–5.—Proximal collateral connection of the femoral artery over the medial circumflex femoral artery to the sciatic artery; subtraction picture. (Courtesy of Anger, V.P., et al.: Fortschr. Geb. Rontgenstr. Nuklearmed. Ergänzungsband 141:318–326, September 1984.)

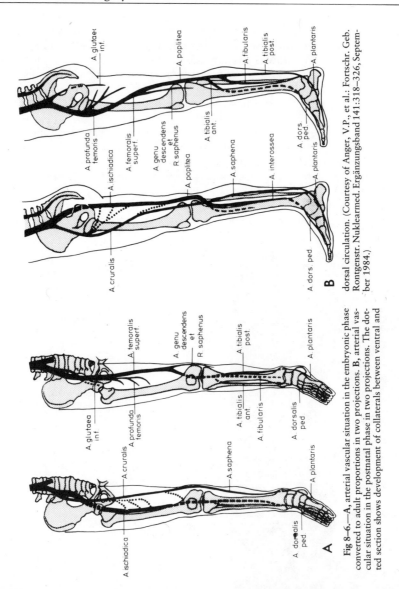

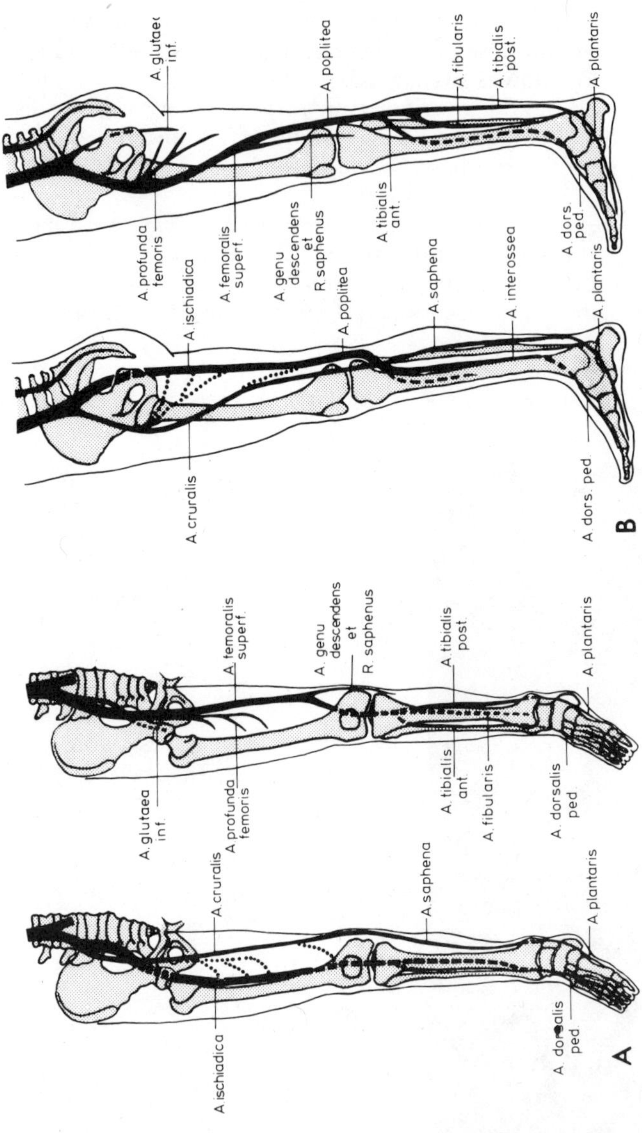

Fig 8–6.—A, arterial vascular situation in the embryonic phase converted to adult proportions in two projections. **B,** arterial vascular situation in the postnatal phase in two projections. The dotted section shows development of collaterals between ventral and dorsal circulation. (Courtesy of Anger, V.P., et al.: Fortschr. Geb. Rontgenstr. Nuklearmed. Ergänzungsband 141:318–326, September 1984.)

known is hypoplasia or aplasia of the superficial femoral artery in combination with a persistent sciatic artery, which normally is present during embryogenesis for only a few days. A typical finding is a large dorsal artery in the thigh accompanied by a hypoplastic superficial femoral artery. For the first time, angiography of this vascular situation is shown in two projections. Complications of persistent sciatic artery include aneurysm (25%) and embolic or thrombotic occlusion. The other two rare variations are duplication of the superficial femoral artery and absence or duplication of the deep femoral artery caused by separately originating branches.

Man, 42, suffered from intermittent claudication. The angiography shows a sudden rupture of a large branch of the right internal iliac artery in the pelvic floor. In the right thigh a hypoplastic superficial femoral artery was found ending in the knee joint area and filling from a collateral of the popliteal artery. Simultaneously a postnatal persistent sciatic artery was seen. The contrast medium filling starts at the proximal thigh through a collateral vessel from the medial circumflex femoral artery (Fig 8–5). The distal sciatic artery fills the popliteal artery. The occluded vessel between the internal iliac artery and the first collateral was bridged with a femoropopliteal venous bypass.

Another patient had a solitary femoral artery which corresponds with a deep femoral artery after separating into various branches.

The development of the extremities begins in the 5-week-old embryo. The blood supply comes from the vessel originating in the umbilical artery (the later internal iliac artery) and is called axial artery; it runs dorsal in close proximity to the sciatic nerve and is also called sciatic artery. It is involuted in favor of a growing vascular stem, the crural or femoral artery (Fig 8–6). It is rare that the involution of the sciatic artery does not start during embryonic development. The persistent sciatic artery is mostly unilateral.

Half of the diagnosed patients are older than age 50 years and one fourth are younger than age 30 years. Frequently in younger patients the condition is combined with malformation or occasionally with vascular changes. In most cases the leg is apparently normal and asymptomatic. A

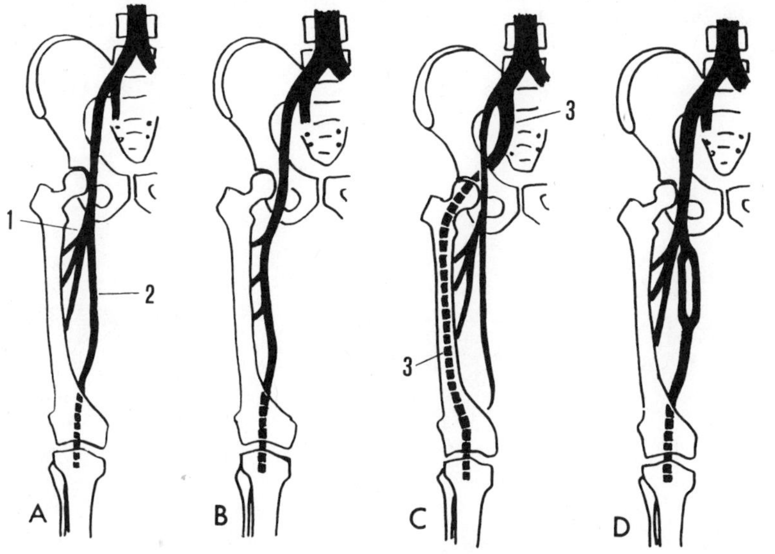

Fig 8–7.—The rare variations of the large arteries of the thigh. **A,** normal findings. **B,** solitary femoral artery with separation into various branches. **C,** hypoplastic superficial femoral artery with persistent sciatic artery. **D,** duplication of the superficial femoral artery (island formation). 1 = deep femoral artery, 2 = superficial femoral artery, 3 = sciatic artery. (Courtesy of Anger, V.P., et al.: Fortschr. Geb. Rontgenstr. Nuklearmed. Ergänzungsband 141:318–326, September 1984.)

persistent sciatic artery in vivo was first recognized angiographically in 1960 in a patient with longstanding intermittent claudication. Angiography is indicated only for patients with vascular complaints. In some cases arteriosclerosis affects the sciatic artery more than the rest of the vascular system. Often a dilated persistent embryonic artery is found; this is either a diffused vascular dilatation (arteriomegaly) or a circumscribed aneurysm. The aneurysm is usually found at the proximal metaphysis of the femur. Besides rupture the complications include thrombi and emboli in the periphery. Hypoplasia and aplasia of the superficial femoral artery are only found in the postnatal persistent sciatic artery. Duplication of the superficial femoral artery is rare. The artery separates, runs parallel for a while, and then unites again; it is also called island formation (Fig 8–7). Mostly it branches off dorsolaterally often together with the lateral and the medial circumflex femoral arteries. The branches that supply the circulation of the missing deep femoral artery originate most frequently from the femoral artery.

Knowledge of embryogenesis of the vessels helps in understanding these artery variations.

▶ Vascular surgeons must know the embryology of the femoral artery and the phenomenon of persistent sciatic artery. In sending such a case to us, a referring surgeon said that he had seen a most unusual arteriogram in that the patient had three femoral arteries. Perhaps this should be the tip-off that a persistent sciatic artery is present. The presence of a persistent sciatic artery is an indication for femorodistal reconstruction to exclude that vessel, its aneurysms, and its enclosed thrombotic material from the arterial stream.

9 Management of Vascular Trauma

The Management of Subclavian Artery Injuries Following Blunt Thoracic Trauma

James T. Sturn, James S. Dorsey, Frederick R. Olson, and John F. Perry, Jr.
(St. Paul-Ramsey Med. Center)

Ann. Thorac. Surg. 38:188–191, September 1984 9–1

The complex anatomy of the superior mediastinum and thorax provides a musculoskeletal tunnel of protection for the subclavian vessels that makes injury to them uncommon but renders surgical exposure of these structures challenging. Data are reviewed on management of 15 patients who sustained subclavian artery injuries after blunt thoracic trauma.

Thirteen injuries were sustained in vehicular accidents; 1 patient had been a pedestrian, and another had a fall. The most common severe associated injuries included long-bone fractures, brachial plexus palsies, hemopneumothorax, and multiple rib fractures. Seven patients had arterial hypotension, 7 had unilateral absence of radial pulse, 8 had ipsilateral brachial plexus palsy, and 4 had supraclavicular hematoma. Findings on chest films included wide mediastinum, apical pleural hematoma, and first rib fractures.

Fourteen patients survived to undergo angiography and operation. Indications for angiography included absent upper extremity pulse in 7 patients, wide mediastinum in 3, persistent arterial hypotension in 2, chest tube hemorrhage in 1, and apical pleural radiodensity in 1. The left subclavian artery was injured in 10 patients, with the site of disruption being near the origin of the vertebral artery in 8 patients, at the junction of the subclavian and axillary arteries in 1, and at the origin of the left subclavian artery from the aorta in 1. The right subclavian artery was disrupted in 5 patients, disruption occurred about 1 cm distal to the innominate bifurcation in 2 patients and near the origin of the vertebral artery in 3. Techniques used for the rupture of the left subclavian artery included the supraclavicular approach in 5 patients, a trap-door incision in 3, an infraclavicular transpectoral incision in the patient with a distal left subclavian tear, and posterolateral thoracotomy for the patient in whom injury occurred at the origin of the artery from the aortic arch. For patients with injuries of the right subclavian artery, a trap-door incision was used in 2 and a supraclavicular approach was used in 2.

Arterial continuity was restored by primary anastomosis in 7 patients, synthetic grafts in 4, and venous interposition grafts in 2. Proximal and distal ligation of a pseudoaneurysm was done in 1 patient with a complete brachial plexus palsy.

Successful revascularization was achieved in 12 patients. Above-the-elbow amputation was performed in 1 patient because of massive injury that precluded restoration of blood flow beyond the brachial artery. Two patients died of postoperative respiratory insufficiency that resulted from severe pulmonary contusions. The most common postoperative complications included pulmonary insufficiency and pneumonitis.

It is concluded that injury to the subclavian artery should be suspected after blunt thoracic trauma when upper extremity pulses are absent, a brachial plexus palsy is present, or an apical radiodensity or a wide mediastinum is seen on chest films. Firm indications for aortography include absent upper extremity pulses, a wide mediastinum, unrelenting thoracic hemorrhage, and persistent hypotension. Relative indications for thoracic angiography include brachial plexus palsy, apical pleural hematoma, and a fractured first rib.

A standard left thoracotomy is used for left-sided injuries that occur at the origin of the left subclavian artery from the aorta. Proximal lesions can be approached through a small left anterior thoracotomy in the third or fourth intercostal space, and a distal injury can be approached by the supraclavicular route. If more exposure is necessary, an upper median sternotomy can be performed to form the trap-door exposure.

Left-sided lesions distal to the vertebral artery may be approached initially through a supraclavicular incision. For lesions on the right side, a supraclavicular incision, extended into a median sternotomy when necessary, provides good exposure for injuries near the origin of the right subclavian from the innominate artery. Lesions distal to the origin of the vertebral artery may be approached by a supraclavicular incision. Exposure can be improved by subperiosteal resection of the medial half of the clavicle.

Management of Arm Arterial Injuries

James V. Sitzmann and Calvin B. Ernst (Johns Hopkins Med. Inst.)

Surgery 96:895–901, November 1984 9–2

Review was made of the data on 102 patients treated in 1971–1981 for 109 arterial injuries involving vessels from the thoracic inlet to the wrist. The 83 male and 19 female patients in the series had an average age of 28 years. Thirty-six arm and 73 forearm arterial injuries were treated. All injuries but 4 followed penetrating trauma.

Most subclavian artery injuries were managed by end-to-end repair after débridement of injured tissue. None of the 13 patients required amputation, and none had disability from the arterial injury itself. Three of 7 patients with axillary artery injuries required saphenous vein interposition grafts. One vein graft thrombosed postoperatively and was corrected by Dacron graft repair. Seven of 16 patients with brachial artery injuries had vein grafting, and 7 had end-to-end repair. Wrist pulses were restored in all cases. Two patients required forearm fasciotomy after restoration of blood flow. Most radial artery injuries were managed by end-to-end repair. Only 1 of 30 patients required vein graft interposition. Arterial ligation was done in 10 cases. Of the 20 patients who underwent arterial reconstruction, 12 had palpable distal pulses postoperatively. No amputations were necessary. Of the 28 patients with ulnar artery injuries, 19 had end-to-end arterial repair. Of the 24 who had any arterial repair, 10 had late disability. None of 6 patients with both radial and ulnar arterial injuries had vascular disability. Both interosseous injuries were managed by ligation.

Arterial injuries in the arm are more life-threatening than forearm injuries, but the latter are more disabling, chiefly because of associated nerve involvement. Suspicion of vascular injury is sufficient indication for arteriography. Most injuries in this study were managed by limited resection with end-to-end anastomosis. Autogenous saphenous vein is preferred when grafting is necessary. One fourth of forearm injuries were managed by arterial ligation without adverse sequelae. Fasciotomy occasionally was necessary after blood flow had been restored.

Open Tibial Fractures With Associated Vascular Injuries: Prognosis for Limb Salvage

Richard H. Lange, Allan W. Bach, Sigvard T. Hansen, Jr., and Kaj H. Johansen (Univ. of Washington)

J. Trauma 25:203–208, March 1985 9–3

Data from 23 patients who were seen between 1977 and 1983 with open tibial fractures and limb-threatening vascular compromise were reviewed in an attempt to clarify the prognosis for limb salvage. The 23 cases, involving 18 men and 5 women with an average age of 36.5 years, represented 6% of all open tibial fractures treated in this period. Significant comminution was present in virtually all cases, and all patients but 1 had significant skin, muscle damage, or both. The most frequently noted vascular injuries were popliteal transection or thrombosis, and disruption at or distal to the trifurcation. In addition to arterial repair, venous reconstruction was attempted in 3 cases. The vascular repairs were covered with local soft tissue or muscle rotation flaps. Two thirds of patients had associated major injuries.

Nineteen patients were followed for an average of 16 months, with an overall amputation rate of 61%. Five primary and 9 delayed amputations were carried out. Excluding 3 limbs that proved viable without revascularization, the final amputation rate was 70%. Crush injury, segmental tibial fracture, and a delay of more than 6 hours before revascularization were associated with a poor outcome. Stable coverage was more readily achieved with primary amputation, but attempted revascularization did not influence the ultimate level of amputation. Patients generally required several operations to obtain satisfactory coverage and a healed tibia.

Indications for primary amputation in these cases are listed in the table. Rapid revascularization is essential in cases of profound ischemia. Provi-

PROTOCOL FOR PRIMARY AMPUTATION FOR OPEN TIBIAL FRACTURES WITH VASCULAR INJURY

A. Absolute Indications
   1. Anatomically complete disruption of the posterior tibial nerve in adults
   2. Crush injuries with warm ischemia time greater than 6 hours
B. Relative Indications
   1. Serious associated polytrauma
   2. Severe ipsilateral foot trauma
   3. Anticipated protracted course to obtain soft-tissue coverage and tibial reconstitution

Primary amputation indicated if: Either of group A or two or three of group B indications are present.

(Courtesy of Lange, R.H., et al.: J. Trauma 25:203–208, March 1985.)

sional skeletal stabilization otherwise is desirable if it can be expedited. Multiple operative procedures must be expected at best, and a long-term commitment to rehabilitation is necessary.

Superior Mesenteric Artery and Vein Injuries From Blunt Abdominal Trauma

Peter A. Courcy, Sheldon Brotman, Mary Lou Oster-Granite, Carl A. Soderstrom, John H. Siegel, and R. Adams Crowley (Maryland Inst. for Emergency Med. Services Systems, Baltimore)
J. Trauma 24:843–845, September 1984 9–4

Records of 13 patients treated for superior mesenteric vascular injury secondary to blunt abdominal trauma during 8 years were reviewed retrospectively. The 10 men and 3 women were aged 18 to 68 years.

Woman, 33, was admitted in profound shock after a motor vehicle accident. Abdominal examination showed diffuse tenderness and guarding. After resuscitation, celiotomy was performed because of increasing abdominal girth and tenderness. Exploration revealed complete transection of the midtransverse colon and small bowel, mesenteric contusions, a proximal jejunal perforation, and a necrotic right colon. The superior mesenteric vein was contused over most of its course, necessitating resection of all but 132 cm of the jejunum and left colon. A jejunostomy 36 cm from the ligament of Treitz and a jejunomidtransverse colostomy were performed. Bowel viability was verified by Doppler examination and intravenous fluorescein injection. A second operation 24 hours after injury revealed small bowel necrosis from the proximal to the distal anastomosis and a thrombosed superior mesenteric vein causing venous gangrene. Necrotic bowel was resected, and 36 cm of jejunum was anastomosed to the midtransverse colon. The patient recovered.

All 13 injuries were caused by motor vehicle accidents. Six patients were in profound shock, 2 in cardiopulmonary arrest, and 5 in mild shock.

Indications for immediate celiotomy included diffuse abdominal tenderness and guarding with associated shock or an expanding abdomen. One patient had a superior mesenteric artery laceration, 7 patients had isolated superior mesenteric vein lacerations, and 5 patients had combined injuries. Associated intra-abdominal injuries averaged 3.2 per patient. Six patients had devitalized bowel as a direct consequence of injury to the superior mesenteric vessels. Blood replacement ranged from 2 to 30 units per patient (average, 11.7). Five lateral arteriorrhaphies and 11 venorrhaphies were performed. Four patients required combined vessel repair, and 1 patient required ligation of both vessels and bowel resection. The 57% mortality was primarily due to free intraperitoneal hemorrhage from superior mesenteric arteriovenous disruption. Intra-abdominal abscesses developed in 3 of 6 survivors and necessitated reexploration and drainage.

Mesenteric arteriovenous disruption after blunt abdominal trauma results in massive hemorrhage from the valveless mesenteric-portal system, which can carry up to 60% of cardiac output. Bowel ischemia and infarction may result if the vessel injury is proximal to the first jejunal branch. Therapy includes immediate celiotomy, digital control of hemorrhage, and avoidance of indiscriminant clamping of bleeding vessels. Revascularization can be accomplished with lateral suture repair techniques. A second operative examination 24 hours after injury should be routine when arteriovenous repair has been performed. Thrombosis at the site of arterial repair, venous contusion, or exposed segments of mesenteric vein predispose the patient to acute postoperative arteriovenous occlusion resulting in intestinal gangrene. Bowel viability should be confirmed by Doppler ultrasound or fluorescein testing.

Determinants of Survival After Vena Caval Injury: Analysis of a 14-Year Experience

Kenneth A. Kudsk, Frederic Bongard, and Robert C. Lim, Jr.

Arch. Surg. 119:1009–1012, September 1984 9–5

More than a third of patients with vena caval injury will die before reaching the hospital, and up to half of those admitted will die despite resuscitation and early surgery—most of exsanguination. The outcome in 70 cases of vena caval injury seen between 1970 and 1983 was reviewed. Most patients were younger than age 40 years. Gunshot wounds caused 40% of injuries, followed by stab wounds; mortality was 21% and 50%, respectively. Blunt injuries were less frequent but carried a mortality of 85%. The overall survival was 55.5%.

Survival was correlated with the blood pressure (BP) noted on admission and with its response to fluid resuscitation. All but 20% of patients with a BP reading below 70 mm Hg died. Both the location and number of caval injuries influenced the outcome (Fig 9–1). All 8 patients with more than two sites of caval injury died. Mortality was lowest in cases involving injury that was isolated to the infrarenal or suprarenal area. Only 7 of 38

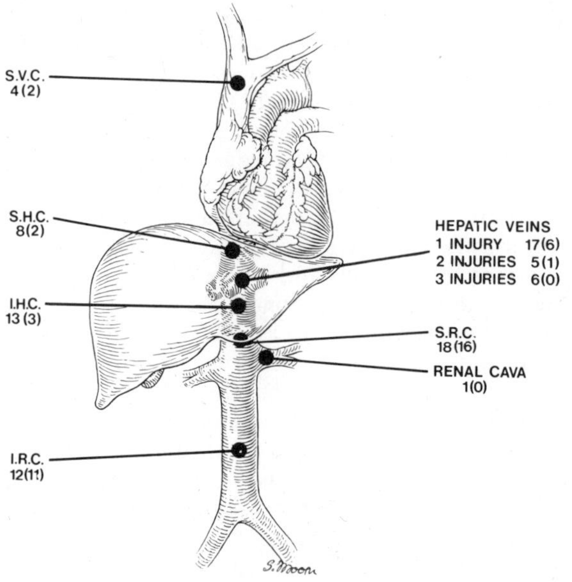

Fig 9–1.—Distribution of vena caval injuries. The number of survivors is in parentheses. (Courtesy of Kudsk, K.A., et al.: Arch. Surg. 119:1009–1012, September 1984; copyright 1984, American Medical Association.)

patients with hepatic vein injury survived. Mortality increased rapidly with the extent of injury; more than half of the patients with associated liver injury died. All but 3 of the 33 deaths occurred during the first 24 hours and were due to uncontrolled bleeding and disseminated intravascular coagulation. Most caval injuries were repaired by lateral venorrhaphy. The infrarenal cava was ligated in 3 surviving patients to arrest bleeding.

Severe associated injuries help explain the high mortality associated with vena caval injuries. Effective resuscitation is one of the most important survival measures in such cases, along with prompt control of bleeding from all sites. Management of injuries to the retrohepatic and suprarenal areas remains a major problem. The prognosis is poor if more than one vein is torn or if there is a second vena caval tear.

▶ Arterial or venous injuries due to blunt trauma, penetrating injury, or fractures continue to present a challenge to vascular surgeons. The indications for primary amputation for open tibial fracture in the article by Lange et al. are worth remembering. Management of subclavian artery injury is often difficult because of exposure. The options described in these articles should clarify proper approaches to subclavian artery injury. The high mortality in superficial mesenteric artery or vein injuries is probably due to bowel infarction and the difficulty in recognizing this condition during the immediate postoperative period. We agree that a second look within 24 hours is needed to ensure that viability of the bowel is preserved. A reliable diagnostic technique to detect postoperative intestinal ischemia is badly needed.

Monitoring Acute Compartment Pressures With the S.T.I.C. Catheter

A. G. P. McDermott, E. Marble, and R. H. Yabsley (Dalhousie Univ., Halifax, Nova Scotia)

Clin. Orthop. 190:192–198, November 1984 9–6

Various intramuscular pressure-measuring methods have been used to diagnose compartment syndromes at an early stage and thus prevent tissue damage. The external transducer and connecting tubing are shortcomings of conventional systems. A solid-state transducer intracompartment (STIC) catheter now is available that combines a multiperforated polyethylene tip with a solid-state transducer. A two-in-one catheter (Fig 9–2) was developed for this study to permit the STIC and conventional catheters to be compared from the same position within the compartment.

Satisfactory correspondence was found between the STIC and conventional systems in animal and human studies, over a pressure range of 0–100 mm Hg and during 12 to 16 hours of monitoring. The hindlimb extensor and forelimb flexor muscle compartments were monitored in dogs, with heparinized saline and then normal saline injected to increase compartment pressures. Clinical studies were done in normal subjects having an STIC catheter inserted in the anterior compartment of the leg, and also in patients with tibial fracture or high tibial osteotomy. The sensitivity of the STIC catheter was such that patency of the tip could be assessed through a cast by movement of the patient's toes. No serious complications attended placement or removal of the catheter.

The STIC catheter is a functionally superior method for monitoring compartment pressure. It is easier than conventional systems to calibrate and maintain, and the findings are more easily interpreted. Use of the STIC as a diagnostic aid is recommended in both acute and chronic compartment syndromes.

▶ Miniaturization of the instrumentation makes this new solid-state device the current state-of-the-art compartment pressure measurement. Recording by strip chart is useful for medicolegal monitoring purposes. In the acute situation, the authors suggested recording pressure over a 2- to 3-hour period to determine the trend and need for fasciotomy in those patients whose pressure

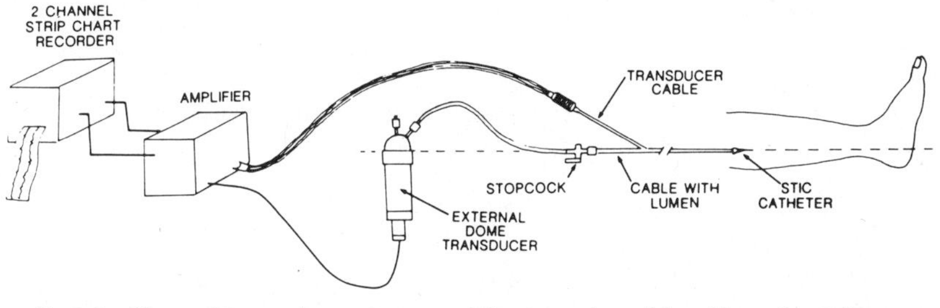

Fig 9–2.—The two-in-one catheter system, permitting comparison of the tubing and transducer components of the conventional pressure-monitoring system with the solid-state transducer intracompartment catheter. (Courtesy of McDermott, A.G.P., et al.: Clin. Orthop. 190:192–198, November 1984.)

reading is initially of the borderline critical level (30 to 40 mm Hg). Chronic compartment syndrome is commonly seen in runners. Compartment pressure measurement will help to guide surgical treatment.

Chronic Compartment Syndrome: Diagnosis, Management, and Outcomes

Don E. Detmer, Kim Sharpe, Robert L. Sufit, and Forrest M. Girdley (Univ. of Wisconsin, Madison)

Am. J. Sports Med. 13:162–170, May–June 1985 9–7

Chronic compartment syndrome (CCS) typically is an exercise-induced condition with a relatively inadequate musculofascial compartment size, resulting in chronic or recurrent pain, disability, or both. The syndrome is seen chiefly in active persons; the history is extremely important. Reduction or cessation of exercise generally leads to symptomatic improvement. The physical findings are unimpressive in nearly all cases. Compartment pressure measurements can confirm the diagnosis. A number of techniques of fasciotomy have been described.

A total of 233 compartments were released in 100 consecutive patients with CCS who were operated on. Most patients were athletes, especially runners. Mean duration of symptoms was 22 months. A large majority of patients had bilateral involvement. The posterior compartment was involved in about half the cases. Eleven patients had operative and postoperative complications. More than 90% of patients were cured or significantly improved symptomatically, functionally, or both, on follow-up a median of 4½ months after operation. The median time to resumption of conditioned running was 3 weeks. A complete functional cure was obtained in 73 patients, and no patient was functionally worse after operation. Recurrences were observed in 5 patients. Overall patient satisfaction with the outcome was high.

Fasciotomy is an effective and safe means of managing patients with CCS. Results are best when operation is performed before severe symptoms have developed or serious functional impairment is present. Fasciectomy is favored in patients who develop new symptoms after a good initial response to fasciotomy. Both procedures can be done with local anesthesia on an outpatient basis.

Percutaneous Transcatheter Embolization for Arterial Trauma

Thomas Panetta, Salvatore J. A. Sclafani, Alan S. Goldstein, and Thomas F. Phillips (SUNY, Downstate Med. Center)

J. Vasc. Surg. 2:54–64, January 1985 9–8

Experience with percutaneous transcatheter embolization (PTE) was reviewed in a series of 242 patients seen between 1977 and 1984 with 328 angiographically documented arterial injuries. One hundred patients were evaluated prospectively and underwent PTE for a total of 107 arterial injuries; 5 patients had two and 1 had three injuries. Sixty embolizations were done with Gelfoam; steel or cotton minicoils and microcoils were used in 28 patients to control bleeding from larger vessels, or if proximal and distal control of isolated injuries was necessary. A combination of Gelfoam and coils was necessary in 12 cases. Intentional intimal dissection with subsequent thrombosis controlled bleeding in 3 cases.

Embolization was successful in 82% of cases. All but 4 of 28 embolizations for retroperitoneal hematoma succeeded, although some patients died of associated injuries after pelvic hemorrhage was controlled. Sixteen of 19 arteriovenous fistulas were successfully embolized. All but 2 of 18 embolizations in patients with penetrating neck injuries were successful. Fifteen of 18 embolizations for peripheral vascular injury succeeded. Eight of 30 attempts in patients with thoracoabdominal trauma failed. Seven failures were in patients with splenic injury who required splenectomy after attempted embolization.

Percutaneous transcatheter embolization is superior to operation in the treatment of selected types of vascular trauma, such as retroperitoneal bleeding secondary to pelvic fracture, and certain parenchymal injuries, such as hematobilia and intrarenal vascular disruption. In other settings PTE can obviate the need for general anesthesia and parenchymal dissection and preclude soft tissue dissection and cosmetic deformity. Interventional radiologic methods now succeed in three fourths or more of cases.

Digital Subtraction Angiography in Extremity Trauma

Philip C. Goodman, R. Brooke Jeffrey, Jr., and Michael Brant-Zawadzki (Univ. of California at San Francisco)

Radiology 153:61–64, October 1984 9–9

Eighty digital subtraction angiographic (DSA) studies were done on 50 emergency patients seen in 1 year with extremity trauma. The medical records of 42 of 44 patients with diagnostic DSA studies were reviewed. Most studies were done by injection into an artery near the area of injury. A dose of 12 ml of Conray 43 was injected at the rate of 6 ml per second into extremity vessels and a 40- to 50-ml volume of Conray 400 into the aorta. Excellent-quality studies were obtained in 57.5% of instances and poor-quality studies in only 7.5%.

Abnormalities were found in 27% of patients with diagnostic DSA studies. Eight patients had small vessel extravasation, 2 had pseudoaneurysms, and 2 had arteriovenous fistulas. Three patients with normal findings at DSA were incidentally found to have small arterial bleeders. No other patient developed signs of bleeding at the site of injury or any pulse deficit in the injured extremity. Angiograms showed bleeding small vessels in 2 patients. In another patient with a similar finding (Fig 9–3), no bleeder was found at operation. Five patients with similar findings were observed and seemed to be well at follow-up. The pseudoaneurysms and arteriovenous fistulas were confirmed at operation.

Digital subtraction angiography reduces the time needed to evaluate the

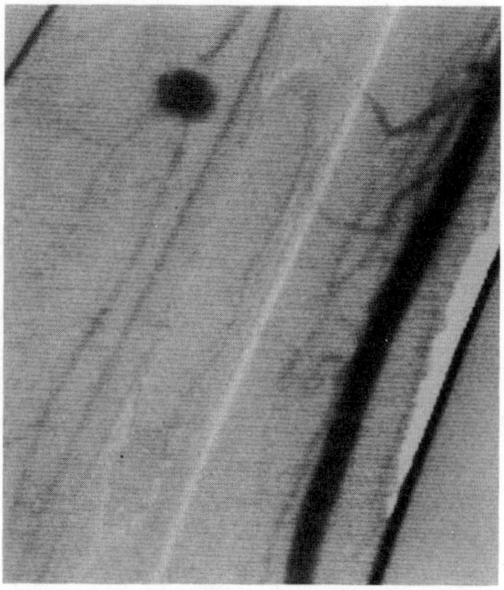

Fig 9–3.—Digital subtraction angiogram of right brachial artery. Large area of contrast extravasation is seen in muscular branch of artery. No bleeding site was discovered at operation. (Courtesy of Goodman, P.C., et al.: Radiology 153:61–64, October 1984.)

arterial system in patients with extremity injury. Less contrast is required, there is less discomfort, and film costs are reduced. The major disadvantage of DSA is the limited field size of the image intensifier. The lower spatial resolution compared with conventional angiography is probably not significant, since most vascular abnormalities related to extremity trauma are not subtle.

▶ Two new diagnostic and therapeutic modalities in vascular disease are now applied to the management of arterial trauma. It is important to remember that only a good quality arteriogram is tolerable. It is a prerequisite in the management of arterial trauma. Therefore, the article on the use of DSA must be interpreted with caution.

Use of percutaneous transcatheter embolization is intriguing. It would appear that the technique is of particular appeal in retroperitoneal bleeding of arteries otherwise difficult to approach surgically, such as the vertebral artery.

Vertebral Artery Transection From Blunt Trauma Treated by Embolization

Marc Kobernick and Raymond Carmody (Univ. of Arizona)

J. Trauma 24:854–856, September 1984 9–10

Although rare, vertebral artery injury resulting from blunt trauma can produce significant morbidity and permanent neurologic deficit. Nonpenetrating traumatic vertebral artery transection was managed by therapeutic embolization in an accident victim.

Man, 22, was admitted to the emergency department unconscious and without blood pressure or pulse after a motorcycle accident. Within 90 seconds of open cardiac massage and cross-clamping of the distal thoracic aorta, supraventricular tachycardia developed and systolic blood pressure was 90 mm Hg. After peritoneal lavage revealed gross blood, splenectomy was performed for a ruptured spleen.

Neurologic examination just prior to laparotomy showed the patient to be unresponsive to deep pain and without spontaneous motor activity. Postoperative CT scanning of the head showed bilateral hemispheric edema with subarachnoid hemorrhage. Because of an expanding hematoma on the right side of the neck, cerebral arteriography was performed. This study revealed complete transection of the right vertebral artery 3 cm distal to its origin, with massive extravasation of contrast material from the proximal segment. Embolization of the proximal portion of the artery with a Gianturco spinal coil successfully stopped the bleeding. Selective left vertebral artery injection revealed no evidence of hemorrhage from the distal right vertebral artery, which was spasmodic. Even though aggressive attempts were made to control cerebral edema and maintain blood pressure, the patient died 12 hours later.

Injuries to the vertebral artery have ranged from minimal intimal tears to dissection, arteriovenous fistula, thrombosis, and transection. Although most blunt vertebral injuries are associated with major trauma, vertebral artery occlusions may occur after seemingly trivial athletic injuries and even after yoga exercises. Clinical findings that may suggest the diagnosis include hematoma of the neck, a bruit, delayed onset of neurologic deficit, and Horner's syndrome. Only angiography provides a conclusive diagnosis, thus awareness of the possibility of vertebral artery injury must be maintained. Angiographic embolization should be considered for patients with complete transection of a vertebral artery. Because the materials available for embolization have individual advantages and disadvantages, the choice of an embolic agent must be tailored to the clinical situation. When performed properly, therapeutic angiographic embolization poses little risk of additional morbidity.

Posttraumatic Vertebral Artery Aneurysm and Arteriovenous Fistula: A Case Report

Pamela R. Roper, Faustino C. Guinto, Jr., and Fred J. Wolma (Univ. of Texas at Galveston)

Surgery 96:556–559, September 1984 9–11

A patient was seen with posttraumatic vertebral artery injury in whom embolization was readily achieved at the time of diagnostic arteriography.

Man, 32, had a pulsatile left neck mass 3 cm in size at the level of the mandible. Two years previously he sustained a stab wound in this area and underwent subsequent neck exploration. A constant thrill and audible bruit were present. The findings on neurologic examination were normal. Ocular plethysmography revealed a relatively decreased flow on the left side compared with the right side. Transfemoral angiography demonstrated marked enlargement of the left vertebral artery, with an aneurysm arising at the level of the third cervical vertebra. An arteriovenous fistula was found at this level, with filling of the plexus of veins that directly connected the aneurysm with the external jugular vein. Right vertebral angiography showed essentially normal posterior fossa circulation, except for an

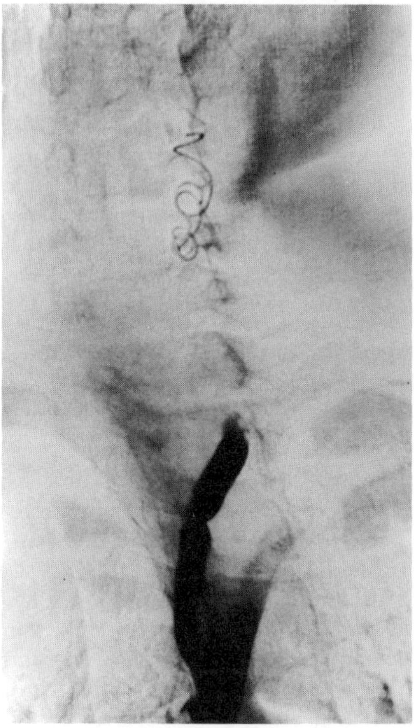

Fig 9–4.—After embolization, the vertebral artery is completely occluded at the level of T1. (Courtesy of Roper, P.R., et al.: Surgery 96:556–559, September 1984.)

abnormal reflux of contrast material down the left vertebral artery to the level of the aneurysm indicating a "vertebral steal" phenomenon. Occluding spring emboli were introduced above and below the aneurysm to embolize the vertebral artery. When extruded into the blood vessel, the emboli took on a coiled configuration, thus blocking flow. Post embolization radiographs taken 5 minutes after positioning of the emboli confirmed occlusion of the vertebral artery and entrapment of the aneurysm and fistula (Fig 9–4).

The clinical diagnosis of vertebral artery aneurysms is frequently difficult. With the advent of selective catheterization techniques, angiography has become the definitive method for diagnosing vertebral artery injuries. Selective evaluation of both the vertebral and carotid systems usually yields sufficient information on which to base therapy. Treatment of vertebral artery injuries by embolization alone is ideal for lesions that are not readily accessible to direct surgical intervention, assuming that the fistula/aneurysm does not involve a critical artery.

Gangrene of the Upper Extremity Following Intra-Arterial Injection of Drugs: A Case Report and Review of the Literature

I. Goldberg, A. Bahar, and Z. Yosipovitch

Clin. Orthop. 188:223–229, September 1984 9–12

A patient was encountered who developed gangrene of the fingers after accidental intra-arterial self-injection of crushed codeine tablets in suspension.

Man, 37, had been addicted to such drugs as opium and codeine for 7 years and recently had used a solution of eight tablets of codeine phosphate dissolved in boiled water by injecting it into the upper limb veins. Severe pain and swelling had immediately followed an antecubital injection 1 week before admission, and darkening and numbness of the fingertips were present 3 days afterwards. Examination showed dry gangrene of the fingers and thumb and mummification of the distal two phalanges of the fingers in the right hand. The fingers were completely anesthetic. Substantial forearm swelling was present, and no brachial or ulnar pulses were felt. The gangrenous area became clearly demarcated 1 week later. Angiography showed complete block of the digital arteries arising from the palmar arch. The hand was amputated through the wrist, and partially organized thrombi were found, with occlusion of the digital arteries.

Studies of codeine phosphate and additives in dogs suggested that microcrystalline cellulose caused development of extremity gangrene. Drugs reported to produce gangrene when injected intra-arterially are listed in the table. Pain is consistently the most prominent symptom in these cases. Massive forearm edema may develop. The pathogenesis of the ischemia and gangrene is unclear. Whether active chemical substances or additives cause the complication is unknown.

Meperidine can be used in large dosage to control pain, and stellate

Drugs Known to Have Produced Gangrene

Generic Name	*Trade Name*
Thiopentone	Pentothal
Quinalbarbitone	Secobarbital, Seconal
Pentobarbitone	Nembutal, Prodormol
Amobarbital	Amytal
Promazine	Sparine
Chlorpromazine	Largactyl, Taroctyl, Thorazine
Mephenesin	Myanesin, Tolosate
Tubocurain	
Meperidine	Pethidin, Dolestin, Demerol Pro-Meperdan
Promethazine	Phenergan
Propoxyphene	Darvon
Hydroxyzine	Atarax
Heroin	
Diazepam	Valium
Amphetamine	Benzedrine, Novydrine
Ether	
Sulfobromophthalein	Bromsulphalein
Methylphenidate	Ritalin
Pentazocine	Talwin
Methohexitone	
5-Hydroxytryptamine	

(Courtesy of Goldberg, I., et al.: Clin. Orthop. 188:223–229, September 1984.)

ganglion block may be effective. Some suggest immediate use of heparin. Vasodilators probably are not helpful. The role of operation is unclear. Antibiotics are given to prevent secondary infection in ischemic tissues. Physiotherapy is indicated as soon as it is tolerated. Frank gangrene is the usual outcome.

▶ The table in this article should provide useful information for those who treat drug abuse, an ever-increasing social and medical problem.

Five-Year Experience With PTFE Grafts in Vascular Wounds

David V. Feliciano, Kenneth L. Mattox, Joseph M. Graham, and Carmel G. Bitondo

J. Trauma 25:71–82, January 1985 9–13

Segmental replacement of injured vessels is increasingly required for civilian injury cases. Satisfactory results have been obtained using expanded polytetrafluoroethylene (PTFE), or Goretex, in elective vascular procedures. A total of 236 PTFE grafts were inserted in vascular wounds in 206 patients in 1978–1983. Most injuries were due to gunshot, shotgun, or stab wounds. Average patient age was 29 years. Nearly 40% of injuries were complete transections, whereas about one fifth each were lateral defects and through-and-through injuries. The open anastomosis technique often was used with 5–0 or 6–0 polypropylene suture material.

The overall mortality was 8%; 1 death resulted from dehiscence of a graft of the superior mesenteric artery, and another from septicemia arising in an area of cellulitis around apparently uninfected grafts. Arterial grafts were most often placed in the brachial or superficial femoral arteries. Graft occlusion was a significant problem with 4-mm grafts in the brachial artery. Long-term patency rates were less than those encountered with saphenous vein grafts. Graft infection did not occur in the absence of graft exposure or osteomyelitis. Venous grafts usually were placed in the superficial vein. Grafts placed in extremity wounds had a high early occlusion rate, but bleeding from blast cavities and fasciotomy sites was reduced.

The PTFE grafts are an acceptable prosthesis for use in arterial wounds, although long-term patency is less than with saphenous vein grafts. Exposed PTFE grafts are more easily managed than exposed vein grafts. The PTFE grafts are excellent temporary conduits when inserted in proximal extremity veins.

Polytetrafluoroethylene Grafts in the Rapid Reconstruction of Acute Contaminated Peripheral Vascular Injuries

Dhiraj M. Shah, Robert P. Leather, John D. Corson, and Allastair M. Karmody (Albany, N.Y.)

Am. J. Surg. 148:229–233, August 1984 9–14

It has been the practice to use autogenous tissue intraposition for vascular reconstructions in contaminated wounds when direct vascular repair is not feasible. Doubt still exists regarding the use of polytetrafluoroethylene (PTFE) grafts for immediate reconstruction of vascular structures in contaminated wounds despite reported successes. Data are presented on 25 vascular reconstructions in contaminated wounds that were performed in 20 patients by using PTFE grafts.

Each patient had life- or extremity-threatening ischemia with severe local tissue damage. Blunt trauma caused injuries to 16 patients, with injury to the axillary artery in 2 patients, the iliac to common femoral artery in 4, the superficial femoral artery in 2, and the popliteal artery in 8. Penetrating trauma caused injuries to the axillary artery in 1 patient, the superior mesenteric artery in 2, and the common femoral artery in 1. All these injuries created extensive vascular defects. In all patients, 6-mm, thin-walled PTFE grafts were used for interposition bypass of arterial injuries; 5 patients underwent concomitant venous reconstruction with the use of 8-mm PTFE grafts.

Surgery involved proximal and distal control of the blood vessels at sites remote from the injuries, debridement of all injured vascular walls, and continuous suture vascular anastomosis by using 6–0 or 7–0 polypropylene monofilament suture. Arterial continuity was established first in patients with concomitant arterial and venous injuries. All patients with leg injuries received mannitol during operation before arterial reperfusion. One patient died after vascular reconstruction was completed. Another patient had one arterial and one venous graft thrombosis at 3 months. All other grafts remained patent up to 2 years of follow-up with no signs of local or systemic infection, distal embolization, or anastomotic disruption.

Use of PTFE grafts was warranted in these severely traumatized patients in whom direct repair was not possible because of extensive vascular injuries. Also, in leg injuries destruction of the saphenous vein meant that the remaining segments were usually of smaller size and quality. In addition, even the largest saphenous veins would have been inadequate in size for reconstruction, and urgency of the clinical situation warranted rapid reinstitution of arterial flow.

Some experimental and human studies have shown that the PTFE grafts are more resistant to infection in contaminated wounds, when compared with excised autogenous vein grafts. This study indicated that if the suture lines are placed in healthy vascular tissue and, particularly, if they are covered by autogenous muscle tissue, the risk of infection is small.

For rapid reconstruction of acute contaminated peripheral vascular injuries, PTFE grafts were an acceptable choice for primary repair in these patients. The ready availability in many calibers, sparing of autogenous vein for future use, and the expedience in vascular reconstruction makes such grafts advantageous for use in multiply traumatized patients without the fear of prosthetic graft infections.

▶ These two reports on the use of PTFE grafts in arterial trauma provide a large number of cases with long-term follow-up (3.5–5 years). It is surprising that infection was not a problem. Coverage of the exposed graft, however, is essential to prevent rupture of any suture line. In patients with multiple injuries and in unstable condition, PTFE grafts may be used to spare the unnecessary time for harvesting saphenous vein. It should not, however, be used for the purpose of sparing autogenous veins for future use.

Fatal Thromboembolic Complications at Aortofemoral Angiography

R. Takolan'ʼr, D. Bergqvist, K. Jonsson, S. Karlsson, and K. Fält (Malmö, Sweden)

Acta Rad.ol. (Diagn.) (Stockh.) 26:15–19, Jan.–Feb. 1985 9–15

Fatal complications of angiography are reported in up to 0.09% of cases, but fatal occlusion of the lumbar aorta after angiography seems to be very rare. Three cases of fatal aortic occlusion associated with extensive microembolization and small vessel thrombosis were encountered. All 3 deaths were due to lumbar aortic occlusion combined with massive peripheral microembolization and macroembolization. The local circulation was surgically restored in all instances, but the affected microcirculation was inaccessible, and profound tissue ischemia and death ensued. It appears that peripheral embolization must be massive to cause clinical problems. A thrombus can form either on the catheter, embolizing on withdrawal, or after subintimal passage of the catheter. Extensive atherosclerotic plaque was not detected angiographically in 1 of the present cases. In another case, the abnormalities were so extensive that slight catheter trauma was sufficient to cause catastrophic embolization.

It seems possible to avoid catheterization of very atherosclerotic arteries by use of intravenous digital subtraction angiography, but this procedure is not feasible for evaluation of gastrointestinal bleeding. Catheter manipulation is a necessary part of percutaneous transluminal angioplasty. Aneurysm or ulcerated plaque can be suspected in a patient presenting with distal microembolization but no ischemia or claudication. Catheter manipulation should be avoided as much as possible in patients with severe atherosclerotic changes in the aorta and iliac vessels. Intra-arterial fibrinolysis might be of benefit in some cases, although it takes several hours to obtain reperfusion in this way. Because widespread damage already existed in the present cases, fibrinolysis would not have been useful.

Iatrogenic Arteriovenous Fistula of the Internal Mammary Artery: Transcatheter Intravascular Coil Occlusion

Tsugihiro Nakamura, Yasuhide Nakashima, Kogi Yu, Yutaka Senda, Osamu Hasegawa, Akio Kuroiwa, and Yoshiki Tsukamoto (Kitakyushu, Japan)

Arch. Intern. Med. 145:140–141, January 1985 9–16

A case of iatrogenic arteriovenous fistula of the internal mammary artery

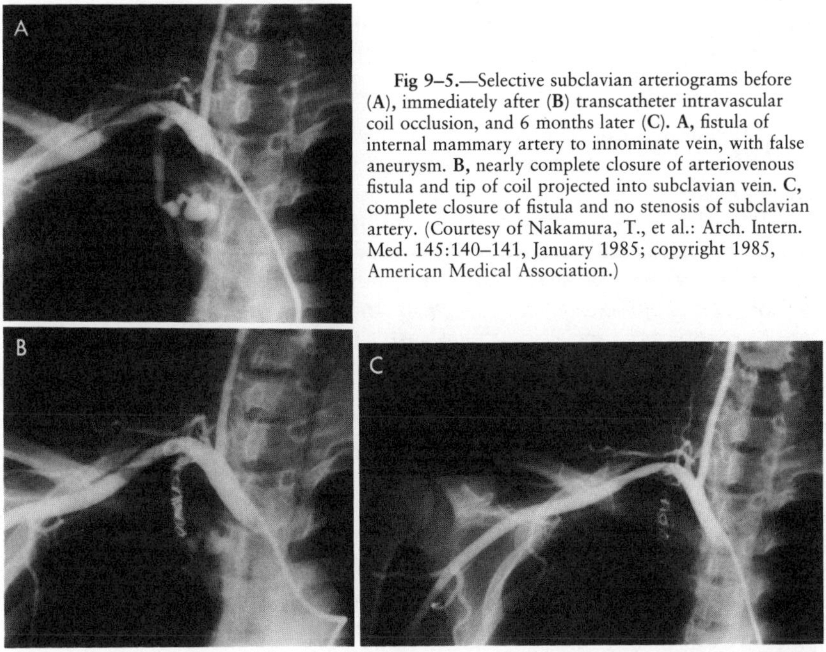

Fig 9–5.—Selective subclavian arteriograms before (**A**), immediately after (**B**) transcatheter intravascular coil occlusion, and 6 months later (**C**). **A**, fistula of internal mammary artery to innominate vein, with false aneurysm. **B**, nearly complete closure of arteriovenous fistula and tip of coil projected into subclavian vein. **C**, complete closure of fistula and no stenosis of subclavian artery. (Courtesy of Nakamura, T., et al.: Arch. Intern. Med. 145:140–141, January 1985; copyright 1985, American Medical Association.)

was encountered, which was complicated by projection of the proximal coil spring after occlusion by the transcatheter intravascular method.

Woman, 20, was admitted with edema and impaired consciousness from uremia. She had received peritoneal dialysis elsewhere and had vomited and developed edema after symptoms of a common cold. Proteinuria had been present since childhood and hypertension for 1 year. The patient was comatose and had a blood pressure of 60/30 mm Hg. A grade 3/6 ejection systolic murmur was heard, as were moist rales. Marked anemia and azotemia were documented. Several attempts were made to insert a central venous pressure catheter by puncturing the right subclavian vein via the infraclavicular approach. Uremia was controlled by peritoneal dialysis and hemodialysis, but a continuous machinery murmur was heard in the right clavicular region on the second day. Right subclavian arteriography showed a fistula between the right internal mammary artery and the innominate vein, with a false aneurysm. Transcatheter intravascular coil occlusion was carried out. The fistula was nearly closed, but the proximal coil spring was seen projecting into the subclavian artery (Fig 9–5). There was no evidence of thromboembolism over 6 months of follow-up. Complete closure of the fistula without subclavian stenosis was documented 6 months later. The continuous murmur was absent on phonocardiography.

Fistula closure was considered in this patient because of possible cardiac complications by shunt flow from the fistula. Ligation appeared to be risky, and conventional transcatheter embolization with small particulate matter can lead to pulmonary infarction. The coil spring projected into the subclavian artery, probably for technical reasons, but embolism of the distal artery did not result during follow-up, and the fistula eventually closed completely. Both thrombocytopenia from chronic renal failure and anticoagulation for hemodialysis may have protected the patient.

▶ In the category of iatrogenic trauma due to diagnostic procedures, we select one abstract on catheter-induced trauma and one rather rare complication of subclavian venous catheterization. The latter abstract indicates the value of small vessel occlusion by transcatheter intravascular coil introduction. The former abstract describes the well-known phenomenon of distal microembolization caused by proximal arterial trauma. Other problems of iatrogenic trauma in the aortoiliac segment include rupture of the iliac artery during percutaneous transluminal dilation and iliac arterial vascular occlusion caused by subintimal introduction of the transfemoral catheter.

Treatment of the Ruptured or Exposed Carotid Artery: A Rational Approach

John J. Coleman III (Emory Univ.)

South. Med. J. 78:262–267, March1985 9–17

Carotid artery bleeding is an uncommon complication of radical head-neck surgery when the wound breaks down and the vessel is exposed to the bacterial flora of the neck or to salivary secretion. Eight patients seen in 1972–1982 had hemorrhage necessitating carotid ligation after treatment for head-neck cancer, and 2 died before surgery. Five other patients had significant exposure of the vessel. Of the 8 patients who underwent emergency ligation, 1 died of sequelae of bleeding, and 1 of subsequent brain abscess. One survivor had a permanent neurologic deficit. Nine of the 10 patients with acute bleeding had had irradiation of the neck, 6 in conjunction with surgery. Vascularized distant tissue was needed for coverage of the neck in 4 of the 6 patients who had bleeding controlled. Exposure of the carotid resulted from orocutaneous or pharyngocutaneous fistulas forming after surgery in 3 cases and from partial loss of a cervical skin flap in 2. Only 1 of these 5 patients had been irradiated. Muscle flap surgery was performed in 4 cases. None of these patients subsequently bled.

The common carotid artery in the middle of the neck and the carotid bulb are at the greatest risk of rupture. A wide McFee flap with horizontal incisions along the clavicle and in the submandibular fold minimizes exposure of the carotid if skin loss occurs after neck dissection. Immediate coverage of the exposed carotid is possible with various well-vascularized thoracic muscle or musculocutaneous flaps. Prevention of fistula formation in irradiated patients will minimize the risk of carotid rupture. Exposure can be managed by débriding necrotic tissue and preventing invasive bacterial infection in nonirradiated patients, followed by definitive closure. In irradiated patients, the exposed carotid must be covered immediately. If débridement necessitates removal of part of the carotid wall, the artery should be ligated proximally and distally and the segment should be excised before muscle coverage. The ruptured irradiated carotid artery should be treated as an infected foreign body. The stumps of the resected carotid artery should be well covered with extracervical muscle.

Emergency Ligation of the External Iliac Artery

Ingemar Blohmé and Hans Brynger (Univ. of Göteborg, Sweden)

Ann. Surg. 201:505–510, April 1985 9–18

Massive bleeding from an infected arteriotomy during renal transplantation can necessitate ligation and resection of an iliac artery. Thirty-five of 1,526 renal transplant procedures performed during a 19-year period in Gothenburg, Sweden, were complicated by gross bleeding from an infected arteriotomy. Nine patients died as a direct result, and all but 3 patients lost their grafts. The external or common iliac artery was resected and ligated in 19 cases. Twelve patients did not undergo arterial reconstruction, and another patient with an autotransplanted kidney and no infection underwent emergency iliac artery ligation.

None of the 13 patients having iliac artery resection without reconstruction had tissue loss. In no case did elective reconstruction become necessary for functional deficit. Eight patients had some degree of weakness, coolness, or intermittent claudication, but these signs were reversed within a few days. Most patients were ambulatory without symptoms within 2–3 weeks. Two patients had persistent claudication, and one might have undergone reconstruction had he survived a myocardial infarction. Among 6 patients followed up 4–10 years after iliac artery ligation, the 5 with well-functioning kidneys were without symptoms of arterial insufficiency in daily activities, although functional deficits could be provoked. Collateral circulation was supplied by different arteries in the patients undergoing angiography.

The iliac artery can safely be ligated without immediate arterial reconstruction in a renal transplant recipient to control massive bleeding from an infected arteriotomy. There is little risk of limb loss, but close follow-up is necessary for the early detection of irreversible arterial insufficiency. The risk of nutritional inadequacy is substantial, and there is also a small risk of gangrene in these cases.

▶ These two abstracts describe forms of iatrogenic trauma and bring up many important points, all of which will be of use to vascular surgeons in large hospitals that do a large volume of head and neck surgery and renal transplantation. In the latter category, the patients in general are younger and have more normal vessels and therefore can stand occlusion of an external iliac artery without tissue loss.

Arterial Complications of Total Knee Replacement

Clyde E. McAuley, David L. Steed, and Marshall W. Webster (Univ. of Pittsburgh)

Arch. Surg. 119:960–962, August 1984 9–19

Arterial complications that develop after total knee replacement can occur on an acute or chronic basis. In a recent patient, arterial occlusion developed either intraoperatively or in the immediate postoperative period. At exploration, the finding of a contused segment of distal superficial femoral artery, as well as a fragment of embolized atheromatous plaque in the distal extracted thrombus, suggested that a disrupting external force had been applied to a chronically diseased vessel. Incomplete luminal occlusion can be caused by kinking of a popliteal artery by a musculofascial constriction. Anterior subluxation of the tibial prosthetic component on the femoral component may occur. A possible explanation for an intimal tear is fracture of a calcified atherosclerotic artery caused by the compressive force exerted by a pneumatic tourniquet. However, it is also possible that fixation of the proximal superficial femoral artery by a tourniquet and stretching the distal artery during intraoperative manipulation of the knee could result in intimal disruption and atheromatous plaque embolization.

In the second patient, a slowly progressive occlusive process led to complete arterial interruption in a leg. This may have been the result of initial intimal disruption with slow development of arterial stenosis. Localized arterial injury also stimulates the development of atherosclerosis at the site of an arterial injury. Because of the frequent association of atherosclerosis and degenerative joint disease in the older patient, and the attendant risk of atheromatous plaque disruption from mechanical arterial compression or stretching, a detailed evaluation of the peripheral arterial system by a vascular surgeon is mandatory prior to total knee replacement if arterial disease is suspected or vessel calcification is present.

Vascular Injury Related to Lumbar Disk Surgery

James M. Salander, Jerry R. Youkey, Norman M. Rich, David W. Olson, and G. Patrick Clagett

J. Trauma 24:628–631, July 1984 9–20

Iatrogenic vascular injury associated with lumbar disk surgery requires timely diagnosis and treatment. Data are reported on 6 patients at Walter Reed Army Medical Center who were operated on from 1949 through 1982 for vascular injury related to lumbar disk surgery.

Two of the 6 patients had previous lumbar disk surgery elsewhere. All neurosurgical interventions were at the L4–5 disk space. Four patients had isolated arterial injuries and 2 had combined arteriovenous injuries. The common iliac artery was involved in all 6 cases, 3 on right and 3 on left. There were no associated intra-abdominal vascular injuries or injuries to the gastrointestinal tract.

A diagnosis of vascular injury was delayed in 3 patients: 2 had minimally symptomatic arteriovenous fistulas, and lateral venorrhaphy and arterial end-to-end anastomoses were performed at 6 weeks and 3 years after injury; 1 who had a known arterial injury presented with back pain and neurologic findings in a lower extremity, and homologous arterial grafting was performed 30 days after injury. Three patients underwent operation immediately upon diagnosis, including 2 who presented with hypovolemic shock and 1 who was diagnosed by angiogram as having an acute false aneurysm. Repair was achieved by lateral arteriorrhaphy in 3 cases. There were no deaths or amputations. Minor complications after operation included hepatitis in 1 patient and transient ejaculatory dysfunction in another. There were no failed venous or arterial reconstructions. Long-term follow-up of 2 patients showed normal vascular findings.

The anterior spinal ligament separates the bifurcation of the aorta and inferior vena cava from the L4–5 disk space. In the presence of a weakened or distorted ligament resulting from chronic disk disease or prior disk surgery or an aggressive exploration of this space, use of an open pituitary rongeur passed blindly into the space and around it can cause injury to the retroperitoneal or intra-abdominal structures.

Most vascular injuries from disk surgery occur within a few centimeters of the bifurcation; however, visceral vessels and external/internal iliac arteries have also been injured. Vascular injury may result in fistula, false aneurysm, or hemorrhage. A single artery is often injured but isolated venous injuries are rare and mostly confined to the inferior vena cava. Late presentation of injuries delays diagnosis and treatment, resulting in increased mortality.

Vascular injury associated with lumbar disk surgery requires timely diagnosis and treatment. Profuse bleeding or shock, or both, can be leading symptoms; however, they may not always be present. The risk of vascular injury may be increased with repeated disk operations; use of the operating microscope can lessen the risk. An angiogram can be a diagnostic adjunct, particularly in a hemodynamically stable patient in whom vascular injury is strongly suspected.

▶ In most general medicine and surgery hospitals, vascular trauma is important. In the various categories of vascular trauma, iatrogenic trauma is reaching almost epidemic proportions. Such trauma can be divided into the injury produced by operations, such as is indicated by these two abstracts, and the trauma introduced by diagnostic procedures. In the former category, these two abstracts speak for themselves.

VENOUS CONDITIONS

10 Occlusive Lesions of the Veins

Leiomyosarcomas of Venous Origin in the Extremities: A Correlated Clinical, Roentgenologic, and Morphologic Study With Diagnostic and Surgical Implications

Örjan Berlin, Bertil Stener, Lars-Gunnar Kindblom, and Lennart Angervall (Univ. of Göteborg, Sweden)

Cancer 54:2147–2159, Nov. 15, 1984 10–1

Many leiomyosarcomas in the extremities seem to have arisen from the wall of a large vein. A correlated clinical, roentgenologic, and morphologic study of 6 cases of leiomyosarcoma of the large veins in the extremities was conducted to define their role in the diagnosis and surgical treatment of such tumors. The leiomyosarcoma was located in the upper extremity in 1 case and in the lower extremity in 5 cases. Preoperatively, phlebography was performed in 1 patient, arteriography in 4, and computed tomography in 2. All tumors were studied by light microscopy; 3 were also studied by electron microscopy.

Patients were initially seen with a firm, enlarging mass on the axilla, in the medial part of the thigh, or in the popliteal fossa (5 cases) or with numbness of the leg before the mass appeared (1 case). The axillary vein was affected in 1 case, the superficial femoral vein in 3, the great saphenous vein in 1, and the popliteal vein in 1. Phlebography in 1 case showed a thrombus in the common femoral vein that apparently was caused by intraluminal growth of the tumor and occlusion of the superficial femoral vein. Angiography in 4 cases showed a highly vascular tumor, with compression of the accompanying artery and narrowing of the arterial lumen where it passed the tumor. Computed tomography in 2 patients showed the topographic relationship of the tumor to the vessels within their common fibrous sheath.

Incisional biopsy was performed in 3 cases and fine-needle aspiration in 2. All tumors grew intraluminally and were highly malignant (5 grade III and 1 grade IV). All tumors showed a strikingly uniform light microscopic appearance that was characteristic of leiomyosarcoma. Tumors cells had a smooth-muscle fiber appearance, with strongly picrinophilic and eosinophilic cytoplasm containing suggestive fibrils. Although they were well differentiated, all tumors showed areas containing tumor cells with large polymorphous and hyperchromatic nuclei and relatively high mitotic activity. Ultrastructural studies showed an abundance of myofilaments of actin type, with focal elongated densities, segments of external lamina, and prominent pinocytotic vesicles. Surgical treatments included 1 interscapulothoracic amputation, 1 extended hip-joint disarticulation, 2 marginal local excisions, 1 radical local excision, and 1 femur amputation. Five of the patients died of metastatic tumor disease, and one is alive with lung metastases.

Leiomyosarcomas of venous origin in the extremities have a tendency to grow intravenously and exert arterial compression. Knowing these characteristics can be helpful in the clinical diagnosis and planning of adequate surgical treatment. The appearance of thrombosis in the common femoral vein on phlebography in 1 patient with helpful in the planning of an operation. Angiographic findings of compression and narrowing of the artery running close to the tumor are suggestive of leiomyosarcoma. The arising of the leiomyosarcoma in the superficial femoral vein is also a possibility when a growing mass is noted in the medial part of the thigh. Symptoms ascribable to the saphenous nerve may suggest the presence of a tumor of the superficial femoral vein. The authors recommend that, after confirmation of the tumor by a fine-needle aspiration, radical local excision of the tumor be performed, including the superficial femoral vessels in the specimen and substituting a vessel graft for the artery.

▶ This detailed study of leiomyosarcomas of venous origin should help vascular surgeons to familiarize themselves with this unusual tumor. Future YEAR BOOKS will deal with the problem of venous leiomyomatosis.

Dynamics of Thrombophlebitis in Central Venous Catheterization via Basilic and Cephalic Veins

I. Curelaru, A. Bylock, B. Gustavsson, E. Hultman, L. E. Linder, T. Stefánsson, and O. Stenqvist

Acta Chir. Scand. 150:285–293, 1984 10–2

The incidence distribution of clinical thrombophlebitis in central catheterization via basilic and cephalic veins was investigated in relation to the duration of catheterization, the catheter material and its surface structures and different stiffnesses and platelet adhesion-stimulating properties in vitro, and effects of heparin coating of the catheters. Two hundred twenty-seven long central venous catheters were inserted in 215 patients. Catheters were made of polyethylene, heparinized polyethylene, silicone elastomer, polyvinyl chloride, soft polyurethane, heparinized soft polyurethane, and relatively harder polyurethane. Catheter lengths varied from 35 to 61 cm.

Catheterization times ranged from 1 to 100 days (mean, 9.4). Of 47 episodes of thrombophlebitis, 44 occurred 1 to 10 days after insertion of the catheter. The incidence distribution of thrombophlebitis had a peak on the fifth day of catheterization and a central tendency between 3 and 8 days; after 10 days the risk of thrombophlebitis fell significantly. The cumulative incidence of thrombophlebitis reached 3.5% after 3 days of catheterization, 19% after 10 days, and 21% after 32 days. The estimated cumulative probabilities of thrombophlebitis, including all catheter types, were 4% after the first 3 days, 26% after 10 days, and 33% between 11 and 100 days after insertion. The incidence of clinical thrombophlebitis and catheter type showed no significant correlation, regardless of material, stiffness, surface roughness, and degree of platelet adhesion in vitro. Only 1 case of suppurative thrombophlebitis and catheter sepsis was found in more than 2,000 catheter-days.

The incidence of clinical thrombophlebitis after central cannulation via basilic or cephalic veins increased with, but was not linearly related to, the duration of catheterization. Thrombophlebitis appeared from 1 to 10 days after insertion of the catheter, suggesting a nonspecific reaction of the vein wall triggered by injury to the vein intima, leakage of chemical substances from the catheter during its insertion and presence, or both. Occasional occurrence of thrombophlebitis after 10 days can be caused by secondary injury to the venous wall triggered by relative hypoxemia at the level of the narrowed vein valve pockets, where laminar blood flow and flotation of the catheter may be impeded. Despite the increased risk of thrombophlebitis 3 days after catheter insertion, the authors believe that central venous catheters inserted via the basilic or cephalic veins should not be removed or changed to counteract the risk of thrombophlebitis, at any rate not when long-term use (at least 10 days) is planned. For conclusive comparisons between catheter materials concerning induction of clinical thrombophlebitis, the catheter should remain in situ for at least 10 days in all patients, unless symptoms of venous reaction arise sooner.

Delayed Soft Tissue Infections in Saphenous Venectomy Limbs of Coronary Bypass Patients

Larry M. Baddour (Univ. of Tennessee) and Waid Rogers (Univ. of Texas)

Infect. Surg. 4:243–250, April 1985 10–3

Recurrent cellulitis is a complication of saphenous venectomy in patients having coronary artery bypass operation. Dermatophytosis has been associated with the disorder in most cases, and treatment of superficial fungal infection has deterred further attacks of cellulitis. The most frequent bacterial cause probably is β-hemolytic streptococci as evidenced by dramatic responses to penicillin. Hypersensitivity to specific fungal antigens may explain some cellulitis-like reactions in coronary bypass patients having tinea infection of the venectomy extremities. Bacterial extracellular toxins also have been implicated. Host immunologic status may be an important pathogenetic factor in recurrent cellulitis. Reactions may be more marked when venous drainage of the extremity is impaired or when lymphatic drainage is compromised.

Subsequent episodes of cellulitis occur unpredictably in these cases. Most patients have a sudden onset of severe symptoms, and most patients appear toxic at presentation. The response to antibiotics is as prompt as the clinical onset, and the cellulitis itself generally resolves completely within 1 week. Penicillin is the antibiotic of choice. Tinea pedis infections should be actively treated in order to prevent further attacks of cellulitis. Topical antifungal therapy is used initially; systemic antifungal agents can be used in refractory cases. Patients who continue to have episodes of cellulitis may receive antistreptococcal regimens similar to those used to prevent rheumatic fever.

▶ Both articles are dealing with new problems caused by an increasing use of respectable procedures. Cellulitis as a result of saphenous vein removal is often mistaken for deep vein thrombosis. The presence of tinea pedis is a diagnostic clue in such patients.

Experimental Deep Venous Thrombogenesis by a Noninvasive Method
John D. Hamer and P. C. Malone (Birmingham, England)
Ann. R. Coll. Surg. Engl. 66:416–419, November 1984 10–4

Stasis itself appears not to be directly responsible for blood clotting and is probably not thrombogenic acting alone. Deep venous thrombosis was produced in dogs by a method causing no injury to the veins or the leg. The endothelium lining the valve pockets in femoral veins of beagle and mongrel Labrador dogs was damaged by hypoxemia and then intermittently reperfused with oxygenated blood. The hindlimbs of some dogs were passively moved at frequent intervals to cause centripetal acceleration of blood flow within the leg veins. Other dogs underwent active movements that were more rapid and greater in amplitude, through manipulation of barbiturate anesthesia.

Thrombi formed much more frequently in the rapid-movement group. All arose from venous valve pockets (Fig 10–1) or from the confluence of tributary veins with the main femoral vein. Most thrombi contained mul-

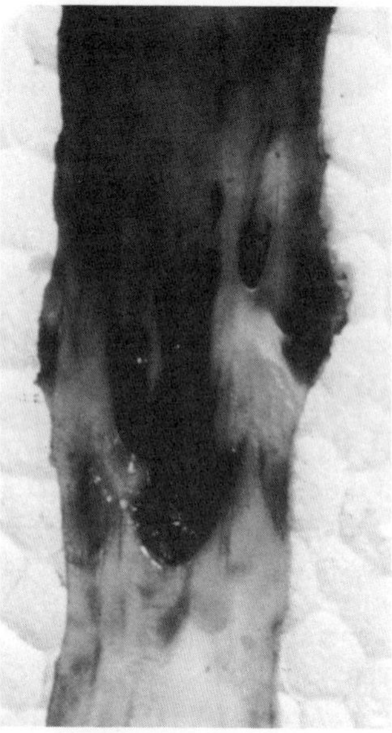

Fig 10–1.—Femoral vein with thrombus arising in valve pocket, attached within pocket and propagating centrally. Dark "shadowings" in orifices of some small tributaries are further thrombi arising at these junctions. (Courtesy of Hamer, J.D., and Malone, P.C.: Ann. R. Coll. Surg. Engl. 66:416–419, November 1984.)

tiple aggregated masses of platelets, each rimmed by a narrow fibrin border and lying within a greater volume of red blood cell thrombus. Much of the structure resembled the propagating parts of femoral valve pocket thrombi in man. The venous intima was sometimes covered by a thin film of granular material containing numerous platelets, some leukocytes, and fibrin threads.

This is the first report of spontaneous deep venous thrombosis in an experimental model the morphological features of which resemble those of deep vein thrombosis in man. The observations suggest that localized venous valve pocket stasis alternating with intermittent restoration of perfusion has a major role in spontaneous clinical thrombogenesis. They also support the use of mechanical methods of prevention in limbs not already harboring venous thrombi. Pharmacologic methods may be necessary if silent thrombi have already formed in the venous system.

Flow Through a Venous Valve and Its Implication for Thrombus Formation

Takeshi Karino and Mineo Motomiya (McGill Univ.)

Thromb. Res. 36:245–257, 1984 10–5

Preferential areas for venous thrombosis are in the deep veins of the lower limbs in older subjects in the form of venous valve pockets, where

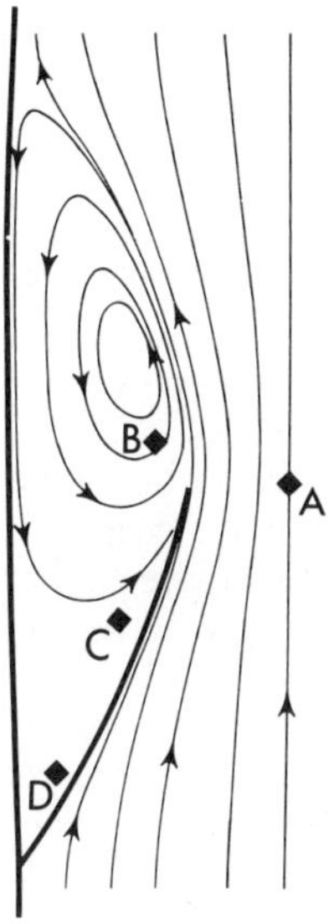

Relative Oxygen Tension, P/P_A

Subject \ Position	B	C	D
Human saphenous vein (10 min) n = 2	0.998	0.985	0.684
Dog femoral vein (10 min) n = 4	0.998	0.993	0.833
Dog femoral vein (90 min) n = 4	0.999	0.361	0.041

Original data from
Hamer et al., Br. J. Surg. 68, 166–170 (1981)

Fig 10–2.—Relative oxygen tension (P/P_A), normalized by value in mainstream, P_A, at various sites in pocket of venous valve, measured by Hamer et al. in human saphenous veins and dog femoral veins under nonpulsatile flow conditions. Numbers in table are means of several measurements indicated by n. Approximate locations of measurements are indicated by *A* to *D* in schematic representation of streamlines through valve obtained in authors' investigation. (Courtesy of Karino, T., and Motomiya, M.: Thromb. Res. 36:245–257, 1984.)

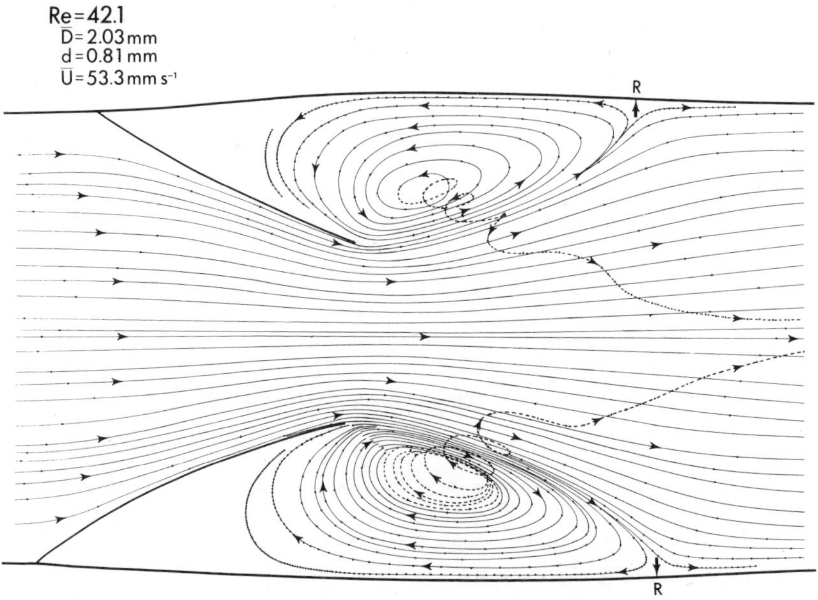

Fig 10–3.—Detailed flow patterns through venous valve in dog saphenous vein 2 mm in diameter as observed along common median plane of valve and vein. Figure shows formation of spiral vortices in pockets of venous valve. Vortex in each pocket in fact consists of pair of vortices located symmetrically on both sides of bisector plane of valve leaflets (normal to common median plane). In lower valve pocket, particle located near bisector plane was traced every two orbits *(solid lines)* then continuously *(broken line)* after it moved away from bisector plane. Broken paths are actually projection of particle path on bisector plane. Arrows at R indicate location of reattachment points. Deep in each valve pocket *(solid area)*, another, smaller, counterrotating secondary vortex was formed. (Courtesy of Karino, T., and Motomiya, M.: Thromb. Res. 36:245–257, 1984.)

stagnant flow and eddies are likely to occur. The possible relation between flow conditions in the pockets and thrombus formation was examined in isolated, transparent veins containing two-leaflet valves prepared from canine hindlimbs. Cinemicrographic techniques were used to evaluate flow in the saphenous veins.

Large, paired vortices were located symmetrically on either side of the bisector plane of the valve leaflets in each pocket under physiologic flow conditions (Fig 10–2). Particles continuously entered the valve pocket from the mainstream and spent considerable time describing a series of spiral orbits while moving away from the bisector plane, eventually leaving the vortex and rejoining the mainstream. Observations with concentrated red blood cell suspensions indicated the presence of a smaller, counterrotating secondary vortex, driven by the large primary one, deep in each valve pocket. Fluid in these regions circulated quite slowly, creating a low shear field that allowed the red blood cells to aggregate.

It is expected that standing vortices form in vivo at sites of venous valves. Stagnation and a lowered hematocrit in the deepest part of the valve pocket could lead to local hypoxia (Fig 10–3). Localized hypoxia may cause endothelial damage and lead to formation of a thrombus on a valve cusp after a short period of nonpulsatile flow. The potential for this type of effect depends on the supply in the mainstream, the tension in the vessel wall, the distances involved, the diffusibility of oxygen, and the levels of consumption of all the structures involved.

Early Events in the Formation of a Venous Thrombus Following Local Trauma and Stasis

R. G. Schaub, C. A. Simmons, M. H. Koets, P. J. Romano II, and G. J. Stewart

Lab. Invest. 51:218–224, August 1984 10–6

Leukocytes contribute to the initiation of venous thrombosis by producing endothelial damage, but the role of platelets is less clear. Early venous thrombus formation was investigated in cats in which a jugular

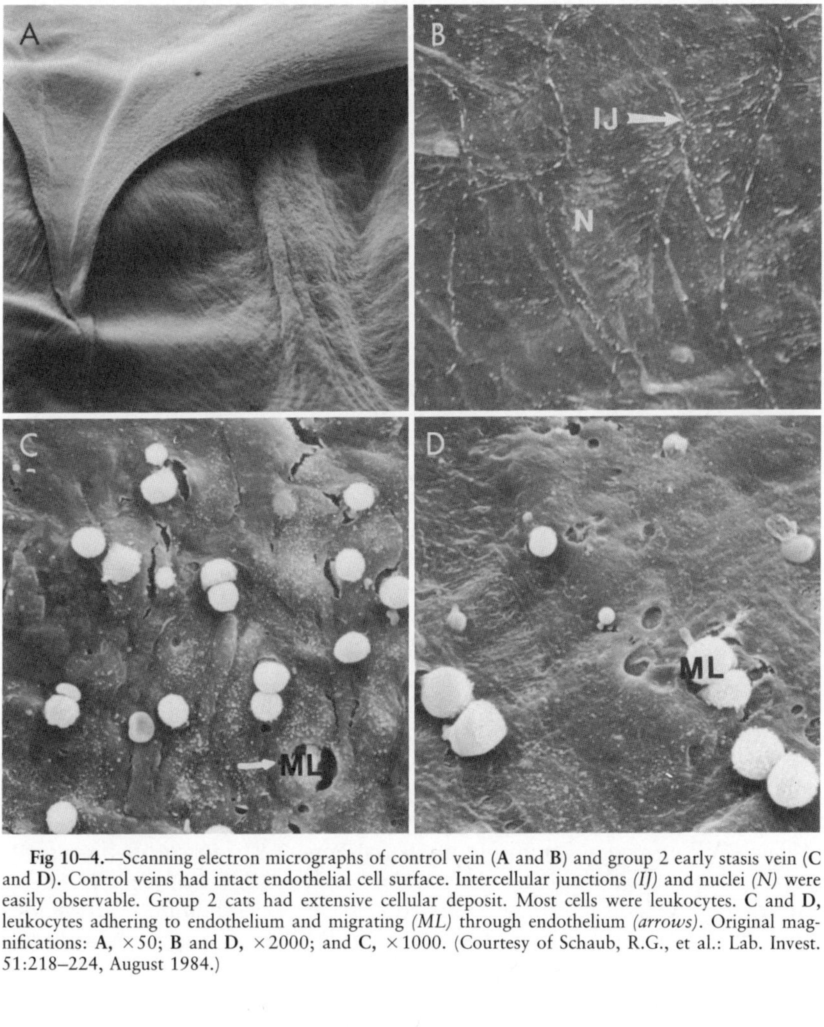

Fig 10–4.—Scanning electron micrographs of control vein (**A** and **B**) and group 2 early stasis vein (**C** and **D**). Control veins had intact endothelial cell surface. Intercellular junctions *(IJ)* and nuclei *(N)* were easily observable. Group 2 cats had extensive cellular deposit. Most cells were leukocytes. **C** and **D**, leukocytes adhering to endothelium and migrating *(ML)* through endothelium *(arrows)*. Original magnifications: **A**, ×50; **B** and **D**, ×2000; and **C**, ×1000. (Courtesy of Schaub, R.G., et al.: Lab. Invest. 51:218–224, August 1984.)

vein was exposed and removed immediately (group 1), after three 5-minute periods of stasis and reflow (group 2), or after occlusion for 24 (group 3) or 72 hours (group 4). The veins in all groups were perfused at physiologic pressure with heparinized saline and immersed in 2.5% glutaraldehyde for fixation.

The findings in early stasis are compared with the control scanning electron microscopic appearances in Figure 10–4. Leukocytes but few erythrocytes or platelets were deposited. Leukocytes were present in association with platelets and red blood cells after venous occlusion. Platelets and erythrocytes were seldom found in the absence of leukocytes. Thrombi were seen on both normal-appearing and damaged endothelium. Most were found at side branches and valve pockets. Leukocytes appeared to be a point of attachment for fibrin and platelets. More consolidated and more complex thrombi were evident in group 4. Leukocytes associated with fibrin were the primary cell type in group 4 thrombi.

The findings indicate that leukocytes have a primary role in the initiation of deep venous thrombi. Platelets may have only a secondary role. Thrombosis appears to begin in valve pockets and to continue through successive fibrin and platelet deposits. The abrupt expansion of blood flow in valve pockets may make these areas especially susceptible to the effects of adherent leukocytes.

▶ The importance of the venous valve pocket as an initiating site for venous thrombosis is further confirmed by the preceding two studies. The mechanism responsible for thrombosis is well shown by hemodynamic, as well as oxygen tension study. This study provides us with a model that mimics human DVT and allows animal research to become relevant to the human condition.

Once again, leukocytes, not just platelets, may play an important role in the pathogenesis of thrombus formation.

Peripheral Venous Pulsatility Detected by Doppler Method for Diagnosis of Right Heart Failure

B. Krahenbuhl, A. Restellini, and A. Frangos (Univ. of Geneva)

Cardiology 71:173–176, 1984 10–7

Peripheral venous flow becomes pulsatile as right atrial pressure increases, but the pulsation is clinically evident only if the pressure is fairly high. A Doppler flowmeter was used to detect pulsatile venous flow at a preclinical stage in 46 patients (35 men) with right heart failure. Mean age was 55 years. Thirty-three patients had coronary heart disease, 17 with recent myocardial infarction, and 9 had valvular heart disease. Twenty-seven patients underwent right heart catheterization. In 19 treated for systemic disease, central venous pressure (CVP) was monitored.

The CVP exceeded 7 mm Hg in 13 patients, 12 of whom had pulsatile venous flow in both femoral veins and a brachial vein. Clinical right heart failure was evident in 7 of these patients, all of whom had pulsatile venous flow (Fig 10–5). One patient with a CVP of less than 7 mm Hg had clinical

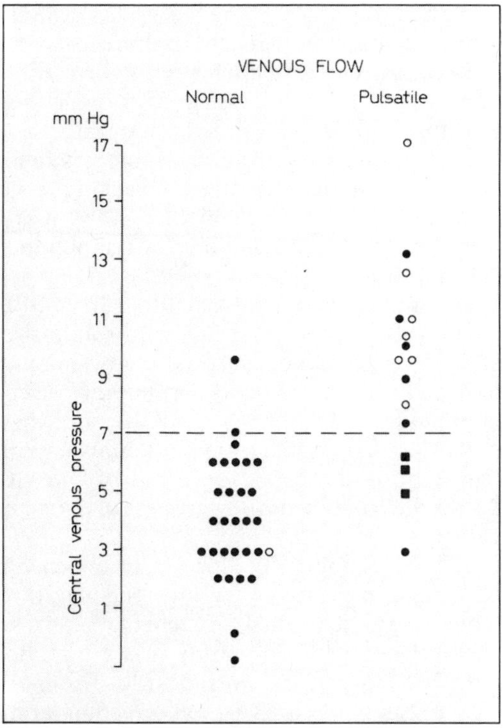

Fig 10–5.—Pulsatility of peripheral venous flow. Open circles denote patients with clinical signs of right heart failure, and solid circles, those without. The three squares indicate patients with valvular heart disease in whom left ventricle ejection fraction was less than 60%. (Courtesy of Krahenbuhl, B., et al.: Cardiology 71:173–176, 1984.)

signs of right heart failure but no pulsatile venous flow. Four others had pulsatile venous flow without clinical signs of right heart failure. The latter had valvular disease; 3 had a left ventricular ejection fraction of less than 60%.

Detection of pulsatile peripheral venous blood flow by the Doppler method is more sensitive than clinical evaluation in detecting right heart failure and probably is more sensitive than CVP monitoring. Examination of three different veins will prevent a false impression of pulsation from systolic movement of a nearby artery in an elderly patient.

Diagnostic Efficacy of Impedance Plethysmography for Clinically Suspected Deep Vein Thrombosis: A Randomized Trial

Russell D. Hull, Jack Hirsh, Cedric J. Carter, Richard M. Jay, Paul A. Ockelford, Harry R. Buller, A. Graham Turpie, Peter Powers, Denise Kinch, Pearl E. Dodd, Gerald J. Gill, Jacques R. Leclerc, and Michael Gent (McMaster Univ.)

Ann. Intern. Med. 102:21–28, January 1985 10–8

Impedance plethysmography combined with leg scanning is a noninvasive approach to evaluating patients clinically suspected of having deep vein thrombosis. Recently referred patients with normal impedance plethysmographic findings were randomly assigned to either serial impedance studies alone or combined impedance plethysmography and leg scanning as a substitute for venography. Plethysmography was first done immediately after clinical evaluation; the occlusive cuff technique with a prolonged cuff occlusion time was used. Anticoagulant therapy was withheld from patients with normal findings. The combined evaluation included leg scanning by the ^{125}I-fibrinogen technique.

Plethysmographic findings were abnormal in 130 of 992 patients with a first episode of clinically suspected deep vein thrombosis. Of those with normal findings, 317 were assigned to serial plethysmography alone and 328 to the combined study. Thrombosis was initially discovered in 1.9% of the former group and in 9.3% of the latter. Most of these patients had calf vein thrombi. No deaths resulted from pulmonary embolism on follow-up. Deep vein thrombosis developed in 1.9% of the plethysmography group and in 2.2% of the combined study group. All patients were followed for at least 1 year.

Serial impedance plethysmography alone is an effective means of evaluating patients clinically suspected of having deep vein thrombosis. If the study is unavailable or cannot be used for technical reasons, anticoagulant therapy should not be withheld. This study was a multihospital regional trial that included a broad range of patients with various comorbid states. The findings therefore can be generalized to both community and hospital-based practices.

A Critical Appraisal of Impedance Plethysmography in the Diagnosis of Acute Deep Venous Thrombosis

Bhagwan Satiani, Don Paoletti, Marge Henry, Roger Burns, and Dennis Smith (Ohio State Univ.)

Surg. Gynecol. Obstet. 161:25–29, July 1985 10–9

Impedance plethysmography (IPG) is a noninvasive alternative to venography for diagnosis of deep venous thrombosis (DVT), but its accuracy in large community hospitals is uncertain. A prospective study of IPG was carried out in a 600-bed community hospital, where all patients referred for noninvasive venous evaluation in a 38-month period were examined with the IPG 200. Indications included possible acute or recurrent DVT, planned saphenous vein stripping, planned withdrawal of oral anticoagulation, and pulmonary embolism.

Abnormal results were reported in 182 of 992 studies and borderline results in 87 others. Comparison of the results with venographic findings in 211 limbs of 143 patients showed 8 false negative results, all in patients with proximal femoropopliteal thrombosis. False positive results were obtained in 24 extremities. The overall accuracy of IPG in detecting calf vein thrombosis alone was 47%.

Impedance plethysmography is not highly accurate in detecting calf vein thrombosis, and contrast venography may be indicated where strong clinical suspicion of DVT exists. When performed, IPG should include sequential tests with prolongation of the filling time to maximize venous filling and ultimately reach a plateau. Patient apprehension or muscle contraction may result in false positive tests. The test is likely to be reliable if an abnormal result is obtained in a suspect limb and the contralateral extremity is clearly normal.

Gastrocnemius Musculotendinous Rupture: A Condition Confused With Thrombophlebitis

James G. McClure (Memphis)

South. Med. J. 77:1143–1145, September 1984 10–10

Twenty-two cases of rupture of the medial head of the gastrocnemius muscle at the site of insertion into the soleus aponeurosis have been encountered by the author in the past 24 years. The condition frequently is confused with rupture of the plantaris or with thrombophlebitis. A middle-

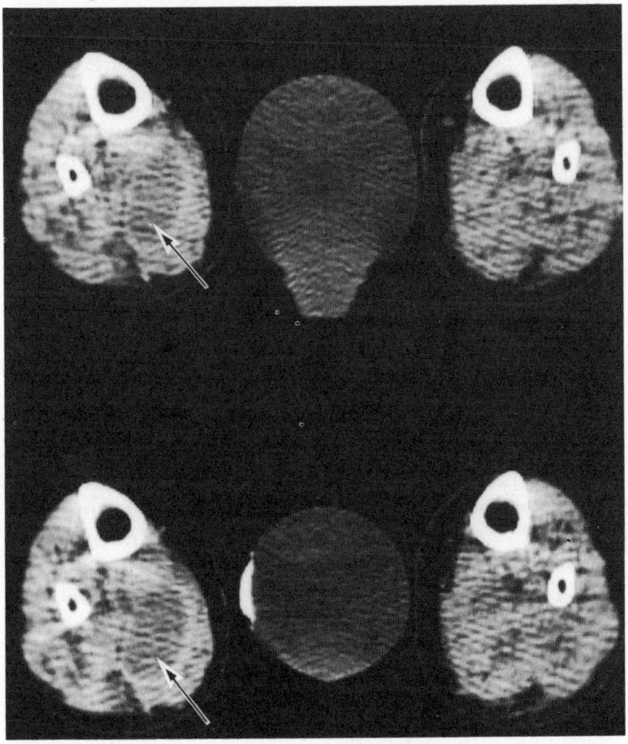

Fig 10–6.—Computed tomography of each leg, showing hemorrhage into the right medial gastrocnemius muscle at the midcalf region *(arrows)*. (Courtesy of McClure, J.G.: South. Med. J. 77:1143–1145, September 1984).

aged person may suddenly experience calf pain when landing on the leg after a jump in the air, or on sudden ankle dorsiflexion with the foot planted. Pain may also occur when stepping off a curb or out of a vehicle. Localized tenderness is present in the medial part of the calf, with varying swelling and tenderness occurring within 24–48 hours, followed later by bluish discoloration of the lower medial aspect of the leg and ankle. A sunken area may be palpated on the medial side of the midcalf and may persist after resolution of the acute process. Venography is the most specific means of ruling out thrombophlebitis, whereas computed tomography may show bleeding into the area of rupture, ruling out rupture of the plantaris tendon (Fig 10–6).

The patient can be permitted limited walking if pain is not severe. Otherwise he should rest in bed for 24 hours, elevating the leg, and apply ice, followed by heat. Crutches or a cane may be needed for a few days. Analgesics and sedatives are used as needed. Surgical repair is not necessary; there is no significant calf weakness when healing is complete. Most patients can resume normal activities in 1 month. It is important to exclude thrombophlebitis to avoid unnecessary anticoagulation therapy and the attendant risk of bleeding.

The occurrence of rupture of the gastrocnemius muscle with minimal trauma in middle-aged persons suggests that it is a degenerative phenomenon analogous to rupture of the long head of the biceps, tendo Achillis, or rotator cuff of the shoulder.

Deep Venous Thrombosis: Detection by High-Resolution Real-Time Ultrasonography

B. Nagesh Raghavendra, Robert J. Rosen, Steven Lam, Thomas Riles, and Steven C. Horii (New York Univ.)

Radiology 152:789–793, September 1984 10–11

High-resolution real-time ultrasonography is useful in detection of venous thrombosis in the inferior vena cava and the jugular, portal, and renal veins. To determine the clinical usefulness of this modality, high-resolution real-time ultrasound examinations were made in 11 patients with clinically suspected deep venous thrombosis of the lower extremity. Findings were correlated with those of contrast venography performed within 24 hours of sonographic examination. The common femoral vein at the groin and the popliteal vein in the popliteal fossa were examined for the presence or absence of an intraluminal soft tissue mass, compressibility of the veins, and response to the Valsalva maneuver and postural changes. The technical adequacy of the method was assessed in 10 healthy persons.

In the 10 healthy persons examined sonographically, the common femoral vein was visualized, easily compressible, free of intraluminal soft tissue mass, and responded promptly and visibly to performance of the Valsalva maneuver. The popliteal vein was visualized in all but 1 of the 10, and was easily compressible and free of intraluminal soft tissue mass. However, its response to the Valsalva maneuver was less consistent, being barely visible or absent, whereas its response to postural changes was rapid and discernible. Five of the 11 patients with clinically suspected deep vein thrombosis were shown to be free of disease by contrast venography. Sonography showed no evidence of thrombus in the common femoral or popliteal vein in these 5 patients. In the remaining 6 patients, both techniques identified deep venous thrombosis. When only the common femoral and popliteal veins were examined, sonography was in complete agreement with the findings on contrast venography. However, contrast venography, but not sonography, demonstrated thrombosis of the superficial femoral vein and calf veins. In all patients in whom sonography detected a thrombus in either the common femoral or popliteal vein, the vein was clearly noncompressible. When the common femoral vein was involved, it did not respond to performance of the Valsalva maneuver. Thus, high-resolution real-time ultrasonography appears promising as a simple, noninvasive method for detection of thrombi in the common femoral and popliteal veins.

Jugular Venous Thrombosis: Diagnosis by Computed Tomography

Elliot K. Fishman, Robert L. Pakter, Bob W. Gayler, Paul S. Wheeler, and Stanley S. Siegelman (Johns Hopkins Med. Inst.)

J. Comput. Assist. Tomogr. 8:963–968, October 1984 10–12

Thrombosis of the internal jugular vein (TIJV) can result from central venous catheter placement, local operation, infection, or intravenous drug abuse. The classic clinical findings of neck pain, swelling, and inflammation are usually present, but clinical diagnosis often is delayed. Computed tomography (CT) was used to diagnose TIJV promptly in 5 patients in whom it was not a primary clinical consideration when CT was carried out. All patients but 1 were examined with contrast enhancement. A high rate of flow of Hypaque 60 was maintained to opacify the vascular structures of the neck.

Four patients had unexplained fever. Three had neck swelling and 1, mediastinal widening. A central venous catheter predisposed to TIJV in 3 patients and neck operations in 2. Two patients had left-sided TIJV after right-sided venous catheterization. The CT findings included enlargement of the thrombosed vein, a nonenhancing filling defect in the lumen of the affected vessel, enhancement of the sharply defined vessel wall by flow through the vasa vasorum, and opacification of collateral venous channels. The collaterals typically appeared as tubular or linear structures that enhanced after contrast administration. The degree of collateral flow depended in part on the age of the thrombus and its location.

Computed tomography is an accurate noninvasive means of evaluating the patency of vascular structures, including the internal jugular vein. It was diagnostically helpful in all patients in this study in whom TIJV was not primarily suspected on clinical grounds.

▶ Both Doppler ultrasound and impedance plethysmography are now standard in many vascular laboratories. It is important to know that venous Doppler velocity tracings can be influenced by cardiac failure, and the finding of pulsatile venous flow tracings offer diagnostic cardiac information in patients with swollen legs. The Doppler tracing is of particular value in patients with bilateral abnormal impedance plethysmograms.

Diagnosis of deep vein thrombosis by impedance plethysmography is not without problems. Serial testing may help to eliminate some of these. The ability of B-mode scan to visualize the femoral and popliteal veins may further help to eliminate some of the diagnostic problems of the impedance plethysmograph.

Muscle tear has been confused with the diagnosis of deep vein thrombosis. Trauma or physical activity prior to the pain should alert the physician to the diagnosis. Noninvasive testing will not help because external compression may yield an abnormal result. A CT scan provides a definitive diagnosis. Also, CT scan is helpful in the diagnosis of jugular venous thrombosis as a result of catheter placement. In the latter, diagnosis by venography is virtually impossible.

Deep-Vein Thrombosis Following Total Knee Replacement: An Analysis of Six Hundred and Thirty-Eight Arthroplasties

Bernard N. Stulberg, John N. Insall, George W. Williams, and Bernard Ghelman (The Hosp. for Special Surgery, New York)

J. Bone Joint Surg. (Am.) 66-A:194–201, February 1984 10–13

To determine the incidence of thromboembolism after total knee replacement and to identify risk factors, data were retrospectively reviewed on 517 patients who underwent a total of 638 procedures for total knee replacement.

All 517 patients had postoperative venograms and 475 had postoperative perfusion lung scans. The results of venographic study showed no thrombosis in 276 cases (43.1%), thrombosis in the calf in 294 (46.2%), and thrombosis in the popliteal veins or thigh in 68 (10.7%). There was no significant correlation between the etiology of the knee condition and the development of deep-vein thrombosis with one exception: 7 patients who underwent revision of a total knee replacement for acute or subacute sepsis had no evidence of deep-vein thrombosis, compared with a 51% incidence for those who underwent revision for nonseptic failure. Of 338 patients who underwent unilateral total knee replacement, 280 were studied by bilateral venography. Nine (3.2%) of the 280 had thrombosis in the contralateral calf and 3 (1.1%) had contralateral popliteal thrombosis.

The incidence of deep-vein thrombosis in each knee after bilateral total knee replacement was similar to that for unilateral replacement. However, when bilateral total knee replacement was performed at the same operative session, the risk of developing deep-vein thrombosis was substantially increased. Thirty-two (26.4%) of 121 patients who underwent bilateral replacement had no evidence of thrombosis in either lower extremity, 72 (59.5%) had thrombosis in the calf, and 17 (14%) had thrombosis in the popliteal veins or thigh.

Forty-one (84%) of 49 patients who inadvertently did not receive prophylaxis for thromboembolism developed ipsilateral deep-vein thrombosis. Incidence of ipsilateral thrombosis in the 468 patients who received some form of prophylaxis was 57%. Fewer than 5% of the clinical examinations suggested the presence of deep-vein thrombosis for a false negative rate of more than 90%.

A total of 475 perfusion lung scans demonstrated segmental defects in 39 patients (8.2%) and one study showed lobar defects. A diagnosis of pulmonary embolism was made clinically in 9 patients (1.7%). There was no correlation between an abnormal perfusion lung scan and the development of thrombosis. Twelve patients were given formal anticoagulant therapy. No fatality resulted from pulmonary embolism.

No specific high-risk population could be identified for the development of deep-vein thrombosis. Although no single prophylactic regimen was found to be significantly more effective than another, it is believed that prophylactic measures should be included in the management of patients who undergo total knee replacement.

Prophylaxis of Deep Vein Thrombosis After Total Hip Replacement: Dextran and External Pneumatic Compression Compared With 1.2 or 0.3 Gram of Aspirin Daily

William H. Harris, Christos A. Athanasoulis, Arthur C. Waltman, and Edwin W. Salzman (Harvard Med. School)

J. Bone Joint Surg. (Am.) 67-A:57–62, January 1985 10–14

Venous thromboembolism continues to be a considerable problem after total hip replacement in older patients who are not protected. The efficacy of a new external pneumatic compression system applied to the calf and thigh, in conjunction with dextran therapy for 3 days, was compared with that of aspirin in daily dosages of 0.3 and 1.2 gm in a prospective study of patients aged 40 and older who were scheduled for total hip replacement. Aspirin was begun a day before operation. Low molecular weight dextran was given in a dose of 10 ml/kg of 10% solution starting during operation; 7.5 ml/kg was given on the next 2 days. Fresh thrombi were detected by the fibrinogen uptake test, cuff impedance plethysmography, and venography.

A total of 135 patients completed the study. Forty-three received low-dosage aspirin, 48 received the higher dosage, and 44 had external compression and dextran therapy. The groups were comparable in demographic and major medical factors. New venous thrombosis developed in 29 patients given 1.2 gm of aspirin and in 26 of the low-dosage group. Only 9 of the 44 patients in the compression-dextran group developed thromboembolic disease. This treatment was superior to aspirin in both men and women. Nine patients in all (6%) had pulmonary emboli; 3 were symptomatic. Compression and dextran therapy effectively reduced the number of thrombi in both the thigh and the calf (table). There were no deaths in the series. Three patients had excessive operative bleeding before the volume of dextran given at operation was limited to 500 ml.

Distribution of Numbers of Calf, Popliteal, and Plantar Arch Thrombi by Size and Prophylactic Regimen

Size of Thrombi	Aspirin, 1.2 g (48 Patients)	Aspirin, 0.3 g (43 Patients)	Boot and Dextran (44 Patients)
Small	22	25	4
Medium	9	6	4
Large	7	8	2
Total	38	39	10

(Courtesy of Harris, W.H., et al.: J. Bone Joint Surg. (Am.) 67-A:57–62, January 1985.)

External pneumatic compression of the calf and thigh with dextran administration provides excellent prophylaxis against calf and thigh thrombi in patients undergoing total hip replacement, even those with previous deep vein thrombosis. Intraoperative bleeding appears not to be a risk when dextran administration is limited to 500 ml in a 4-hour period.

▶ Whereas it may be true that no one prophylactic regimen proved superior to any other, no prophylaxis was associated with an 84% incidence of deep vein thrombosis in orthopedic patients. Such an alarming incidence calls for routine use of some prophylactic regimen in these patients.

Protein C Deficiency: Risk Factor for Venous Thrombosis

H.-G. Klingemann, A. W. Broekmans, R. M. Bertina, R. Egbring, and E. A. Loeliger

Klin. Wochenschr. 62:975–978, Oct. 15, 1984 10–15

Protein C is a vitamin K-dependent protein produced in the liver. Activated protein C has an anticoagulant effect by inactivating clotting factors V and VIII. The authors report on a young female patient who suffered from recurrent thrombosis of the deep calf and pelvic veins with pulmonary embolism. Superficial thrombophlebitis also occurred repeatedly. The authors found reduced plasma levels of protein C antigen (0.62 units/ml) and activity (0.42 units/ml). Investigation of other family members revealed a protein C deficiency in the father, sister, and son. During anticoagulant treatment with Marcumar, the patient developed a coumarin-induced skin necrosis, to which complication a protein C deficiency is evidently predisposed. Marcumar was discontinued and heparin (10,000 units twice daily) was administered. Neither a new thrombosis nor pulmonary embolus developed. Marcumar was started again with simultaneous administration of heparin (6,000 units twice daily). After the adjustment period the patient was treated with Marcumar alone, and no complications developed. Skin necrosis could have been prevented if heparin had been given simultaneously during the adjustment period.

None of the family members examined had taken anticoagulants of the coumarin type. There was also no evidence of damage to the liver cells or increased consumption of coagulating factors.

When in relatively young patients thrombi and pulmonary emboli as well as thrombophlebitis appear, a hemostatic defect should be considered. This may reveal an imbalance of coagulation and fibrinolysis favoring thrombophilia. Antithrombin III deficiency is the best known cause, which can be congenital or acquired. Since the clear representation of protein C, it is possible to develop a monospecific antiserum. In patients treated with coumarin it is advisable to consider, in addition to the protein C antigen, the quotient protein C/factor II-antigen as well as the protein C/factor X-antigen. In general, a level of less than 0.5 shows a protein C deficiency. Patients with congenital protein C deficiency are treated lifelong with coumarin derivatives. However, observation is important since these patients frcqucntly develop coumarin necrosis as was reported in the patient of this study. Commercial prothrombin complex preparations also contain protein C, and their use is being discussed. However, as long as no depurated concentrate is available, it should not be given to patients with tendency to thrombosis. Besides congenital protein C deficiency, there exists the acquired types in which the meaning of protein C deficiency with simultaneous changes of other coagulation parameters is not yet assessed. In healthy young patients with sudden thrombi or thrombophlebitis, protein C deficiency should be considered. Diagnosis with available commercial test methods should soon be possible.

Recurrent Venous Thromboembolism in Patients With a Partial Deficiency of Protein S

Philip C. Comp and Charles T. Esmon (Oklahoma City)

N. Engl. J. Med. 311:1525–1528, Dec. 13, 1984 10–16

Defects and deficiencies of certain plasma proteins may cause pathologic thrombus formation. Protein S, an antithrombotic plasma factor, serves as a cofactor of the anticoagulant effects of activated protein C, which in turn inhibits blood clotting at the levels of factors V and VIII in the blood-clotting cascade. The authors postulate that patients deficient in protein S could be predisposed to recurrent thrombosis in a manner similar to patients with congenital deficiency of protein C. The authors developed a functional protein S assay based on the ability of protein S to serve as cofactor of activated protein C. The prolongation of the factor Xa one-stage clotting time by the activated protein C is dependent on the protein S content of the test plasma. With this assay, the protein S activity of normal persons ranges from 63% to 160%.

Of 120 patients with recurrent thrombosis assayed for protein S activity, 6 unrelated persons showed substantially decreased functional levels of protein S, ranging from 15% to 37%, while these patients were not receiving heparin or warfarin anticoagulation. Determining immunologic levels by Laurell rocket immunoelectrophoresis was difficult; protein S levels ranged from 21% to 118% and did not correlate closely with the functional levels. Lack of correlation may be due to the separation of bound protein S from the C4b-binding protein, which is one form of protein S in the plasma, aside from free protein S. Supplementing the plasma of protein S-deficient patients with purified protein S resulted in normal anticoagulant effect of the plasma to activated protein C. Four of these 6 patients had family histories of recurrent venous thrombosis. Markedly reduced levels of protein S and recurrent deep-vein thrombosis was present in the father of 1 patient examined; however, despite markedly reduced levels of protein S, the mother of another patient examined showed no history of thrombotic disease.

The data suggest that determination of the functional protein S levels will be useful in the evaluation of patients with recurrent thrombosis. Use of immunologic techniques alone for protein S measurement may be deceptive, since the Laurell rocket electrophoretic analysis does not distinguish between free and functional protein S and the nonfunctional form that is bound to C4b-binding protein.

The Role of the Fibrinolytic System in Deep Vein Thrombosis

B. Wiman, B. Ljungberg, J. Chmielewska, G. Urdén, M. Blombäck, and H. Johnsson (Karolinska Hosp., Stockholm)

J. Lab. Clin. Med. 105:265–270, February 1985 10–17

It has been suggested that impaired fibrinolysis may sometimes play a role in the development of deep venous thrombosis (DVT). Specific methods of measuring tissue plasminogen activator (t-PA) activity and antigen before and after venous occlusion as well as the fast inhibitor to t-PA were used to evaluate the fibrinolytic system in 37 patients with recent symptomatic DVT, confirmed by plethysmography and thermography and by phlebography where necessary, and in 20 healthy subjects. The respective mean ages were 57 to 58 and 41 years. The estimates of t-PA activity and inhibitor activity utilized a one-chain human melanoma cell t-PA.

Thirteen patients with DVT (35%) had t-PA activity of less than 0.5 international units (IU)/ml after venous occlusion, whereas the lowest value in the control group was 0.56 IU/ml. Preocclusion values were similar in the patient and control groups. Patients had significantly higher t-PA antigen values before venous occlusion, but postocclusion values did not differ significantly. Inhibitor values were substantially higher in the patient group, particularly in patients who had low t-PA activity in postocclusion plasma samples. Release of t-PA antigen was significantly less in these patients than in healthy subjects.

Decreased fibrinolytic activity in patients with DVT is a result of an increased plasma concentration of a fast inhibitor of t-PA combined with impaired release of t-PA. Decreased fibrinolytic activity may have a pathogenetic role in DVT in these cases. Impaired fibrinolysis may be more frequent in association with thromboembolic disease than has been recognized.

Heparin-Induced Thrombocytopenia and Recurrent Thromboembolism in Siblings

Rodney E. Kosfeld, Allan M. Lansing, Zahi Masri, and Yong K. Liu (Louisville)

Am. J. Hematol. 18:421–423, April 1985 10–18

Thrombocytopenia with or without thromboembolism can complicate heparin therapy, probably from immune-mediated platelet destruction. Heparin-induced thrombocytopenia associated with peripheral arterial and venous thromboembolism was encountered in 2 middle-aged brothers, both with diabetes. The patients had multiple arterial and venous thromboembolic episodes affecting peripheral vessels. Heparin-dependent antiplatelet antibody was detected in both cases by platelet aggregometry. Heparin initially was given during aortocoronary bypass operation. Platelet counts increased after heparin was discontinued. One patient improved clinically, but the other became worse and died. The latter patient also had received heparin during peritoneal dialysis.

Increasing platelet counts after withdrawal of heparin in these cases supports a diagnosis of heparin-induced thrombocytopenia. The presence of heparin-dependent serum platelet-aggregating activity supports this diagnosis. Findings in animals suggest that specific immune responses to various antigens are controlled by specific genes. The present cases in siblings may be coincidental, but familial occurrence of susceptibility to heparin-induced thrombocytopenia must be considered because of the potentially serious outcome of the reaction to heparin.

▶ In addition to diminished antithrombin III, low levels of protein C and its cofactor protein S have been identified as a risk factor in deep vein thrombosis. In young adults with multiple recurrent and unexplained venous thrombosis, these two vitamin K-dependent proteins, produced by the liver, may be responsible.

A new technique to measure tissue plasminogen activator also shows defects in the fibrinolytic system that may play a role in the pathogenesis of deep vein thrombosis.

Arterial thrombosis due to heparin-induced thrombocytopenia is now a recognized clinical entity. It would appear that this heparin-induced complication may also be a factor in venous thrombosis.

A Randomized Study of a Semisynthetic Heparin Analogue and Heparin in Prophylaxis of Deep Vein Thrombosis

S. Törngren, K. Kettunen, J. Lahtinen, K. Koppenhagen, P. Brücke, P. Hartl, O. Hutter, U. Haller, G. Lahnborg, and B. Forsskåhl

Br. J. Surg. 71:817–820, November 1984 10–19

Low doses of heparin prevent thromboembolic complications in patients having major elective abdominal surgery, but they also increase the risk of wound hematomas. The thromboprophylactic effects and complications

FREQUENCY OF DEEP VEIN THROMBOSIS IN THREE GROUPS OF PATIENTS

	SSHA 50 mg	SSHA 37·5 mg	Heparin 5000 units
No. of patients	138	141	148
DVT			
Positive fibrinogen uptake test*	16 (11·6%)	21 (14·9%)	21 (14·2%)
Verified by phlebography	10	13	10
Bilateral	1	7	6

*$P = .70$.
(Courtesy of Törngren, S., et al.: Br. J. Surg. 71:817–820, November 1984.)

of administering heparin in a dose of 5,000 units twice daily were compared with those of administering the semisynthetic heparin analogue SSHA in doses of 37.5 or 50 mg twice daily.

The prospective double-blind, international trial included 440 patients older than age 40 years who were admitted for major general or gynecologic surgery and lacked a history of risk factors for deep vein thrombosis (DVT) and pulmonary embolism. Deep vein thrombosis was diagnosed by the ^{125}I-fibrinogen uptake test.

The three treatment groups were well matched for age, sex, body surface area, and risk factors for thromboembolism. Presence of DVT was diagnosed by the uptake test in 58 patients and confirmed by phlebographic study in 33, with no significant differences among the groups (table). Wound hematoma and postoperative bleeding also were similarly frequent in all groups, and measured operative blood losses did not differ among the 3 groups. One patient in each group had a pulmonary embolism; 1 patient in the heparin-treated group died.

This prospective study showed no differences in prophylaxis of DVT or in bleeding complications when SSHA or low-dose heparin was used. There were fewer patients with DVT in the group that received 50-mg doses of SSHA than in the heparin-treated patients, but the difference was not significant.

Incidence of Preoperative Deep Venous Thrombosis in Abdominal Surgery

J. J. Rodzynek, J. Damien, M. Huberty, C. Abramowicz, J. L. Garcez, and J. P. Govaerts (Free Univ. of Brussels)

Br. J. Surg. 71:731–732, September 1984 10–20

Some of the cases of deep venous thrombosis (DVT) discovered after operation may be present before surgery. The incidence of preoperative and postoperative DVT was determined by phlebographic study in 51 consecutive patients who had major abdominal surgery without prophylactic anticoagulant therapy. Bilateral phlebography was done with the use of Telebrix 30 Meglumine before and 9 days after operation. The most frequent diagnoses were cholelithiasis-cholecystitis, gastrointestinal cancer, and gastroduodenal ulcer; the most common operations were cholecystectomy, colectomy, and subtotal gastrectomy. The 29 women and 22 men had a mean age of 61 years.

Deep venous thrombosis was found on preoperative phlebography in 8 patients (16%). A high risk of pulmonary embolism was considered present in 2 cases. Two patients had bilateral DVT and 2 had iliofemoral involvement. No patient had a past history of DVT. Three of the 8 patients had cancer. Four had been confined to bed for longer than 5 days before examination. After operation DVT was demonstrated in 28 patients (55%), including the 8 with abnormal preoperative findings. Incidence of surgery-related DVT was 39%. Surgery led to extension of preexisting DVT in 3 instances. Six patients had clinical signs of pulmonary embolism after operation, which were confirmed by lung scintigraphy. No deaths resulted from pulmonary embolisms in the postoperative period.

A substantial number of patients in this study had asymptomatic preoperative DVT that was related to cancer, confinement to bed, or the presence of varicose veins. Prophylactic anticoagulant therapy seems indicated for patients who are having major abdominal surgery, and it should be instituted before operation.

Long-Term Anticoagulant Therapy in Patients With Venous Thrombosis

Russell Hull and Jack Hirsh (McMaster Univ.)

Arch. Intern. Med. 143:2061–2063, November 1983 10–21

Patients with acute proximal vein thrombosis are commonly treated by a course of heparin and then oral anticoagulation for weeks to months. Three randomized trials have been done to determine the appropriateness of long-term anticoagulation for venous thrombosis. Fixed low-dose subcutaneous heparin, adjusted intermediate-dose subcutaneous heparin, and conventional oral anticoagulation with warfarin sodium were evaluated. Warfarin was used to prolong the thromboplastin time to either 1½ to two times normal or about 1¼ times normal. Initially, heparin was given intravenously in all studies. Fixed low-dose subcutaneous heparin was ineffective, but heparin therapy adjusted to keep the activated partial thromboplastin time at 1½ times control effectively prevented recurrent venous thromboembolism. The treatment was well tolerated by most patients. Oral warfarin therapy was also effective, and the less-intense regimen was associated with much less bleeding than conventional warfarin therapy.

Adjusted-dose subcutaneous heparin therapy seems to be appropriate for pregnant patients and patients living in remote areas where long-term monitoring is impractical. Osteoporosis must be watched for in patients managed in this way. In other settings, less-intense oral warfarin therapy is effective and relatively safe. Patients with calf vein thrombosis may not require long-term treatment, but this must be confirmed before being adopted in clinical practice. Longer treatment is indicated for patients with recurrent venous thrombosis and those at continued risk. The latter should be treated until risk factors are reversed. Patients with recurrent venous thrombosis probably should be treated for at least 1 year, and those with irreversible risk factors should undergo anticoagulant therapy indefinitely.

Intensive Initial Oral Anticoagulation and Shorter Heparin Treatment in Deep Vein Thrombosis

Sam Schulman, Dieter Lockner, Kurt Bergström, and Margareta Blombäck

Thromb. Haemost. 52:276–280, December 1984 10–22

The results of conventional anticoagulation for deep vein thrombosis (DVT) were compared with those of an initial constant high-dose regimen involving a shorter period of heparin administration. A total of 129 consecutive patients with confirmed DVT of the lower extremity received heparin by infusion, followed by low-dose warfarin therapy in daily doses of 15, 7.5, and 7.5 mg or less on the first 3 days, and then individualized maintenance dosages. The high-dose group received 15 mg of warfarin daily until the prothrombin time (PT) fell to less than 30% with Simplastin A (Sp-A). Heparin was discontinued when the Sp-A value was 19% or less for 2 consecutive days. Another 40 patients were followed by coagulation factor assays and repeated venography after being randomized.

In the initial study, low-dose recipients reached a stable PT after 4.3 days and high-dose recipients did so after 3.3 days. Heparin was discontinued after 6 and 5 days, respectively. No differences in significant bleeding were observed, and there was no evidence of progression of DVT. In the second part of the study, a stable PT was reached after 4.4 days in the low-dose group and 3.7 days in the high-dose group, and heparin was discontinued after 5.4 and 4.4 days, respectively. No clinical bleeding occurred. Coagulation factor values were the same in both groups when heparin was discontinued. There were no thromboembolic complications in either group.

More intensive initial oral anticoagulation with briefer heparin administration appears to be a safe approach to the treatment of DVT. Use of this regimen could limit hospitalization and reduce costs considerably in view of the frequency of DVT.

▶ A 15.7% venographic evidence of thrombosis prior to surgery is a surprise. It must be related to bedridden patients with cancer. Prophylaxis in such patients probably should be in order. Controversy continues about the length of anticoagulant therapy in patients with established deep vein thrombosis. The editorial by the McMaster group should clarify the confusion. The myth of less bleeding tendency of new heparin analogues was not substantiated by the multicenter trial. So much for new forms of heparin.

Venous Gangrene of the Upper Extremity

Bruce M. Smith, Gregory W. Shield, Douglas H. Riddell, and James D. Snell (Vanderbilt Univ.)

Ann. Surg. 201:511–519, April 1985 10–23

So-called venous gangrene is an uncommon sequel of venous occlusive disease related to overwhelming venous outflow obstruction that eventually compromises arterial inflow. Associated disorders are frequent and severe, and mortality is high. Gangrene of the hand associated with acute upper-extremity venous insufficiency was encountered in 4 limbs of 3 patients, all of whom had life-threatening illness associated with decreased tissue perfusion, hypercoagulability, and venous injury. One patient required above-the-elbow amputation, but venous thrombectomy and thrombolytic therapy prevented major tissue loss in the other patients. All 3 eventually died of their underlying illness.

Sixteen patients with venous gangrene of the upper extremity, including the authors' 3 cases, are summarized in the table. Mean age was 42 years. Both arms were involved in 2 patients. Patients most often were initially seen with pain, swelling, and cyanosis, which progressed to phlegmasia cerulea dolens. Six patients had hematologic abnormalities. Three had heparin-induced thrombocytopenia. A serious disorder possibly producing low cardiac output was present in 6 patients. Three patients had pulmonary embolism. Treatment varied widely. Half of the patients required amputations. Overall mortality was 50%.

Gangrene of the hand associated with acute upper-extremity venous insufficiency appears to result from global circulatory stasis, subclavian or axillary venous occlusion, and peripheral venous thrombosis. Early, aggressive restoration of adequate cardiac output and thrombectomy or thrombolytic therapy or both are indicated. The latter measures, compared with anticoagulation alone, may reduce the risk of long-term sequelae.

▶ An excellent summary of the literature on venous gangrene of the upper extremity.

The Risks of Pulmonary Arterial Catheterization

H. Mathilda Horst, Farouck N. Obeid, Deepak Vij, and Brack A. Bivins (Detroit)

Surg. Gynecol. Obstet. 159:229–232, September 1984 10–24

An emphasis on specific life-threatening complications of pulmonary artery catheterization has led to an underestimation of overall risks of the procedure. Risks were examined in a prospective series of 937 surgical patients seen in the intensive care unit at Henry Ford Hospital in 1982. One hundred thirty-six (14.5%) patients had a total of 211 pulmonary artery catheters inserted. There was more than one clinical indication for insertion in most instances, most frequent being determination of fluid status and cardiac function.

Collected Series of Venous Gangrene Reports*

Patient	Author	Age	Sex	Side Involved	Predisposing Causes	Associated Illness	Venogram	Extent of Gangrene	Treatment	Amputation Level	Outcome
1	Present Report	53	F	Left	IV Infusion	Hodgkin's Disease	ND	Arm	Elevation	Above Elbow	Died @ 6 mo.
2	Present Report	25	M	Left	Trauma HIT IV Infusion	MI CHF, Sepsis	ND	Fingers	Thrombectomy Elevation	None	Died
3	Present Report	19	F	Bilat.	IV Infusion DIC	Viral myocarditis, CHF, sepsis Renal Failure	Negative for Thrombus	Fingers	Streptokinase Elevation	None	Died
4	Coon (13)	?	M	Left	Trauma Cryoglobu-linemia	None	ND	Forearm	Unspec.	Above Elbow	LTFU
5	Fountain (21)	42	F	Right	None	Status Asthmaticus Sepsis	ND	Forearm	Heparin Elevation	None	Died
6	Adams (1)	57	M	Right	None	Suspected carcinoma of lung	ND	Hand	Anticoagulation	None	Died
7	Paletta (32)	71	M	Bilat.	IV Invsion HIT	Carcinoma of lung	Positive for Subclavian & axillary vein Thrombus	Forearm	Fasciotomy	Right Below Elbow	Died @ 1 mo.

8	Haimovici (23)	36	M	Right	IV Infusion	None	ND	Fingers	Unspec.	Finger	Recovered
9	Haimovici (23)	44	M	Side Unspec.	IV Infusion	None	ND	Forearm	Unspec.	None	Died
10	Haimovici (23)	57	F	Right	None	None	"Positive"	Fingers	Sympathectomy	None	Recovered
11	Haimovici (23)	37	M	Right	Penetrating wound-axilla	None	ND	Forearm	Unspec.	Above Elbow	Recovered
12	Haimovici (23)	45	M	Left	None	Carcinoma of lung	ND	Hand	None	None	Died
13	Haimovici (23)	8	M	Left	"Trauma"	None	ND	Forearm	Unspec.	Above Elbow	Recovered
14	Moore (31)	67	F	Left	Subclavian venous catheter HIT	Pyelonephritis Sepsis	ND	Forearm	Unspec.	Above Elbow	Recovered
15	Hans (25)	56	F	Left	Polycythemia	Cirrhosis CHF	Postoperatively Normal	Hand	Heparin Elevation Thrombectomy	None	Recovered
16	Ravitch (36)	7	F	Left	IV Infusion	Rhabdomyosarcoma Exchange Transfusion	ND	Arm	Unspec.	Unspec.	Unspec.

*Unspec., unspecified; LTFU, lost to follow-up; ND, not done; MI, myocardial infarction; CHF, congestive heart failure; DIC, disseminated intravascular coagulation; and HIT, heparin-induced thrombocytopenia.

(Courtesy of Smith, B.M., et al.: Ann. Surg. 201:511–519, April 1985.)

Complications resulted from 52% of all catheter insertions. Cardiac dysrhythmias were the most frequent technical complication and occurred during insertion of 16 catheters. There was 1 case each of hemothorax, air embolism, pulmonary artery disruption, and catheter embolization. Eighty-four mechanical complications were attributed to equipment malfunction. The most common was rupture of the catheter balloon. Nine technical complications were considered to be potentially immediately life threatening. Six patients had ventribular tachycardia, and 1 progressed to intractable fibrillation and death. Another death resulted from disruption of the pulmonary artery. Overall catheter-related mortality was 0.9% of insertions.

Nine of 16 autopsies showed abnormalities that possibly were related to use of a pulmonary artery catheter. Three patients had pulmonary emboli, and 3 had thrombosis of the superior vena cava. These findings were not clinically apparent before death.

New modifications of pulmonary artery catheters that allow transvenous cardiac pacing and His bundle electrocardiography promise to increase the use of these catheters. Serious complications and death may be more frequent than previously recognized, and a pulmonary artery catheter should be used only for defined indications when there is a reasonable chance of benefit from the data obtained.

Complications of Superior Versus Inferior Vena Cava Occlusion in Infants Receiving Central Total Parenteral Nutrition

Sean J. Mulvihill and Eric W. Fonkalsrud (Univ. of California, Los Angeles)

J. Pediatr. Surg. 19:752–757, December 1984 10–25

Parenteral nutrition is now a major adjunct in infants and children with gastrointestinal disorders. Superior vena cava catheterization has been associated with many serious complications, but some have avoided venous access to the inferior vena cava via the saphenous vein from fear of infection or vena cava thrombosis. The sequelae of long-term catheterization for total parenteral nutrition were examined in 204 infants younger than age 1 year in whom a total of 294 Broviac central venous hyperalimentation catheters were inserted between 1975 and 1983. Infant-size catheters were used in most instances. Access was via the saphenous vein in 267 patients, the internal jugular vein in 16, the external jugular vein in 7, and the cephalic and right atrial veins in 2 each. Sixty-eight infants were given parenteral nutrition at home. The most frequent indications were malabsorption syndrome and short bowel syndrome.

The catheters functioned for a mean of 112 days. Vena cava thrombosis occurred in 7% of infants. Five percent of saphenous catheterizations resulted in inferior vena cava thrombosis. Removal of the catheter alone appeared to be adequate. No infant developed chronic lower limb edema, and in no case did thrombosis extend to the renal or hepatic veins or to the right atrium. No symptomatic pulmonary embolism occurred, although only 2 patients received heparin. Two saphenous catheters broke off during attempted removal. Five infants developed superior vena cava thrombosis, 3 in association with inferior vena cava thrombosis. All the latter infants died of pulmonary insufficiency within 6 months of superior vena cava occlusion. One infant died after cardiotomy to remove right atrial thrombus. The 2 infants with superior vena cava occlusion alone had mild to moderate edema; 1 developed pleural effusion.

Combined superior and inferior vena cava thrombosis is associated with serious morbidity and high mortality. Inferior vena cava catheterization is an easier procedure that does not require an operating room or general anesthesia. Significant complications were infrequent after inferior vena cava thrombosis in this study, supporting continued use of inferior vena cava catheterization via the saphenous vein to administer intravenous alimentation.

▶ Catheters are now being used more often, especially for parenteral nurturing in infants. It is important to know that extensive thrombosis involving the vena cava can occur. Similarly, pulmonary artery catheterization is not without morbidity. The 52% reported morbidity should remind users to reconsider their indication for pulmonary artery catheterization. These two articles, each with large numbers of patients, re-emphasize the importance of selective use of catheterization.

A New Vena Caval Filter for Percutaneous Placement and Retrieval: Experimental Study

Gunnar Lund, Joseph A. Rysavy, Erich Salomonowitz, Andrew H. Cragg, Frank Kotula, Wilfrido R. Castaneda-Zuniga, David W. Hunter, Carol C. Coleman, and Kurt Amplatz (Univ. of Minnesota Hosp.)

Radiology 152:369–372, August 1984 10–26

When anticoagulant or fibrinolytic therapy is contraindicated or fails, transvenous placement of vena caval filters is an effective procedure for treatment of pulmonary thromboembolism. A vena caval filter was designed that can be inserted percutaneously through an angiographic catheter. The spider-shaped filter, composed of an inert metal, is secured by controlled penetration of the caval wall to 2 mm. A hook at 1 end allows percutaneous retrieval by a snare. In canine studies, the filter securely engaged the wall of the vena cava, though in a somewhat tilted position in 6 of the 11 animals. Filling defects in the open cone of the filter, representing firmly attached organized thrombi, were found in 6 dogs, but in no case was flow obstructed. No filter migrated cranially. The filters were easily removed without bleeding, although 1 that was in place for 5 weeks could not be dislodged. In vitro tests showed the filter to be highly effective and less dependent on positioning than the Greenfield filter is. These preliminary findings suggest that the described filter is suitable for prophylactic placement in patients at high risk for the development of pulmonary thromboembolic disease.

Surgical Approaches to Thromboembolism

L. J. Greenfield and M. R. Langham (Med. College of Virginia)

Br. J. Surg. 71:968–970, December 1984 10–27

Besides verifying the diagnosis and the extent of embolic occlusion, pulmonary angiography allows direct measurement of pulmonary artery (PA) pressures, which facilitates classification of a patient on the basis of the hemodynamic effects of the embolic load in that patient. Major pulmonary embolism is defined as that degree of acute pulmonary vascular occlusion producing systemic hypotension, either transient (class III, mean PA pressure of more than 20 but less than 25 mm Hg) or sustained and requiring vasopressor support (class IV, mean PA pressure of 25 to 30 mm Hg). Class V patients have chronic, recurrent thromboembolism (mean PA pressure, more than 40 mm Hg). A total of 313 patients with angiographically confirmed pulmonary thromboembolism were managed on the basis of this physiologic classification. Patients who were given heparin before operation were maintained on oral anticoagulant therapy for at least 4 months after operation. Follow-up studies included confirmation of filter position by x-rays films, radionuclide venogram-lung scan or contrast venacavogram, and noninvasive venous measurements.

Pulmonary embolectomy was performed on 31 patients. Patients in shock (class IV) were managed by catheter embolectomy (26 patients), with 27% mortality rate, or by open embolectomy during active resuscitation (6), with a 33% mortality rate. Emboli were extracted by catheter from 23 patients (88%). Access was from the right common femoral vein in 16 and the right internal jugular vein in 10. Class III patients with significant risk of recurrent embolism were managed by anticoagulation and filter insertion. The most common indication for filter placement was a contraindication to anticoagulation (37%) and recurrent embolism despite anticoagulation (30%). Filter placement was obtained through the jugular vein in 245 patients, the femoral vein in 55, and the right atrium in 3. Filter placement was infrarenal in 268 patients (86%) and intentionally suprarenal in 19 (6%). Misplacement of the filter (3%) occurred in 5 iliac veins and 3 renal veins and once in the heart, but it has not occurred since the guidewire technique for insertion was developed. The 30-day mortality for patients receiving filters was 14% and was usually due to other causes. Only 1 death was due to suspected recurrent embolism. Follow-up studies up to 99 months in 110 patients showed long-term patency of 97% in 110 venacavograms performed. Recurrent pulmonary thromboembolism occurred in 5 patients (2%) but caused no deaths.

Anticoagulation with heparin, unless contraindicated, is the basic therapy for pulmonary thromboembolism. However, class IV patients who are in hemodynamically unstable condition can benefit from catheter manipulation of the thrombus or open embolectomy with cardiopulmonary bypass. In patients in whom anticoagulation fails to prevent recurrent embolism or is contraindicated, vena cava filter placement is necessary. Positioning the guidewire in the inferior vena cava before insertion of the filter carrier-catheter makes passage through the heart easier and misplacement unlikely, and it minimizes the time that the carrier remains in contact with blood. Intermittent or continuous infusion of heparinized saline also retards thrombus formation.

A 30-Year Survey of Pulmonary Embolism Verified at Autopsy: An Analysis of 1,274 Surgical Patients

D. Bergqvist and B. Lindblad (Univ. of Lund)

Br. J. Surg. 72:105–108, February 1985 10–28

The extent to which pulmonary embolism causes death in surgical patients is unknown. A retrospective study was undertaken of all surgical patients in Malmö, Sweden, between 1951 and 1980 in whom pulmonary emboli were found at autopsy. Autopsy rates ranged from 73% to 100% during the review period. Urologic patients were included with general surgical patients between 1951 and 1964.

Pulmonary emboli were found in 23.6% of the 5,477 autopsies. The number of patients with contributory and incidental emboli increased during the 30-year review period, but the number with fatal emboli declined in the last 5 years. A total of 349 embolic episodes were considered to be fatal, whereas 353 contributed to death. Fifty-one percent of patients were not operated on. Pulmonary embolism was less frequent in patients younger than age 50 years. The proportion of females increased during the study period. Twenty-four patients had major embolism arising from thrombi about central venous catheters. In the most recent 5-year period, three fourths of patients with fatal or contributory embolism who were operated on received some form of prophylaxis against thromboembolism. Most patients received dextran.

Pulmonary embolism continues to be a major cause of death in surgical patients. In this large series it was as common a cause of death in both patients who were and who were not operated on. Clinically relevant embolism declined in the most recent years, despite a tendency toward an older age. The occurrence of pulmonary embolism within 10 days after operation was unchanged. A large proportion of patients with clinically relevant embolism who were operated on had benign disease or underwent remedial operations for malignancy.

Surgical Management of Chronic Pulmonary Embolism

W. Randolph Chitwood, Jr., H. Kim Lyerly, and David C. Sabiston, Jr. (Duke Univ.)

Ann. Surg. 201:11–26, January 1985 10–29

Patients who develop significant pulmonary hypertension from chronic embolism have a poor outlook with medical management, although embolectomy appears to be helpful in selected cases. Fourteen of 25 such patients seen between 1968 and 1983 were selected for embolectomy for chronic pulmonary arterial obstruction. The 9 men and 5 women had a mean age of 38 years. All patients had received long-term anticoagulation therapy with warfarin. Six patients had no known predisposing factors for phlebitis or pulmonary embolism. Dyspnea developed insidiously in 4 patients who had no preceding symptoms. In those who had been symptomatic, symptoms usually were progressive. The PaO_2 at admission on room air averaged 56.5 mm Hg. On average, 62% of total pulmonary blood flow was obstructed by emboli; in 5 cases, an entire lung was not perfused. Bronchial angiography was done in 9 cases to assess the patency of the distal pulmonary arteries. Peripheral venography findings were positive in 9 of 12 cases. The average mean pulmonary artery pressure was 43 mm Hg. Right ventricular compromise was evident in 4 patients.

Patients who have proximal labor or main pulmonary artery embolic occlusion with perfusion of distal vessels via bronchial collaterals are good candidates for embolectomy. Of the patients described herein, cardiopulmonary bypass was used in 7. One patient died intraoperatively of hemorrhagic lung syndrome and another patient with intractable right ventricular failure died 3 days postoperatively. Pulmonary arterial pressures fell significantly in the surviving patients, however, with an increase in the group PaO_2 and correction of respiratory alkalosis. A substantial improvement in New York Heart Association functional class occurred during an average followup period of 5½ years. The conditions of all of the unoperated patients deteriorated clinically during the follow-up period; and 3 died.

Pulmonary embolectomy can produce considerable symptomatic and functional improvement and an increased life expectancy in patients with chronic pulmonary embolism who have severe respiratory insufficiency, hypoxemia, and chronic pulmonary hypertension. Patients with emboli in distal vessels or with massive obesity or right ventricular failure are unsuitable for surgery at the present time.

▶ Once again, we are reminded that pulmonary embolism is a common autopsy finding in the surgical population. It was thought that pulmonary emboli were uncommon in upper extremity thrombosis. Frequent use of the catheter has changed this opinion. As demonstrated in the article by Bergqvist and Lindblad, 24 patients had major embolism arising from thrombi about the central venous catheter. An excellent patency rate of 95% by venogram, reported by Greenfield, further establishes this filter as the choice for vena cava interruption. Similar to percutaneous balloon pump insertion, the development of percutaneous placement of a vena cava filter will revolutionize the technique of vena cava interruption but, hopefully, not the indications.

11 Venous Stasis Disease

Sclerosant Treatment of Varicose Veins and Deep Vein Thrombosis
Russell A. Williams and Samuel E. Wilson
Arch. Surg. 119:1283–1285, November 1984 11–1

There is concern that the chemically induced reaction in sclerotherapy may extend into the deep venous system, producing deep vein thrombosis and exposing the patient to the risk of pulmonary embolism or postphlebitic syndrome. Sixty-seven legs treated with compression sclerotherapy in 50 patients (mean age, 53 years) were examined with impedance plethysmography (IPG) and the Doppler ultrasonographic probe to determine whether the chemical thrombophlebitis extended to involve the deep veins of the leg. Indications for sclerotherapy included unacceptable appearance, pain, cramps, and stasis ulcer.

All injection sites were below the knee. The varicosities were emptied and fingertip pressure was applied to selected control points of the collapsed veins, especially over the perforating veins. If pressure over these points controlled reappearance of the varicosities upon standing, the veins were precisely marked for injection of 0.5 ml of 3% sodium tetradecyl sulfate with a 26-gauge disposable needle. Local compression was obtained with a dental swab taped over the injection site. The leg was then firmly wrapped with elastic bandages from the distal part of the foot to below the knee. Blood flow studies in the deep veins were performed before and 1 and 2 weeks after injection treatment.

Each leg received an average of six injections (range, 3 to 11). In each leg, results of venous studies 1 and 2 weeks after treatment were unchanged from preinjection results. In 9 extremities, delayed venous emptying was found on IPG and persisted after sclerosis. This was interpreted as evidence of previous deep vein thrombosis.

There is no evidence that deep vein thrombosis follows sclerotherapy. With a properly executed technique, proper compression, and a small volume of sclerosant injected into the empty vein, this method is highly unlikely to be complicated by deep vein thrombosis.

Incompetent Perforating Veins: Comparison of Varicography and Ascending Phlebography
M. Lea Thomas and John N. Bowles (St. Thomas' Hosp. Med. School, London)
Radiology 154:619–623, March 1985 11–2

Ascending phlebography is frequently inaccurate in evaluating incompetent perforating veins and in visualizing some communicating veins. A technique of varicography was compared with ascending phlebography in

50 patients with recurrent varicose veins in 61 legs, 28 women and 22 men with a mean age of 49 years. Ascending phlebography was done to assess the deep veins and detect incompetent perforators. Varicography then was performed to determine the extent and connections of the varicose veins.

Contrast is injected under fluoroscopic control directly into a prominent varicose vein with the patient standing. As with ascending phlebography, the veins are cleared of contrast at the end of the study to minimize the risk of thrombophlebitis.

Forty-one of 55 incompetent perforating calf veins were visualized by ascending phlebography and 46 by varicography. The latter study showed the veins better much more often than did ascending phlebography. Varicography only showed incompetent perforators in 14 legs and ascending phlebography only in five. All 17 incompetent gastrocnemius veins were shown by varicography, but only three of them by ascending phlebography. Five of six incompetent perforating veins of the midthigh were visualized by ascending phlebography and four by varicography.

Varicography is as accurate as ascending phlebography in detecting incompetent perforating veins in the calf, and it is much more accurate in demonstrating incompetent gastrocnemius veins. It is easily and rapidly carried out, but ascending phlebography is still necessary where incompetent communicating veins are likely present but are not visualized by varicography.

New Ideas in Surgery of Varicose Veins

E.-D. Schwilden

Chirurg 56:81–89, February 1985 11–3

The fundamental principle of surgical treatment of primary varicose veins consists of removal of pathologic reflux between the deep and superficial venous system and subsequent extirpation of superficial varicose veins. Today it is of great importance in cases of incomplete varicosis to remove only the incompetent part of the saphenous vein, thus preserving the normal saphenous for reconstructive operations on the arterial system.

The operation begins with the exposure of the termination of the great saphenous vein into the femoral vein. The recommended placement of the incision is related to a fixed point of the pubic tubercle. A high incision into the groin prevents damage to the lymph vessels and has a cosmetic advantage. The resection of the venous star is essential as faulty technique here is the highest cause of varicose recurrences. This depends upon exact exposure of the termination of the great saphenous vein as well as all of its side branches which must be ligated and extirpated. Besides the saphenous termination, the femoral vein must be skeletonized over a distance of 0.5–1 cm above and below the saphenous junction in order to recognize any variants and their removal. The distal exposure of the great saphenous vein for passing of the stripper is usually at the medial internal malleolus. Fundamentally the introduction of the stripper should follow the complete distal and proximal division of the vein. Presumably the stripper is in a correct position. The main risk is possible saphenous nerve damage. To prevent tearing of the nerve and permanent disturbance of sensation a downward stripping of the great saphenous vein is preferred. The surgical principle of the partial preservation of the great saphenous vein consists of removal of the pathologic reflux if any at the junction of the femoral vein, the perforator reflux, and the subsequent stripping of only the insufficient segment.

The main problem of lessor saphenous varicose veins is the relatively high recurrence rate. An exact preoperative and intraoperative diagnosis must be established in order to recognize the many relevant anatomical variants. The resection of the lessor system starts with the proximal exposure of the lessor saphenous in the hollow of the knee. The distal exposure is accomplished through a transverse or vertical incision between the lateral malleolus and the Achilles tendon. The stripper is introduced from distal to proximal while the extraction is done in the reverse direction. Competent segments of the lessor saphenous vein should also be preserved.

To achieve the best permanent results, the removal of insufficient perforating veins should be an essential component of surgical therapy of primary varicose veins. The opinions of surgeons in the field of phlebology are widely diverse in regard to methods of selective ligation of perforating veins. The most radical but most effective method of perforans reconstruction is subfascial ligature.

Exact knowledge of the anatomy of the venous system and its tributary structures especially the countless anatomical variants should guide the selection of a surgical procedure as radical as necessary and as sparing as possible. A standard procedure does not always justify these requirements.

Long Saphenous Incompetence as a Cause of Venous Ulceration

K. K. Sethia and S. G. Darke (Royal Victoria Hosp., Dorset, England)

Br. J. Surg. 71:754–755, October 1984 11–4

Management of venous ulceration in the leg must involve assessment of the superficial, deep, and perforating vein function. To assess the role of primary long saphenous incompetence in venous ulceration, 417 consecutive patients with significant chronic venous disorders of the lower extremity were studied. In 299 cases there were uncomplicated primary varicose veins with saphenous incompetence. The other 118 patients presented with a history of pain or swelling with current or previous ulceration. Ascending and descending venography and Doppler studies were performed on these patients. Measurements of foot vein pressure were performed on 12 patients in whom the only venous abnormalities detected were a long saphenous and calf perforator incompetence. Pressures were recorded after heel-raising exercises, after a midthigh tourniquet was inflated to 160 mm Hg, and after surgery.

Venous ulcerations were found in 60 patients (14.4%), 59 of whom had calf perforator incompetence. Of the 17 patients (28.3%) with long saphenous and calf perforator incompetence alone, only 8 showed long saphenous incompetence on both venography and Doppler studies, another 8 showed incompetence only on Doppler study, and 1 showed incompetence only at venography. Among the 12 patients who have had surgery mean preoperative fall in preexercise and postexercise foot vein pressure was 12.9% and then 35.6% with the thigh tourniquet inflated. After accurate groin ligation and stripping of the long saphenous vein to the knee, mean fall was 31.9%.

The apparent discrepancy between Doppler studies and venography in the diagnosis of saphenous incompetence casts doubts on the sensitivity of both studies. Validation of the presence of saphenous incompetence derived from measurements of foot vein pressure, irrespective of the means by which the original diagnosis was established, confirms previous reports which indicated this technique is an established quantitative means of testing venous hemodynamics of extremities. A high postexercise pressure which returned to relatively normal levels after surgery that was confined to the long saphenous system would seem to indicate a relevant contribution from saphenofemoral incompetence in pathogenesis of ulcers. The results also confirm that thigh tourniquet test occludes superficial veins and produces a similar reduction in foot vein pressures that may be predicted to follow surgery. The role of calf perforator incompetence as a cause of venous ulceration seems less certain.

The authors recommend that in patients with ulcers in whom long saphenous and calf perforator incompetence are the only identifiable venous abnormalities, surgery should be confined to the long saphenous system and should be expected to result in healing of ulcers.

The Acute Ischemia Syndrome of the Leg After Sclerotherapy

A. Oesch, P. Stirnemann, and F. Mahler (Univ. of Bern)

Schweiz. Med. Wochenschr. 114:1155–1158, Aug. 25, 1984 11–5

The inadvertent injection of the sclerosant into an artery is a rare complication of sclerotherapy. Four cases are presented. In all cases, the posterior tibial artery was involved with resulting necrosis of the center of the heel. All patients had about the same case history, which was similar to other cases described in literature. There is chronic venous insufficiency with recurring small ulcers in the area of the internal malleolus. In one case a below-knee amputation was necessary. The necrosis depends mainly on the amount of the injected sclerosant. The injection is given in the area of the ulcer in order to block a vein leading to it. However, occasionally the injection is given inadvertently into the distal posterior tibial artery. Already during the injection, pain sets in at the puncture site and travels into the heel and forefoot region within a few seconds; the foot becomes pale. In more severe cases the pulse at the posterior tibial artery disappears. The most frequent ulcer localization is in the area of the medial malleolus.

A noteworthy improvement due to specific therapy seems rare and was seen in one of the authors' cases. In this instance regional fibrinolysis was performed, whereas in a second case, this approach proved detrimental. The many published methods used only in single cases is evidence of the uncertainty and inadequacy of relevant therapeutic experiments. The following rules are recommended: *(1)* decrease of blood viscosity and clotting (heparin, dextran, hemodilution), *(2)* antiinflammatory agents (high-dose steroids, phenylbutazone), and *(3)* dilation of the periphery through lumbar sympathectomy, periarterial injection of local anesthesia and vasoactive medications. Experiences with other intra-arterially applied substances show that the initial severely damaged tissue section often recovers and finally after demarcation only a small necrosis remains. Therefore, in lighter cases, one should forego potentially dangerous therapies.

The prevention of this severe complication should be possible with available knowledge of the critical points and preventive measures in the sclerosing technique. The essential points are as follows: *(1)* puncture with a thick needle; *(2)* elevation of the leg with the resting cannula above the level of the thorax; *(3)* injection in this position of emptied veins with an easily movable syringe; and *(4)* careful injection of maximal 0.5 ml of the sclerosing substance. With these measures an intra-arterial injection becomes immediately evident. In the case of increased resistance or definite pain, the injection is to be discontinued immediately.

▶ Surgical care of patients with varicose veins may be bettered by these articles from abroad. Traditionally, venous ulcer was always thought to be of deep venous origin. Sethia and Darke dispel this misconception and prove their point by venous pressure study, before and after stripping. Another technique may help to eliminate the recurrence of varicose veins after stripping. This is the selective use of varicography. Varicography is a better technique to visualize incompetent perforating veins in the thigh than ascending venography. Failure to ligate an incompetent perforating vein in this region may cause recurrent varicose veins.

Recently, sclerosing therapy has received more attention in the United States, and many vein clinics are now in practice to administer sclerosing therapy. The availability of noninvasive tests helps to assure that deep veins are not affected by sclerosing therapy. Even so, sclerosing therapy is not without its problems; in particular, arterial ischemia due to injection of a sclerosing agent into the posterior tibial artery is disastrous.

Muscle Changes in Venous Insufficiency

Syde A. Taheri, Reid Heffner, James Williams, Louis Lazar, and Steve Elias (Buffalo)

Arch. Surg. 119:929–931, August 1984 11–6

Patients with venous valvular insufficiency or venous hypertension, or both, often have swelling of the affected extremity, muscular pain, and limitation of movement, all of which could be related to damage of skeletal muscles. To determine the nature and extent of pathologic changes in muscle that may result from venous disease, biopsy specimens from the gastrocnemius muscles of 53 patients were studied. All patients had varicosities and venous hypertension of the lower extremities, but no clinical signs or symptoms of occlusive arterial disease. The diagnosis of venous insufficiency and hypertension had been established by using standard diagnostic methods.

Autogenous vein valve transplant had been used in these patients to relieve venous valvular insufficiency. Eleven patients with occlusive arterial disease but no evidence of venous insufficiency or hypertension served as a control group.

Biopsy specimens from 21 patients showed atrophy of type 2 muscle fibers. Thirteen of the 21 had moderate to severe atrophy of type 2 muscle fibers only, whereas the remaining 8 patients also exhibited associated pathologic changes. Four of the 8 had atrophy of both type 1 and type 2 fibers. A second group of 21 patients showed evidence of denervation atrophy, including type grouping of fibers that was most likely indicative of chronic denervation with reinnervation. A third group of 20 patients exhibited myopathic abnormalities, including fiber degeneration or necrosis, fiber regeneration, and inflammation. Five of the patients in this group also showed features of denervation. (Among the three groups there was overlap of pathologic changes in 12 patients.)

Biopsy specimens from patients with arterial insufficiency displayed an atrophic pattern similar to that seen in specimens from patients with venous insufficiency and histologic features of denervation. The atrophic process was of equal severity and involved type 1 and type 2 fibers. However, neither type grouping nor target fibers were observed. Selective type 2 fiber atrophy was not observed in patients with arterial insufficiency. Necrosis of muscle fibers was as prevalent as in specimens from patients with venous disease whose biopsy specimens showed myopathic changes.

The three types of morphological injury observed suggest that disuse, denervation, and ischemia may each be partially responsible for damage in skeletal muscle in patients with venous insufficiency and hypertension. Thus, injury to skeletal muscle is a likely explanation for the higher preoperative level of serum creatine kinase in many patients and may account for the postoperative failure of venous pressures to return to normal levels.

Direct Venous Surgery for Venous Valvular Insufficiency of the Lower Extremity: Updated Experience

Willard C. Johnson, Donald C. Nabseth, Harry L. Bush, and Warren C. Widrich (Tufts Univ.)

Contemp. Surg. 26:35–43, January 1985 11–7

Venous operations were performed on 11 extremities with severe deep venous insufficiency producing stasis, swelling, and present or past ulceration. Dynamic venous pressure measurements were made before and after operation and in conjunction with exercise. Valve incompetence was tested with a transcutaneous directional ultrasound flowmeter. Valve transposition was performed if the superficial femoral venous valves were incompetent but competent valves were present in the proximal part of the greater saphenous vein or the profunda femoris vein. Alternative procedures include femoral vein valvuloplasty, valve transplantation from the brachial vein if valvuloplasty is not feasible, and superficial femoral vein ligation.

Postoperative venography showed all anastomoses to be patent and reflux into previously incompetent venous systems to be absent. No patient has had venous thrombosis or pulmonary embolism, but 2 patients have had persistent ulceration. Three patients had lymph drainage from the femoral incision, but infection was not documented. Secondary colonization by staphylococci occurred in two extremities.

Generally favorable hemodynamic results were obtained by various direct venous operations in these patients with venous valvular insufficiency in the lower extremity. Many patients with venous ulceration may have abnormal valve leaflets, making them susceptible to stretch injury, but valvuloplasty, vein transposition, and even autogenous valve transplantation may have limited value in this setting. Nonautogenous transplantation or prosthetic valve replacement may be indicated.

▶ Muscle changes in venous insufficiency may explain muscle pump failure in these patients. It would be of interest to correlate degrees of muscle pump dysfunction with hemodynamic studies and with types of morphological change by muscle biopsy.

The role of the incompetent venous valve and its correction by direct surgery continues to be controversial. Could valve replacement with a preserved or prosthetic valve help? Study of the mechanical properties of valves by the St. Thomas group is the first step in this direction. Further work, especially the use of B-mode scan to evaluate valve movements after surgery, is needed to establish the validity of venous valve surgery.

Leg and Foot Ulcers: An Epidemiologic Survey

Eva Andersson, Carita Hansson, and Gunnar Swanbeck (Univ. of Göteborg)

Acta Derm. Venereol (Stockh.) 64:227–232, 1984 11–8

Leg and foot ulcers are common among the elderly. They are taken care of by practitioners in various medical disciplines. Records of patients from hospital wards and clinics in Göteborg were reviewed to estimate the incidence of leg and foot ulcers and determine where they were treated.

An estimated 1,377 patients with leg and foot ulcers were found, 61% of whom were women. Median ages were 76 years for women and 70 years for men. Age-specific frequencies did not differ between men and women. The cause of the ulcers could not be determined from the records alone. Thirty percent of patients had ulcers on the feet only. The ratio between men and women was 1:1. Men got their foot ulcers 5 to 10 years earlier than women. Seventeen percent of all patients had ulcers on the medial side of the calf only; 70% of these were women. The patients were mostly seen as outpatients by dermatologists, followed by general practitioners, general surgeons, orthopedic surgeons, and geriatric physicians.

The prevalence of leg and foot ulcer patients in Göteborg is between 0.2% and 0.4%, and the percentage increases exponentially with age. Arterial insufficiency may be becoming a more common causal factor in the disease as suggested by the finding that ulcers were found only on the feet of 30% of the patients. In contrast, the number of leg ulcers caused by venous insufficiency may have decreased, since only 17% of the patients had ulcers on the medial side of the calf alone. Since leg and foot ulcer patients seek help from varied medical disciplines, utilizing the special expertise of each branch can yield optimal results in management of these patients.

Chronic Ulceration of the Leg: Extent of the Problem and Provision of Care

M. J. Callam, C. V. Ruckley, D. R. Harper, and J. J. Dale (Edinburgh)

Br. Med. J. 290:1855–1856, June 22, 1985 11–9

Chronic ulceration of the leg continues to be puzzling. Little is known of the extent of the problems or its clinical course. A mail survey was undertaken in two health board areas of Scotland, encompassing a population of about 1 million. A total of 1,477 cases of chronic ulceration of the leg were reported by more than 500 general practitioners. Women predominated by 2.8 to 1. Median ages were 74 years for women and 67 years for men. Five percent of patients were treated in the hospital, 12% were managed jointly by the primary care team and outpatient department, and 83% were managed entirely in the community.

Attempts to improve the management of chronic leg ulceration should focus on primary health care. The clinical course is characterized by episodes of recurrence followed by periods of healing. The disorder affects both the elderly and younger persons and in the latter may result in substantial loss of work time. The problem is expected to increase with further aging of the population.

▶ Unlike arterial occlusive disease, there is virtually no information on epidemiologic surveys of venous ulcer. A study similar to these two reports is badly needed in the United States.

12 Reconstructive Surgery of the Peripheral Veins

Long-Term Patency of Venous Repairs Demonstrated by Venography
Travis J. Phifer, Amil J. Gerlock, Jr., Normal M. Rich, and John C. McDonald
J. Trauma 25:342–346, April 1985 12–1

Indications for venous reconstruction after trauma are uncertain, partly because of doubt about continued patency. Review was made of data on 31 patients who were seen during a 20-year period with femoral venous

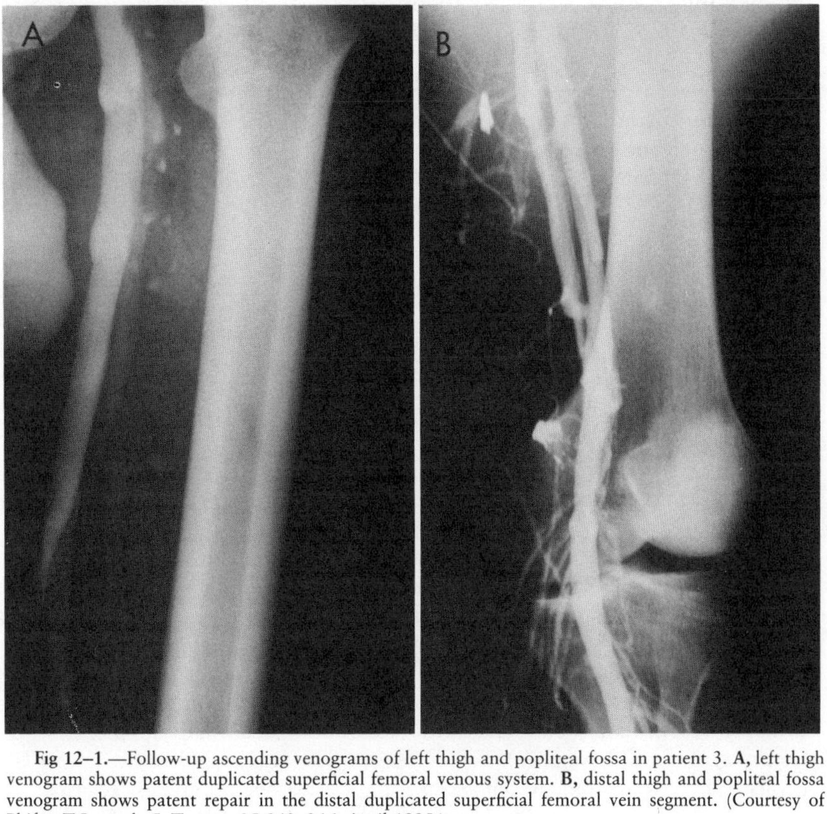

Fig 12–1.—Follow-up ascending venograms of left thigh and popliteal fossa in patient 3. **A**, left thigh venogram shows patent duplicated superficial femoral venous system. **B**, distal thigh and popliteal fossa venogram shows patent repair in the distal duplicated superficial femoral vein segment. (Courtesy of Phifer, T.J., et al.: J. Trauma 25:342–346, April 1985.)

injuries, 24 of whom underwent reconstruction. Five patients having 6 reconstructions were contacted. Three injuries had been caused by 0.22-caliber missiles, 2 by 0.38-caliber missiles, and 1 by a 12-gauge shotgun blast. Only the superficial femoral vein was injured in 4 cases. One patient had also recevied a common femoral vein injury on a separate occasion. Interpositional Teflon and saphenous vein grafts and an autogenous vein patch graft were performed, as well as an end-to-end anastomosis and a lateral suture repair. The only significant complication was persistent edema in 1 case.

Five of the 6 repairs were patent on follow-up venography, carried out 6–20 years after operation. The interpositional Teflon graft repair was occluded in a patient who had dysfunctional valves in the entire deep venous system. The other patients had normal valve function on exercise venography. The findings in 1 case are shown in Figures 12–1A and 12–1B.

The outcome in this small series supports reconstruction rather than ligation in cases of vein injury. All but 1 of the 6 femoral venous repairs followed were still patent on long-term evaluation. The absence of valves in remaining tributaries in the patient with an occluded graft suggested at least partial recanalization following early thrombosis.

Use of Intermittent Pneumatic Compression of the Calf in Femoral Venous Reconstruction

Robert W. Hobson II, Bing C. Lee, Thomas G. Lynch, Krishna Jain, Richard Yeager, Zafar Jamil, and Frank T. Padberg, Jr. (New Jersey Med. School, Newark)

Surg. Gynecol. Obstet. 159:285–286, September 1984 12–2

Progress in venous reconstructive procedures in the lower extremities has been hampered by problems such as venous graft occlusion. Data are presented on 7 cases in which intermittent pneumatic compression of the calf was used to increase the velocity of blood flow in the deep venous system of the lower extremity. One is described below.

Boy, 14, sustained a stab wound to the left medial thigh and developed an expanding hematoma at site of injury. Distal pulses were palpable. After resuscitation with fluids, exploration revealed extensive laceration of the left superficial femoral vein and repair was accomplished by using the contralateral saphenous vein as an interposition graft. After operation the patient had edema of the calf and ankle, with a Doppler systolic pressure of 75 mm Hg at the left ankle. A venogram confirmed occlusion of the interposition venous graft. Venous hypertension developed and an in situ saphenopopliteal bypass was performed. Intermittent pneumatic compression of the calf was used for 72 hours after operation. Edema of the extremity subsided, with restoration of normal Doppler systolic pressure at the ankle. Augmentation of venous flow was audible over the bypass on each calf compression. A venogram 4 days after operation showed a patent bypass. Doppler ultrasonic testing confirmed patency 30 months later. The patient had no physical restrictions and no edema in the lower extremity.

Intermittent compression of the calf was also used in 6 other venous reconstructions of lower extremities: 2 after superficial femoral and 4 after common femoral venous injuries. No complications occurred and patency was confirmed in all cases.

Application of intermittent compression of the calf can be a useful adjunct to maintaining patency of femoral venous reconstructions after trauma by increasing the velocity of blood flow in the deep venous system of the lower extremity. Previous reports show its use as a prophylaxis of postoperative deep venous thrombosis. The authors recommend its use in instances of femoral and popliteal venous reconstructions, particularly when an interposition or bypass graft has been used.

▶ The use of intermittent pneumatic compression in venous reconstruction eliminates the need for continuation of heparin infusion during the postoperative period, thus avoiding the complication of hematoma. Long-term patency of venous repair, demonstrated by Phifer and his colleagues, further supports reconstruction rather than ligation as the treatment of choice in venous injury.

Evaluation of Superior Vena Cava Syndrome by Axial CT and CT Phlebography

Rogelio Moncada, Richard Cardella, Terrence C. Demos, Robert J. Churchill, Manuel Cardosa, Leon Love, and Carlos J. Reynes

AJR 143:731–736, October 1984 12–3

Because the superior vena cava (SVC) syndrome is often produced by neoplastic involvement of the mediastinum, but may also result from benign processes, it is important to define its cause and exact level of venous blockage, as well as to map the collateral circulation. Transverse axial CT combined with CT digital phlebography was used to evaluate findings in 9 patients with SVC syndrome.

The cause of SVC syndrome was malignant involvement of the mediastinum in 5 patients, fibrosing mediastinitis in 2, and intraluminal SVC thrombus in 2. The combined CT examination demonstrated the abnormal morphology in all 9 patients, showing external compression, encasement by tumor, or intraluminal thrombosis. Opacification of collateral venous channels was clearly demonstrated in 8 patients. The CT findings directed successful biopsy procedures in 3 of the 5 patients with malignant mediastinal involvement. Thrombi within the lumen of the superior vena cava were demonstrated in 2 patients, thereby avoiding thoracotomy. In 1 of these 2 patients, the thrombus was a paraneoplastic feature of an adenocarcinoma of the colon. Thoracic CT disclosed intraluminal SVC thrombosis with no abnormal mediastinal mass, and CT phlebography showed nonfilling of the SVC with opacification of extensive chest wall and paravertebral collaterals. The second patient had a gastric adenocarcinoma and an associated SVC thrombus with extensive collateral circulation; CT demonstrated a few mediastinal nodes that were not compressing the major veins. Conventional superior vena cava angiography was also performed in 1 patient and radionuclide cavography in 2 others, but neither provided information other than that obtained with the combined CT approach.

This combined technique is a rapid, informative, and cost-effective method for evaluation of SVC syndrome. However, the CT digital phlebogram is limited in its ability to opacify the normal SVC consistently and optimally because of the limited amount of contrast material used, the dilution effect of the nonopacified inflow from the jugular and azygous veins, and the lack of image enhancement from the CT digital scanograms. Even so, the successful demonstration of high-level obstruction of the SVC in this series was sufficient to satisfy the referring physician and preclude the morbidity and expense accompanying the use of a conventional phlebogram.

Supradiaphragmatic Renal Cell Carcinoma Tumor Thrombus: Indications for Vena Cava Reconstruction With Pericardium

Fray F. Marshall and Bruce A. Reitz (Johns Hopkins Univ.)

J. Urol. 133:266–268, February 1985 — 12–4

Vena cava reconstruction may sometimes be indicated after successful removal of renal cell carcinoma with a supradiaphragmatic tumor thrombus. A recent patient undergoing extirpation of renal cell carcinoma with a large tumor thrombus had vena cava reconstruction with a pericardial patch.

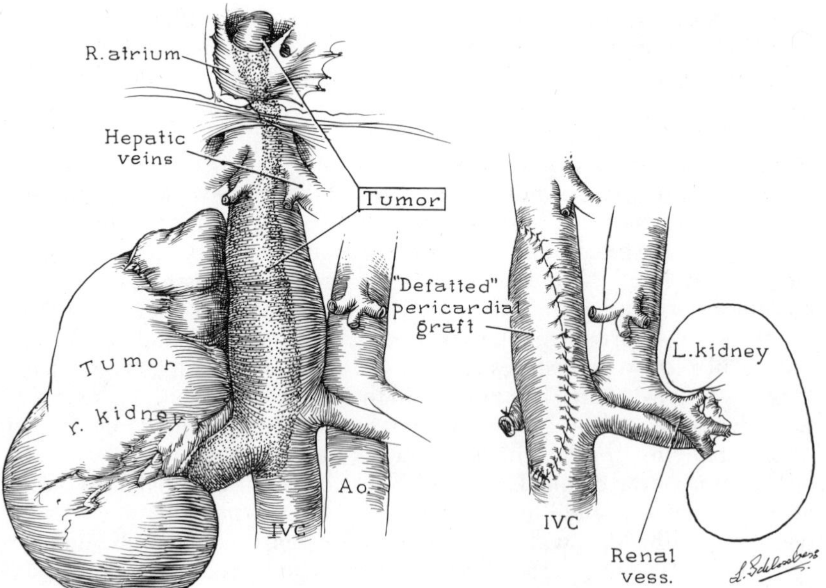

Fig 12–2.—Extension of tumor thrombus from right renal cell carcinoma extending above hepatic veins, and reconstruction of vena cava, after resection, with defatted pericardial graft. (Courtesy of Marshall, F.F., and Reitz, B.A.: J. Urol. 133:266–268, February 1985.)

Woman, 54, had had intermittent gross, painless hematuria for 2 years and was found to have a nonfunctioning right kidney with an apparent mass, confirmed by computed tomography. Inferior venacavography showed tumor thrombus extending above the hepatic veins, without total occlusion. A superior venacavogram showed thrombus extension just below the right atrium. Right radical nephrectomy was performed, with excision of part of the inferior vena cava and resection of the tumor thrombus with hypothermia, cardiac arrest, and temporary exsanguination. A pericardial patch was used to reconstruct the vena cava wall (Fig 12–2). Tumor thrombus was found in the central adrenal vein and in vessels in the periadrenal soft tissue. A patent vena cava was present 3 months after operation. Renal function was normal 1 year later, but hematuria led to exploration, which showed recurrent tumor in the distal part of the ureter and iliac node involvement.

Up to 10% of patients with renal cell carcinoma have tumor thrombus in the vena cava. Ligation of the left renal vein can lead to irreversible renal failure if the vena cava must be completely resected and collateral venous drainage has not fully developed. Pericardium can be used to reconstruct the vena cava in these instances. Saphenous vein might be considered if the pericardial patch is small. Vena cava reconstruction might also be performed in cases of left-sided tumor with massive vena caval involvement in which the venous drainage of the right kidney must be preserved. Renal autotransplantation and anastomosis of the right renal vein to the portal vein are other options.

▶ Once again, CT scan shows us diagnostic information unobtainable by contrast venography. The use of pericardium offers an alternate technique in vena cava reconstruction.

Endothelial Seeding of Venous Prostheses

G. Plate, L. H. Hollier, R. J. Fowl, J. R. Sande, and M. P. Kaye (Mayo Clinic and Found.)

Surgery 96:929–936, November 1984 12–5

Thrombogenicity of graft material and low flow in the venous system have been shown to cause prosthetic graft failures when implanted in the venous system. To evaluate the potential benefits of endothelial seeding of venous prostheses, 20 dogs were subjected to iliocaval venous reconstruction with expanded polytetrafluoroethylene grafts that were protected by an arteriovenous fistula. Grafts seeded with enzymatically derived endothelial cells were compared with control grafts that were sham seeded with blood mixed with culture medium. The patency rate and mean thrombus-free surface area in the 2 groups were calculated. Microscopic evaluations of endothelialization were performed on specimens from thrombus-free surface areas.

Early patency was determined in 6 of 10 seeded and 8 of 10 sham-seeded grafts. When the grafts were harvested 4 to 6 weeks after implantation, 2 seeded and 1 sham-seeded graft had a luminal surface completely free of mural thrombus. Mean thrombus-free surface area was 80% in the seeded group and 71% in the sham-seeded group. Light microscopy study of the thrombus-free area showed a monocellular surface lining in all grafts. Scanning electron microscopy study demonstrated a thin cellular lining covering 50% to 100% of the surface area in 4 seeded and 5 sham-seeded grafts. Transmission electron microscopy revealed these cells exhibited characteristics typical of endothelial cells. The subcellular layer was equally thin in both groups.

The authors conclude that endothelial seeding of polytetrafluoroethylene grafts implanted in the venous system does not improve the early patency rate. Seeding of grafts with enzymatically derived endothelial cells provides a good endothelial cover with a thin subendothelial layer but not to a greater extent than does sham seeding of the venous prostheses.

This is in conflict with previous clinical and experimental studies of Sauvage et al. and Graham et al., which showed that vascular prostheses implanted in the arterial and venous system of both animals and human beings essentially never obtained an internal endothelial lining. Reendothelialization may possibly have been due to transformation of blood elements harvested from the jugular vein in the preparation of the endothelial cells or, possibly, the nonheparinized blood and culture medium used for sham seeding of the grafts also played a role in reendothelialization. This raises the possibility that a proper culture medium and surface condition may permit early and complete endothelialization of vascular grafts.

▶ Major vein reconstruction is being done rarely. We must understand that these are still experimental procedures. Whether endothelial seeding will aid in ensuring patency of these procedures is yet to be determined.

PORTAL HYPERTENSION

13 Variceal Hemorrhage

Portal Venous Thrombosis: Correlative Analysis of Sonography, CT, and Angiography

Bala R. Subramanyam, Emil J. Balthazar, Richard S. Lefleur, Steven C. Horii, and Donald H. Hulnick (New York Univ.)

Am. J. Gastroenterol. 79:773–776, October 1984 13–1

The noninvasive findings in portal venous thrombosis were assessed in 17 patients diagnosed radiologically. Thrombosis was due to malignant liver tumor with venous extension in 9 cases. Seven patients had hepatocellular carcinoma, and 1 each had metastatic adenocarcinoma and cholangiocarcinoma. Nonneoplastic thrombosis was due to cirrhosis in 4 cases, pancreatic disease in 2 cases, and complications of splenectomy and cavernous transformation of the portal vein in 1 case each. Ultrasound studies were done with a contact B scanner or real-time sector scanner. The computed tomography (CT) was done after intravenous contrast administration in all cases. Noncontrast scans also were obtained in 11 patients suspected of having focal liver disease.

Ultrasound study correctly identified portal venous thrombosis in all cases but 1. The thrombosed vein was distinguished by its echogenic wall. Other contiguous veins were seen to be involved in most cases. The vein draining the neoplastic liver segment was involved in cases of tumor. The CT diagnosed portal vein thrombosis in 13 cases for a false negative rate of 24%. Tumor extension into the portal vein was visualized in 6 cases. The involved vein was adjacent to the liver tumor. Angiography missed tumor thrombosis in 1 case. It detected arterioportal shunting in 3 tumor cases.

Sonography is a sensitive means of detecting and evaluating portal vein thrombosis, but it is limited in the presence of obesity or excessive bowel gas. Computed tomography is less sensitive in evaluating the extent of thrombosis. Angiography remains very useful in depicting the detailed vascular anatomy in patients who may be surgical candidates.

▶ Abdominal CT is teaching us that mesenteric venous thrombosis is more common than was formerly understood. Perhaps portal venous thrombosis is also more common. Certainly, the CT is the best way of assessing mesenteric and portal venous circulation.

Results in 100 Consecutive Patients With Stapled Esophageal Transection for Varices

R. A. J. Spence and G. W. Johnston (Belfast)

Surg. Gynecol. Obstet. 160:323–329, April 1985 13–2

Stapled esophageal transection was performed in 100 consecutively seen patients with varices between 1976 and 1985. Cirrhotic patients who were considered unsuitable for shunt surgery, as well as those with extrahepatic obstruction who lacked suitable veins, were included. The 55 men and 45 women had a mean age of 55 years; 20 patients older than age 70 years. Twelve patients in the series had extrahepatic portal vein obstruction, whereas 88 had intrahepatic disease. Most patients had been admitted once or twice previously for variceal bleeding. The Russian gun was used in earlier cases, and the EEA stapler more recently. Twenty-five patients had emergency surgery.

Fourteen patients required dilation for dysphagia postoperatively. Two patients had esophageal leaks, but not from the esophageal anastomotic line. Late portosystemic encephalopathy was not a significant problem. Three patients rebled shortly after emergency transection. Twenty-six of 85 discharged patients had recurrent bleeding from various sites, 11 of them from varices. Two died after variceal hemorrhage. More than 80% of patients remained free of variceal rebleeding 5 years after treatment, and just over 60% at 7 years. More than 90% of the extrahepatic group remained free of bleeding. The hospital mortality was 15%; 28% in emergency cases.

Esophageal stapled transection is a useful elective procedure for patients with varices who cannot undergo shunt surgery for any reason. Increased rebleeding rates are expected with longer follow-up periods, and injection sclerotherapy probably is preferable where available. Transection does not preclude subsequent surgery for portal hypertension, but splenic artery ligation might best be avoided where a distal splenorenal shunt is a possibility.

▶ The results of this 100-patient study are at great variance from experience in North America. Perhaps the difference is in the state of the patient population; the Irish patients being much more favorable than the ones who received this operation in America.

Sclerotherapy After First Variceal Hemorrhage in Cirrhosis: A Randomized Multicenter Trial

The Copenhagen Esophageal Varices Sclerotherapy Project

N. Engl. J. Med. 311:1594–1600, Dec. 20, 1984 13–3

Recent trials have favored sclerotherapy over established medical treatment for bleeding esophageal varices, but they have included patients with better-than-average prognoses. In this trial, conducted from 1978 to 1982, all patients with upper gastrointestinal bleeding who required transfusion for an initial episode of variceal hemorrhage were randomized as soon as possible to evaluate the effects of intensive sclerotherapy, used as a supplement to the medical regimen. A total of 187 unselected cirrhotic patients were randomized to medical treatment that included either balloon tamponade ("medical-regimen group") or intensive paravariceal sclerotherapy ("sclerotherapy group") and were followed for 9–52 months. Sclerotherapy was performed at least 3 times at intervals of about 3 days until bleeding stopped. The sclerosant used was polidocanol.

After the first 2 months, when about half of the patients had died, the sclerotherapy group had more survivors than did the medical-regimen group. The overall survival curves, however, did not differ significantly, although the beneficial effects of sclerotherapy was apparent most of the time during follow-up. When mortality was corrected for the degree of encephalopathy and ascites, the rate in the sclerotherapy group was 63% of that in the medical-regimen group. Sclerotherapy has no significant effect on the duration of initial hemorrhage or on immediate mortality. The sclerotherapy group also had a much lower incidence of recurrent bleeding after the first 40 days, with reductions in both the number of patients having rebleeding and the number of episodes. Endoscopic perforation of the esophagus was confirmed in 4 cases from the sclerotherapy group. There was 1 esophageal rupture in each group.

Overall survival was not significantly improved by sclerotherapy in this series of patients with variceal bleeding caused by cirrhosis, but a significant effect was apparent when the degree of encephalopathy and ascites were taken into account. Sclerotherapy can be recommended over medical treatment alone for cirrhotic patients with bleeding esophageal varices. Further efforts are needed to improve survival shortly after the onset of bleeding.

The Esophagus After Endoscopic Injection Sclerotherapy: Acute and Chronic Changes

Farooq P. Agha (Univ. of Michigan)

Radiology 153:37–42, October 1984 13–4

Endoscopic injection sclerotherapy (EIS) has become an increasingly popular treatment for esophageal varices, especially in patients with Child class C portal hypertension and bleeding varices or in whom the anatomy is unsuitable for splenorenal shunt placement. Esophageal changes that followed EIS were assessed in 10 patients who underwent esophagography 33 times after EIS for varices. Age range was 21 to 66 years. All patients had hepatic cirrhosis, portal hypertension, and recurrent variceal bleeding. Two patients had had recurrent bleeding after an esophagogastric devascularization procedure. Sclerotherapy was administered with a flexible fiberoptic endoscope, 5% sodium morrhuate solution, and local anesthesia with intravenous sedation. One to five treatments were necessary to inject up to 65 ml of sclerosant solution. All patients had at least one double-contrast study of the esophagus.

Early changes after EIS included mucosal ulceration, luminal narrowing, intramural defects, sinus and fistula formation, and perforation. Five patients had ulcerations within 30 days of the procedure, and 7 had various degrees of luminal narrowing. Two patients had intramural sinuses and dissection (Figs 13–1 to 13–3). Two had an esophagoesophageal fistula (double-barrel esophagus). One perforation occurred without mediastinal abscess formation. Four patients later developed esophageal strictures, including both who had had previous devascularization procedures. Seven

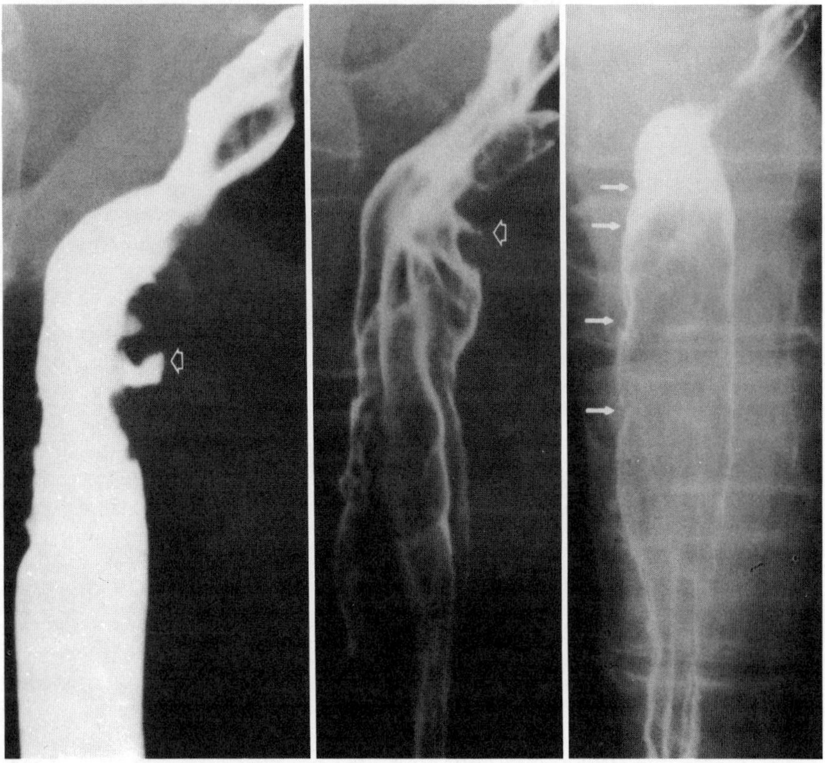

Fig 13–1 (left).—Barium esophagogram 2 weeks after two courses of EIS given 1 week apart shows diffuse ulceration in distal third of esophagus and one intramural sinus tract *(arrow)*.

Fig 13–2 (center).—Double-contrast esophagogram 1 month later shows residual mucosal ulceration and intramural sinus tract *(arrow)*.

Fig 13–3 (right).—Double-contrast esophagogram 2 months later shows nodular and notched contour defects *(arrows)* in distal part of esophagus. Ulcerations and intramural sinus tract have completely resolved. Contour defects are due to sclerosed varices confirmed at endoscopic examination.

(Courtesy of Agha, F.P.: Radiology 153:37–42, October 1984.)

of the 10 patients had some contour abnormality on esophagography. Three patients has significant dysmotility as a late manifestation, ranging from an atonic dilated esophagus to severe tertiary contractions.

An appreciation of the esophageal changes after EIS is important in following patients, especially those for whom a relevant history is unavailable. The most important early complication is esophageal perforation and necrosis. Later, both luminal narrowing and motility disturbance may be evident.

▶ Many surgeons treating portal hypertension have welcomed endoscopic sclerotherapy for treatment of the patient who is a Child's class C bleeder, commonly referred to as a "late Friday afternoon." The prospective study abstracted here provides much valuable information, as does the study showing esophageal changes after endoscopic sclerotherapy.

14 Portal Shunts

Nonselective Left Gastric-Caval Shunt: Indication, Technique, and Results

E. Moreno Gonzáles, A. Calle Santjuste, G. Garcia Blanch, I. Landa Garcia, and I. Garcia Garcia (Madrid)

Chirurg 55:575–578, September, 1984 14–1

A total of 104 patients with bleeding esophageal varices were treated surgically between 1976 and 1982. Indication for nonselective gastric-caval shunt was determined by strict criteria: *(1)* adequate lumen of the left gastric vein firmly established by angiography, *(2)* absence of anterograde portal flow, and *(3)* presence of pharmacologically intractable ascites. Ascites estimated between 4 to 61 was observed in 2 patients. Anemia, leukopenia, platelet counts below 85×10^9/L were found in all patients.

This gastric-caval shunt without splenectomy was performed in 3 patients, two suffering from liver cirrhoses of toxic or posthepatitic origin respectively. The third patient had a thrombosis and cavernous transformation of the portal vessel. According to the criteria established by Viamonte et al. (1970), liver panangiography confirmed phase II or phase I of the illness (Fig 14–1). Surgical procedure was performed 3–7 weeks after the last episode of hemorrhage. Diameter of the gastric vein was 2, 2.5, and 2.5 cm, respectively. The vessel demonstrated from about 10 cm

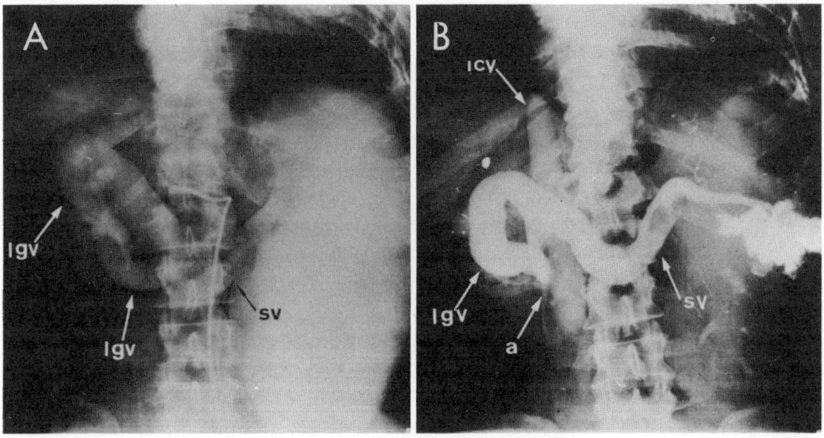

Fig 14–1.—A, indirect arterial splenoportography in posthepatitic liver cirrhoses. VL = v. linealis, VCV = wide v. coronaria ventriculi. The portal vessel is not depicted. **B,** indirect arterial splenoportography 3 years after shunt. The gastric vein (VCV) anastomosed with the v. cava inferior. An = anastomosis. (Courtesy of Gonzáles, E.M., et al.: Chirurg 55:575–578, September 1984; Berlin–Heidelberg–New York: Springer.)

from its outlet into the portal vein up to its origin at the lesser gastric curvature where it was then severed between two ligatures. It was then looped around the outer lateral edge of the hepatoduodenal ligament. After opening the outer anterolateral segment of the vena cava inferior, an end-to-side gastric-caval shunt was realized with 4 × 0 individual sutures.

Ascites and esophageal varices disappeared in the 3 patients between 1 and 3 weeks after the operation. The shunts were confirmed open between 8 months to 8½ years after operation. All 3 patients are still living.

Selective Variceal Decompression in Portal Vein Thrombosis

J. M. Henderson, W. J. Millikan, J. T. Galambos, and W. D. Warren (Emory Univ.)

Br. J. Surg. 71:745–749, October 1984 14–2

Bleeding from gastroesophageal varices secondary to portal vein thromboses usually occurs in younger patients. The normal liver in these patients differentiates them from most patients with variceal bleeding. Management should be directed at correcting the pathologic component, the high gastroesophageal venous pressure, without disturbing the physiologic adaptation of collateral portal venous perfusion of the liver.

An evaluation was made of the use of distal splenorenal shunts (DSRS) in the management of bleeding gastroesophageal varices in 32 patients with congenital portal vein thrombosis; 17 had an intact spleen (group 1), and 15 were splenectomized (group 2). In group 1, 13 patients received DSRS and 4 underwent splenectomy and devascularization because no veins were suitable for DSRS. Nine of the 15 group 2 patients had endoscopic sclerosis, 4 underwent devascularization, and 2 received total shunts. The follow-up period ranged from 6 months to 7 years (mean, 3.1 years).

There were no deaths in either group. In group 1, there was 1 shunt thrombosis and 1 patient had transient rebleeding despite a patent shunt. This single episode of rebleeding occurred at 1 week secondary to renal vein hypertension and was managed expectantly with no further bleeding at 4 years. Recurrent bleeding episodes developed in 6 patients in group 2. Although clinically significant, these episodes were not life-threatening except in 1 patient. Within a mean follow-up of 3.1 years, rebleeding occurred in 1 patient treated by DSRS and in 8 patients managed by sclerosis/devascularization ($P < .05$). Detailed study of 7 patients before and 1 year after DSRS showed an increase in platelet count and maintenance of hepatocyte function, portal perfusion, liver blood flow, and liver size. The size of the spleen, which was 5 times normal before shunting, was reduced significantly by transplenic decompression ($P < .025$). The use of DSRS provides an excellent method by which long-term control of bleeding can be achieved without compromising liver function or hemodynamics.

Simplified Portoazygous Disconnection (Tanner's Operation) Combined With Operative Sclerotherapy for Bleeding Varices

Ralph S. Chung and Daniel S. Camara

Am. J. Surg. 148:389–392, September 1984 14–3

The authors describe a simplified technique of portoazygous dissection that uses the linear stapler and operative sclerotherapy and report the results of its application in six patients, all of whom were in Child's class C and had alcoholic cirrhosis.

TECHNIQUE.—An upper midline incision is made from the xiphoid to the umbilicus, and the left lobe of the liver is elevated and held in place by a self-retaining device, giving excellent exposure of the cardioesophageal angle. The angle of His is dissected bluntly and the lower part of the esophagus encircled with a Penrose drain. Between stay sutures, the anterior wall of the stomach is entered through a 1-cm gastrostomy 3 cm distal to the esophageal junction (Fig 14–2). Diathermy is used. The anterior wall of the stomach is divided toward the right by a single application of a GIA Auto-Suture stapler, producing a hemostatic incision of the anterior gastric wall up to the lesser curvature. The transection is completed by a

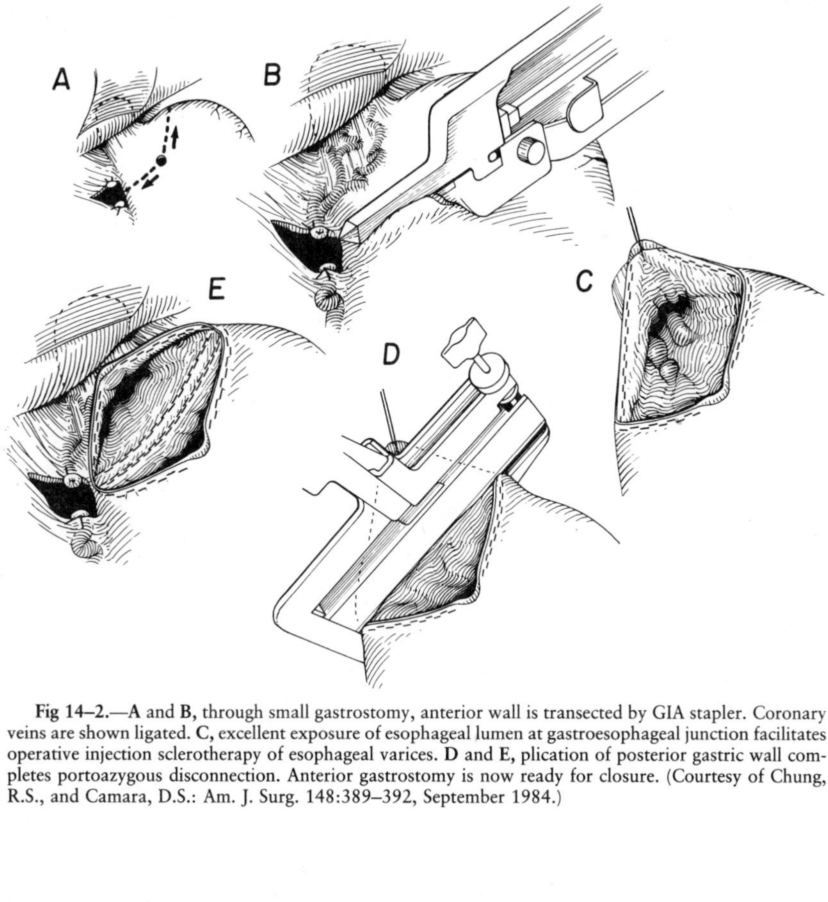

Fig 14–2.—**A** and **B**, through small gastrostomy, anterior wall is transected by GIA stapler. Coronary veins are shown ligated. **C**, excellent exposure of esophageal lumen at gastroesophageal junction facilitates operative injection sclerotherapy of esophageal varices. **D** and **E**, plication of posterior gastric wall completes portoazygous disconnection. Anterior gastrostomy is now ready for closure. (Courtesy of Chung, R.S., and Camara, D.S.: Am. J. Surg. 148:389–392, September 1984.)

second GIA application directed to the left. All blood clots are now evacuated and the area searched for active bleeding sites. Any bleeding gastric varices are ligated by underrunning with continuous fine polyglycolic sutures. Bleeding from esophageal varices can be managed by intraoperative sclerotherapy. The vessels on the lesser curvature at the gastroesophageal junction in the space between the esophagus and the left side of the vertebral column are then encircled and divided between ligatures, with preservation at minimum of the anterior vagal trunk. This divides the coronary veins and the ascending branch of the left gastric artery and clears 1 cm or more of the lesser curvature. Through this clearing, the posterior fundic wall is stapled in continuity, in effect plicating the posterior gastric wall with four suture lines. If there are venous collaterals to the left of the esophagus, they also should be divided between ligatures. The divided anterior wall of the stomach is then resutured with a continuous running polyglycolic suture.

The indications for this procedure included failure of sclerotherapy for esophageal variceal bleeding and a diagnosis of ruptured gastric varices as the source of bleeding. The 6 patients were followed from 2 to 28 months. One died in the postoperative period and another died of hepatic failure 8 months after operation. No patient has rebled. In 2 patients, all varices were found to have been eradicated 12 to 18 months after operation.

This approach combines sclerotherapy and portoazygous disconnection, each of which tends to compensate for the deficiencies of the other.

▶ As endoscopic sclerotherapy becomes more generally available, operative decompression of portal hypertension becomes less important to general and vascular surgeons. Nevertheless, surgeons must know the various alternatives as indicated by these three abstracts.

Two-Stage Surgical Management of the Budd-Chiari Syndrome Associated With Obstruction of the Inferior Vena Cava

W. Dean Warren, John R. Potts, J. Timothy Fulenwider, William J. Millikan, Jr., and J. Michael Henderson (Emory Univ., Atlanta)

Surg. Gynecol. Obstet. 159:101–107, August 1984 14–4

The authors describe a case of Budd-Chiari syndrome complicated by obstruction of the inferior vena cava that was successfully managed by a new, staged, surgical approach.

Woman, 20, developed jaundice and ascites 5 weeks after she had started to take oral contraceptives. A liver biopsy and hepatic venography confirmed the preliminary diagnosis of Budd-Chiari syndrome. Six weeks after the appearance of symptoms, she underwent a mesocaval interposition graft using the left internal jugular vein. The ascites failed to resolve. Angiography revealed thrombosis of the mesocaval shunt and inferior vena cava obstruction. At this time, she was in moderate distress with jaundice, tense ascites, and marked edema of the lower part of the body. Venography demonstrated compression of the suprarenal inferior vena cava, but there was no evidence of extensive vena cava thrombosis. Mean pressure of the infrarenal vena cava was 23 mm Hg, with a right atrial pressure of 5 mm Hg. Two weeks after the initial shunt, a mesoatrial shunt was performed, using 20 mm of reinforced polytetrafluoroethylene (Gore-Tex). Six liters of ascites were removed from the abdomen during the procedure. Postoperatively, diuresis was immediately established, with the patient's weight falling from 91.3 to 80.5 kg within 24 hours and to 75 kg at the time of discharge 14 days later. Patency of the mesoatrial shunt was demonstrated by postoperative angiography. Four months later, the patient was readmitted for elective takedown of the mesoatrial graft and side-to-side portacaval shunt. A side-to-side portacaval shunt was made with ease in the presence of a decompressed portal system. After completion of the anastomosis, the intra-abdominal portion of the mesoatrial shunt was removed and the remaining graft oversewn. Examination of the graft lumen disclosed a grossly visible, laminated thrombus. Liver biopsy at the time of the second operation showed moderate chronic inflammation with some increased bridging fibrosis, focal regenerative activity, and no evidence of parenchymal necrosis or congestion.

The presence of vena caval obstruction is a contraindication to any form of portacaval shunting. The staged approach adopted in this patient produced an excellent result and represents a surgical alternative in patients with Budd-Chiari syndrome complicated by obstruction of the inferior vena cava. Because of the possibility of eventual thrombosis of the mesoatrial graft, secondary portacaval anastomosis is advocated after reduction of hepatic volume and angiographic documentation of resumed caval flow.

▶ The Budd-Chiari syndrome is an interesting variant on the portal hypertension theme. Its rarity causes a number of procedures to be employed; thus, no standard operation has emerged as the best. This report from a very experienced group is of great value.

15 Ascites

Peritoneovenous Shunts: Predictive Factors of Early Treatment Failure

John J. Gleysteen and Thomas W. Klamer (Med. College of Wisconsin)

Am. J. Gastroenterol. 79:654–658, August 1984 15–1

Although palliation of refractory ascites with peritoneovenous shunts has received enthusiastic support, other investigators have reported high mortality, serious perioperative complications, and early shunt malfunction with recurrent ascites. Preoperative clinical, biochemical, and operative variables were evaluated in 39 consecutive alcoholics, aged 29 to 73 years, who had peritoneovenous shunts for intractable ascites, to identify factors that might predict early death or shunt malfunction during the first 4 postoperative months. There was no standardized protocol for operative exclusion. Seventeen LeVeen and 22 Denver shunts were inserted.

Early treatment failure occurred in 23 patients (59%), including 18 deaths and 5 shunt malfunctions. Preoperative encephalopathy was observed in 12 patients who died. Elevated total bilirubin concentrations characterized patients who died significantly better ($P < .005$) than did serum creatinine elevations. Hepatorenal disease, expressed as total bilirubin plus creatinine concentrations of more than 4 mg/dl, correlated significantly with mortality ($P < .001$). Abnormal coagulation indices did not predict early failures except for an elevated prothrombin time, which characterized 61% of patients who died. Failure to drain ascitic fluid was associated with more hospital deaths ($P < .05$), and operative documentation of venous catheter placement in a central location reduced early shunt malfunction ($P < .001$). Although the malfunction rates were 33% with Denver shunts and 67% with LeVeen shunts, the difference was not significant.

The overriding predictive factor for avoidance of early shunt failure after peritoneovenous shunting for intractable alcoholic ascites is hepatorenal disease, both obvious and occult. This criterion is both sensitive (83%) and specific (81% of patients who survived had total bilirubin plus creatinine sums of less than 4 mg/dl). Although the type of shunt inserted did not significantly alter the outcome, the Denver shunt has the theoretical advantage of a valve in a subcutaneous fluid-filled chamber, permitting external manipulation to flush debris into the central venous system. Early occlusion is detected by resistance of the chamber to compression, and patency can be restored by nonoperative forceful manipulation. The importance of operative documentation of the venous catheter should be emphasized.

Control of Malignant Ascites by Peritoneovenous Shunting

Ian R. Gough (Univ. of Queensland)
Cancer 54:2226–2230, Nov. 15, 1984 15–2

Malignant ascites is a frequent cause of distress in patients with advanced cancer. Experience with 16 LeVeen and 4 Denver shunts in 17 patients with intractable malignant ascites was reviewed. The 10 women and 7 men were aged 41 to 73 years. They were expected to live at least 1 month and could not be adequately managed by diuretics and intermittent, infrequent paracentesis. Ovarian and gastrointestinal malignancies were most frequent. Twelve patients had received systemic chemotherapy, hormonal therapy, or both, and 5 had received cytotoxic agents intraperitoneally. Most shunts were inserted via the external jugular vein.

Nine patients had complications; shunt blockage and uncontrolled ascites were most frequent. Three patients required continued diuretic therapy for control of peripheral edema and 2 when shunts were inadequate. Six patients had improvement in severe hypoalbuminemia within 2 months of successful shunting. The median duration of shunt function was 12 weeks, and the median survival was 13 weeks. Ascites was controlled until death in 13 patients. One patient remained alive with a functioning shunt at 14 weeks.

Performance status improved or remained stable after peritoneovenous shunt insertion in most of these patients with malignant ascites. Ascites was controlled in most. The success rate of peritoneovenous shunting in selected patients is about 75%. The procedure should be considered for patients with uncontrollable malignant ascites who are likely to survive longer than 1 month. Complications of shunting are relatively frequent but usually not severe.

Surgical and Pathologic Complications Associated With Peritoneovenous Shunts in Management of Malignant Ascites

Robin G. Souter, Clive Wells, David Tarin, and Michael G. W. Kettlewell (Univ. of Oxford)
Cancer 55:1973–1978, May 1, 1985 15–3

Thirty-three patients with malignant ascites underwent 43 LeVeen peritoneovenous shunt procedures. Most of them were thought to be in the last 3 months of life. All patients had undergone paracentesis, and most had received chemotherapy for systemic effects or by intracavitary administration. The Stortz Denver system has occasionally been used in recent years. The most frequent primary malignancies were ovarian and breast cancers.

Three patients had mild early postoperative heart failure that was readily controlled by diuretics. One death resulted from massive pulmonary edema within hours of shunt insertion. Ascites was temporarily relieved in all cases, and half of the patients required no further paracentesis. Shunt blockage occurred in 10 patients with a LeVeen shunt and after 8 Denver procedures. Nine patients did not have their shunts replaced, for varying reasons. Most of the 12 autopsies done showed complications associated with treatment that had contributed to total or partial shunt blockage.

The peritoneovenous shunt procedure controlled ascites at least temporarily in all patients in this study and did not adversely affect the prognosis, except for the death caused by pulmonary edema after the operation. Viable cancer cells are disseminated after peritoneovenous shunting and sometimes grow within a new capillary bed or interstitially. Tumor embolism is not, however, a major clinical hazard in patients with malignant ascites.

Patient Selection and Survival After Peritoneovenous Shunting for Nonmalignant Ascites

Robert E. Smith, Timothy T. Nostrant, Frederic E. Eckhauser, Joanne P. Wilson, James A. Knol, and William E. Strodel (Univ. of Michigan)
Am. J. Gastroenterol. 79:659–662, August 1984 15–4

Despite wide acceptance of peritoneovenous shunting (PVS) to relieve ascites, some investigators have reported that unreserved application of this technique may result in significant complications. Data on 30 patients, aged 27 to 70 years, who underwent 44 PVS procedures for nonmalignant ascites over a 5-year period, were reviewed to demonstrate the impact of patient selection on long-term survival. Indications for PVS included refractory ascites alone (RA) in 14 patients, refractory ascites complicated by hepatorenal syndrome (HRS) in 10, and nonrefractory but recurrent ascites (NR) in 6. Thirty shunts contained a LeVeen pressure-activated valve; the other 14 shunts used a Denver pump-type valve.

Mean survival was 265 days. Patients with NR survived significantly longer (mean, 767 days) than patients with RA (mean, 256 days) or patients with HRS (mean, 28 days). One-year survival was significantly greater among patients with NR (67%) than patients with RA (14%) or patients with HRS (0%) ($P < .005$). Combined in-hospital mortality was 30%; it was significantly greater in patients with HRS (70%) than in patients with RA (14%) or with NR (0%). Overall, 34% of shunt procedures were associated with serious postoperative complications, including disseminated intravascular coagulation, sepsis, peritonitis, congestive heart failure, and gastrointestinal bleeding. Mean duration of shunt function was 37 days. Patients with HRS had significantly briefer shunt function (mean, 15 days) than in patients with RA (45 days) or with NR (64 days). Twenty-two (56%) of 39 shunts malfunctioned, and another 5 (13%) ended in shunt ligation or removal. Mechanical malfunction was significantly more common in LeVeen shunts than in Denver shunts.

Patient selection significantly influences survival after PVS. Patients with NR are most likely to survive longer after PVS. Divergent results reported by others may be influenced by the varied criteria for patient selection.

The LeVeen Shunt in the Elective Treatment of Intractable Ascites in Cirrhosis: A Prospective Study on 140 Patients

Claude Smadja and Dominique Franco (Villejuif, France)

Ann. Surg. 201:488–493, April 1985 15–5

Later reports on the peritoneovenous LeVeen shunt emphasized complications and a high operative mortality. Experience was reviewed with 140 consecutively seen patients with chronic liver disease, all referred since 1967 with intractable ascites and subjected to the LeVeen shunt. Most patients had alcoholic cirrhosis. Medical measures had been pursued for a mean of 4 months before referral. Severe liver failure was present in 24 patients and moderate failure in 50 others at the time of surgery.

Operative mortality within 2 months of surgery was 10%. Mortality was higher in patients with severe liver failure and lower where ascites was drained at operation. Ascites recurred in 30.5% of surviving patients,

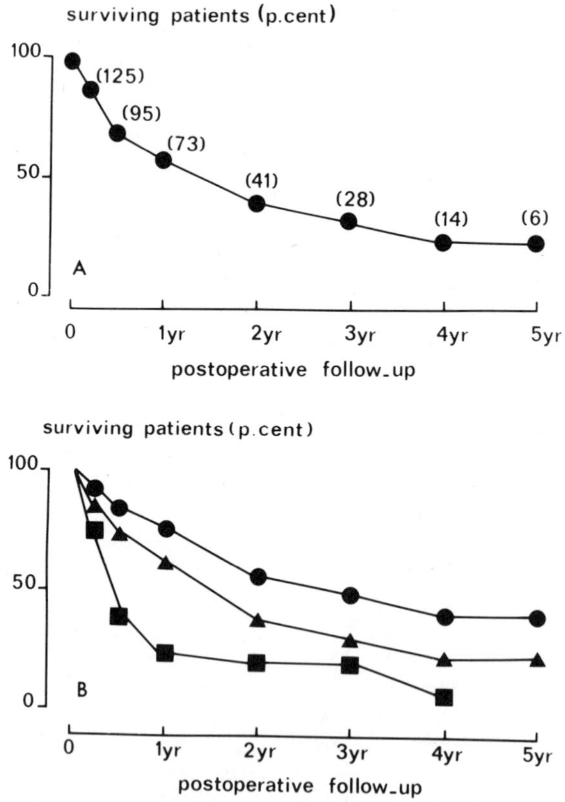

Fig 15–1.—**A,** postoperative actuarial survival curve of 140 cirrhotic patients with intractable ascites treated by peritoneovenous shunt (PVS). **B,** postoperative actuarial survival curve of cirrhotic patients with good liver function *(black circles),* moderate liver failure *(black triangles),* and severe liver failure *(black squares)* after PVS for treatment of intractable ascites. (Courtesy of Smadja, C., and Franco, D.: Ann. Surg.: 201:488–493, April 1985.)

regardless of the severity of liver failure. Obstruction at the level of the venous tubing and valve obstruction by fibrin deposits were the most frequent causes. Upper gastrointestinal bleeding occurred in 13% of patients. The rate of infection was 9%. Peritoneal fibrosis developed in 3 patients. Survival is related to liver function in Figure 15–1. All surviving patients had normal renal function and a normal nutritional status.

The peritoneovenous shunt procedure is a simple approach to intractable cirrhotic ascites. Mortality is low, and the risk of late complications is small. Long-term survival is similar to that reported after portal diversion in similar patients. Portosystemic shunting is indicated only in patients with a history of variceal bleeding and in those with recurrent ascites related to superior caval thrombosis.

▶ Endoscopic sclerotherapy may stop hemorrhage from varices in patients with portal hypertension, but ascites remains a problem treatable only by surgical means when medical means fail. Surgeons must know the value of peritoneovenous shunting in malignant ascites and how to manage patients who have nonmalignant ascites as well. Hence, the selection of this relatively large number of abstracts for a relatively small subject in vascular surgery.

MISCELLANY

16 New Developments

An Absorbable Anastomotic Device for Microvascular Surgery: Experimental Studies

Rollin K. Daniel and Michael Olding (McGill Univ.)

Plast. Reconstr. Surg. 74:329–336, September 1984 16–1

Suturing time is an especially important factor in replantation surgery, and a means of achieving acceptable patency rates in a rapid manner would be of value. The absorbable anastomotic coupler (Fig 16–1, top left) combines the classic cuffing principle with modern injection-molding tech-

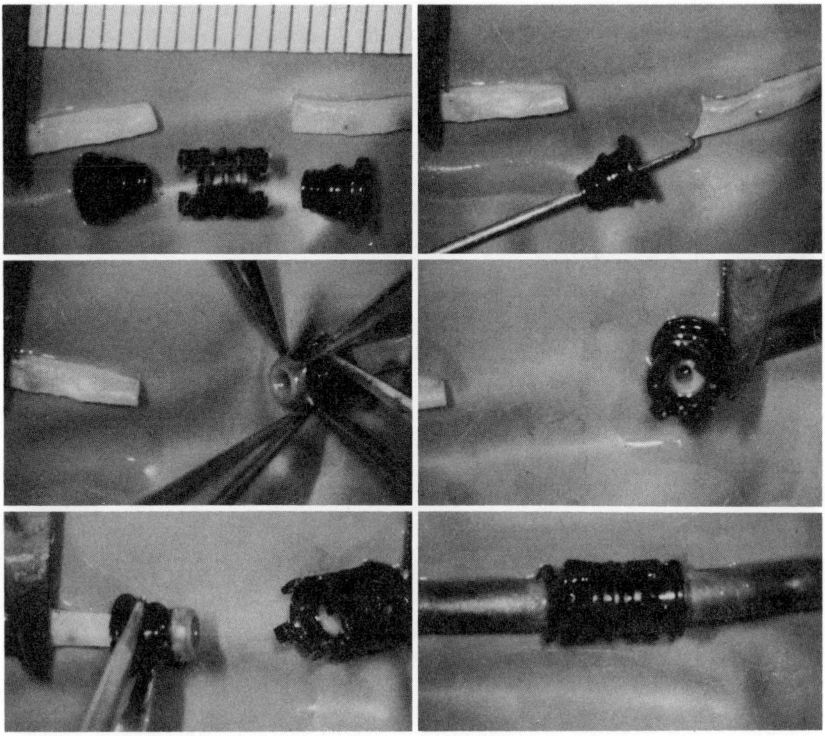

Fig 16–1 (top left).—Initial preparation of vessel for insertion of 1.5-mm coupler.
Fig 16–2 (top right).—Cut end of vessel is pulled through cuff.
Fig 16–3 (center left).—Vessel end is everted over cuff and stabilized.
Fig 16–4 (center right).—Cuff and collar are snapped together, completing first half of anastomosis. Note well-circumscribed lumen and presence of intact intimal layer.
Fig 16–5 (bottom left).—Preparation for second half of procedure, with eversion of vessel and approximation of the two parts.
Fig 16–6 (bottom right).—Completed patent anastomosis with flow.
(Courtesy of Daniel, R.K., and Olding, M.: Plast. Reconstr. Surg. 74:329–336, September 1984.)

niques. Made of the polymer polyglactin (Vicryl), the device is absorbed by hydrolysis in 50–70 days. The cuff is "loaded" on a hook, and the outer wall of the severed vessel end is snared and pulled through the cuff (Fig 16–2, top right), after dilation of the vessel if necessary. The vessel is everted over the cuff and stabilized at two points (Fig 16–3, center left) before the interconnecting collar is docked with the cuff (Fig 16–4, center right). A similar maneuver is performed on the other end of the vessel (Fig 16–5, bottom left). A watertight intima-to-intima seal is obtained, with no intraluminal foreign body present (Fig 16–6, bottom right). The device is available in sizes of 2.0, 1.5, and 1.0 mm.

The 1.5-mm device was evaluated in the rabbit carotid artery and posterior facial vein. All 16 arteries and all but 2 of 16 veins remained patent in a 12-day study. Patency was confirmed by assessing blood flow after vessel severance and by histologic study of the vessels. A patency rate of 94% was achieved in a 360-day study; the rate was 88% for 24 arteries and 100% for 24 veins. A recent 70-day study yielded a 100% patency rate for both arteries and veins. The mean length of vessel consumed per coupled anastomosis was 3.3 mm, with a range of 2–5 mm. The mean time needed for coupler insertion was 5 minutes; only 3 minutes has been needed in recent cases. The maximum vessel-size discrepancy accommodated was 1.9 mm for arteries and 2.0 mm for veins when superficial inferior epigastric groin flaps were transferred to the neck.

This device provides a consistently high patency rate when used to join small vessels. Additional sutures and glue are unnecessary. The device is completely absorbed within 70 days. More vessel is used than with a pinned-ring device, however, and a skilled assistant is needed to maintain vessel eversion. Significant vessel-size discrepancy precludes use of the absorbable anastomotic coupler. The device is expected to be helpful in replantations where multiple vein grafts must be done and in some free-tissue transfers where complications make rapid revascularization necessary.

▶ This device should be of interest to microvascular surgeons. It is fascinating to note that intimal hyperplasia remains a feature in the healing process even when sutures are not used for the anastomosis.

Laser Ablation of Human Atherosclerotic Plaque Without Adjacent Tissue Injury

Warren S. Grundfest, Frank Litvack, James S. Forrester, Tsvi Goldenberg, H. J. C. Swan, Leon Morgenstern, Michael Fishbein, I. Stuart McDermid, David M. Rider, Thomas J. Pacala, and James B. Laudenslager

J. Am. Coll. Cardiol. 5:929–933, April 1985 16–2

An attempt was made to deliver ultraviolet laser energy in nanosecond pulses potentially to excise atherosclerotic plaque without causing thermal injury to the vessel wall. Seventy specimens of human cadaver atherosclerotic aorta were irradiated in vitro with a pulsed 308-nm xenon chloride excimer laser. Sixty segments were also irradiated with an argon ion and an Nd:YAG (neodymium:yttrium-aluminum-garnet) laser operated in the continuous mode. Exposed tissues were fixed in formalin for sectioning and microscopic study.

Tissues irradiated with the Nd:YAG and argon lasers had a central crater with irregular edges and concentric zones of thermal and blast injury. Excimer laser-irradiated tissue, in contrast, exhibited deep incisions with minimal or no thermal injury.

Nanosecond-pulsed ultraviolet laser irradiation can ablate biologic tissue more precisely and with less thermal and blast damage than use of conventional argon and Nd:YAG lasers. Pulsed ultraviolet lasers that can be transmitted through fiberoptics would seem to be well suited to a variety of medical applications, including ablation of bone or cartilage fragments at arthroscopy, destruction of stones and tumors in the biliary and urologic tracts, and excision of neural tumors. The long-term effects of excimer laser energy on tissues remain to be determined.

Conditions for Effective Nd-YAG Laser Angioplasty

Herbert J. Geschwind, Georges Boussignac, Bernard Teisseire, Nicole Benhaiem, Renée Bittoun, and Daniel Laurent

Br. Heart J. 52:484–489, November 1984 16–3

Experiments have established the efficacy of the laser in removing thrombi and atheromatous plaques in test tubes, human cadaver arteries, and animal arteries. To determine the optimal conditions for recanalization of obstructed arteries without damage to the vessel walls, a Nd-YAG (neodymium-yttrium, aluminum, garnet) laser coupled to an optic fiber 0.2 mm in diameter was used in experiments on 10 thrombi in test tubes 5 mm in diameter, 10 atheromatous plaques removed from obstructed fresh human cadaver arteries, 20 totally occluded fresh human cadaver coronary arteries, and 10 totally occluded popliteal and tibial arteries in freshly amputated limbs. Percutaneous transluminal Nd-YAG laser angioplasty was used in obstructed femoral and popliteal arteries in 3 patients.

The main laser beam was used with continuous emission, and duration of exposure varied from 2 and 50 seconds. Peak emission was also used for variable durations with automatic firing in bursts at the rate of one emission every 5 seconds. The optic fiber was inserted into an inflated balloon catheter to maintain the coaxial position of the fiber, and both were advanced against the atherosclerotic plaque or thrombus. For coronary arteries, both the optic fiber and the balloon catheter were inserted into the guiding catheter; in test tubes the laser beam was directed through the open end. Fluid was circulated in both the guiding and the balloon catheters; blood (hemoglobin concentration, 15 gm/dl), saline, or a mixture of blood and saline (hemoglobin concentration, 3 gm/dl) was used. The rate of perfusion was adjusted to 10, 20, and 50 ml per minute. The effects of laser emission were evaluated grossly and microscopically and by angiography for amputated limb arteries.

Retraction of thrombi occurred in all cases and reduction in size by 50%–70% was obtained with 200 joules. Vaporization of atheromatous plaques was consistently obtained with energies of 360–600 joules and a diluted blood perfusate with a hemoglobin concentration of 3 gm/dl, a temperature of 22 C and a perfusion rate of 20 ml per minute. No effect was obtained when later emission was used in bursts. When the coaxial position was maintained with the inflated balloon catheter, no damage to the arterial wall occurred, and no leak of contrast medium was seen at repeat angiography during recanalization of the amputated limb arteries (Figs 16–7 to 16–9). Histologic findings included thermal injury, fissures, retraction, and dissection of the atheromatous plaques with the various hemoglobin concentrations used; however, no perforation of the vascular wall occurred with the dilute hemoglobin perfusate.

Percutaneous transluminal Nd-YAG laser angioplasty performed on 2 patients with either a totally occluded femoral or popliteal artery and a third with a femoral stenosis 5 mm long and 1 mm in diameter showed recanalization of the occluded femoral and popliteal arteries at three firings of 600 joules each and enlargement of the femoral artery stenosis to 4 mm at three firings of 360 joules each. No perforation of the arterial wall occurred. The only side effect was a burning sensation in the limb during laser emission.

The experiments showed that laser energy carried by optic fibers is effective when lasing is used with diluted blood perfusion (hemoglobin concentration of 3 gm/dl at the rate of 20 ml per minute). The arterial wall is protected from thermal injury by inserting the optic fiber into an inflated balloon catheter and by cooling the system with the perfusate. Clinical studies showed the method to be feasible, effective, and harmless, although further studies are required to improve penetration of the obstruction and increase the diameter of the tunnel.

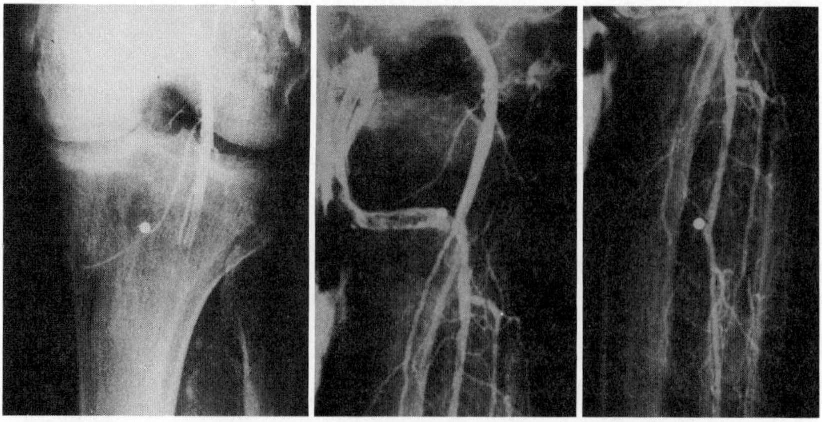

Fig 16–7 (left).—Angiogram of obstructed popliteal artery in freshly amputated limb.

Fig 16–8 (center).—Angiogram showing recanalization of popliteal and tibial arteries after laser treatment. Note retrograde opacification of previous obstructed bypass *(arrow)*.

Fig 16–9 (right).—Angiogram showing repermeation of distal vessels in same limb.

(Courtesy of Geschwind, H.J., et al.: Br. Heart J. 52:484–489, November 1984.)

► In the coming years, we will see more use of lasers in vascular surgery. The effect of the laser on arterial walls is closely related to the type of laser energy used. The excimer laser appears to be less damaging than Nd-YAG and argon lasers. Further work on the effect of laser energy on arterial walls is needed prior to applying this technique to vaporization of atherosclerotic plaques.

Application of Antibiotic Bonding to the Treatment of Established Vascular Prosthetic Infection

Ralph S. Greco, Stanley Z. Trooskin, Anthony P. Donetz, and Richard A. Harvey (Rutgers Med. School)

Arch. Surg. 120:71–75, January 1985 16–4

Vascular prosthetic infection is infrequent but has serious consequences, including loss of limb and of life. It has been proposed that anionic antibiotics such as penicillins and cephalosporins be noncovalently bound to Dacron and polytetrafluoroethylene (PTFE). Surfactant-mediated antibiotic bonding has now been used in treatment of established vascular prosthetic infection in an animal model. The infrarenal aorta of dogs was replaced with a PTFE graft contaminated locally with *Staphylococcus aureus*, and these grafts then were replaced with grafts of either control PTFE or PTFE bonded with benzalkonium chloride and penicillin G tagged with radioactive carbon or PTFE bonded with tridodecylmethylammonium chloride (TDMAC) and tagged penicillin G. Grafts replaced 2-cm segments of infrarenal aorta. The treated grafts contained 4 to 5 mg of penicillin G per cm of graft.

All but 1 of 9 dogs in which infected grafts were replaced with control grafts had at least one positive culture. One of 9 dogs given a penicillin-benzalkonium chloride graft had a positive culture, a highly significant difference. When penicillin-TDMAC-bonded grafts were placed, only 4 of 18 cultures for *S. aureus* were positive. Patency was significantly improved in dogs with benzalkonium chloride-bonded grafts, but TDMAC appeared to be relatively thrombogenic. A cationic anchor study indicated that TDMAC-treated PTFE adsorbs parenterally administered antibiotic for some time after implantation, compared with control PTFE.

These findings suggest that antibiotic-bonded grafts might be used in treatment of clinical vascular prosthetic infections, but models resembling human infection more closely will have to be devised. Benzalkonium chloride would seem to be well suited for use in prosthetic grafts in smaller vessels below the inguinal ligament, where thrombosis is frequent. The thrombogenicity of TDMAC might be obviated by high blood flow in the human aorta.

► It will be a real challenge to replace an infected graft with an antibiotic-bonded graft in humans. The authors state that they have approval for clinical application of these grafts in humans. We look forward to a controlled, perhaps a multicenter trial, to establish the value of such an antibiotic-bonded graft in well-established graft infection.

Mechanical Fatigue in an Arterial Prosthesis

M. Batt, M. King, R. Guidoin, O. Goëau-Brissonnière, C. Michetti, M. Marois, C. Gosselin, A. Garton, and P. Le Bas
Press. Med. 29:1997–2000, September 1984 16–5

Durability of a material becomes all important in the case of prostheses placed in young and active patients after trauma.

Man, 18, presented with a contusion of the left iliac fossa after a cycling injury. Arteriography revealed a left external iliac thrombosis. At operation the thrombosed segment was replaced by a De Bakey standard knitted Dacron graft. The patient recovered completely but, in spite of advice to the contrary, resumed competitive cycling. Five years later, he presented again with left leg claudication. Angiography revealed a slight increase in diameter of the graft and marked lengthening with a stenosing kink. A surgical procedure confirmed the lengthening of the prosthesis subtended by the greatly hypertrophied psoas muscle. There was complete absence of encapsulation of the prosthesis and no evidence of deterioration. The kink was resected and analyzed. The patient recovered and, this time, accepted advice to discontinue cycling.

Textile analysis revealed a considerably stretched prosthetic knit with a diminution of 32% in the density of the mesh. The fiber diameter had increased by 5.6% and density had decreased by 0.12%. This physical degradation was accompanied by chemical degradation. Apparently, the mechanical forces to which the prosthesis was exposed had accelerated chemical changes in the material.

Recent studies suggest that very compact woven grafts may have an advantage even though they may be rigid upon implantation and may ravel at the ends since the constraints of mechanical degradation there are less. Long-term results are now considered satisfactory.

The placement of an arterial prosthesis should be a definitive procedure. Technical data now lead to a preference for a woven polyester when an arterial graft must be placed in an iliac or aortic position because of trauma in a young and active subject. If possible, a failing knitted polyester graft should be completely replaced with a woven model.

Arterial Regenerative Activity After Prosthetic Implantation

Howard P. Greisler, Dae Un Kim, John B. Price, and Arthur B. Voorhees, Jr.
Arch. Surg. 120:315–323, March 1985 16–6

Arterial regeneration has been observed over absorbable woven polyglycolic acid (PGA) prostheses implanted in the rabbit aorta. The factors modifying the regenerative process were examined by replacing adult rabbit aortas with either PGA or nonabsorbable Dacron prostheses. The prostheses were 3.5 mm in internal diameter and 24 mm long and were woven to identical specifications of pore size, wall thickness, and elastic modulus. Specimens were obtained at intervals of up to 1 year from 48 rabbits with PGA prostheses and 20 with Dacron prostheses.

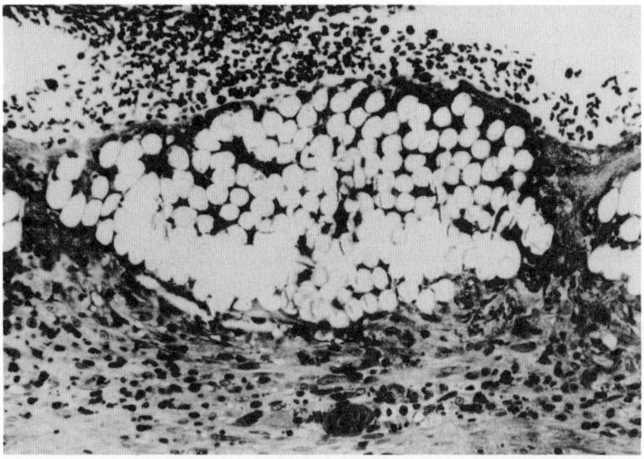

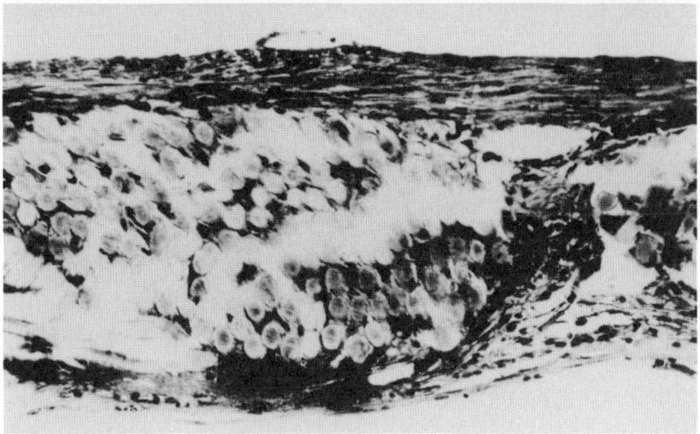

Fig 16–10 (top).—Midportion of Dacron specimen at 2 weeks showing outer capsular inflammatory reaction including macrophages, giant cells, and polymorphonuclear leukocytes, with paucity of cells in prosthetic interstices or inner capsule. Inner capsule composed of fibrin coagulum. Hematoxylin-eosin; original magnification ×250.

Fig 16–11 (bottom).—Midportion of PGA specimen at 2 weeks showing similar outer capsular inflammatory reaction but with invasion of cells into interstices and inner capsule. Inner capsule composed of myofibroblasts beneath spindle-shaped cellular luminal surface. Hematoxylin-phloxine-saffron; original magnification ×250.

(Courtesy of Greisler, H.P., et al.: Arch. Surg. 120:315–323, March 1985; copyright 1985, American Medical Association.)

The PGA prostheses were replaced by tissue forming a conduit with the original 3- to 4-mm diameter in 75% of instances. Moderate aneurysmal dilatation was seen in 10% of specimens and marked neointimal hyperplasia with stenosis in 15%. The inner capsule was greatly thickened within 2 weeks in the PGA group, but it remained relatively thin in the Dacron group. Both materials elicited a surrounding inflammatory reaction containing macrophages (Figs 16–10 and 16–11). This transgressed the interstices of only the PGA prostheses. Myofibroblasts proliferated in the inner capsule of PGA implants within 4 weeks of placement, producing a neointima more than three times as thick as that in the Dacron implants.

The myofibroblasts developed from ultrastructurally primitive cells. The final luminal surface in the PGA implants resembled endothelium, whereas that in the Dacron implants was fibrinous. All specimens withstood saline infusion at three to five times systolic pressure without neointimal disruption.

Great aterial regenerative potential was demonstrated in these studies. Myofibroblast activity is much more evident in PGA than in Dacron implants in the rabbit aorta. Lipid and calcium deposit in the inner capsule has been much more extensive in Dacron than in PGA implants.

Quantification of Deposition of Neutrophilic Granulocytes on Vascular Grafts in Dogs With ^{111}In-Labeled Granulocytes

Mrinal K. Dewanjee, Eduardo Solis, Scott T. Mackey, Steve Socher, Sushital Chowdhury, Fu Ping Wu, and Michael P. Kaye (Mayo Clinic)
Mayo Clin. Proc. 60:173–179, March 1985 16–7

Noninvasive semiquantitative and invasive quantitative techniques have been developed for estimating the deposition of neutrophilic granulocytes on Goretex and saphenous vein grafts in a canine model. Nine dogs underwent bilateral femoral artery resection and reconstruction with grafts of Goretex and femoral vein. Pure granulocytes separated from whole blood were labeled with ^{111}In-tropolone in plasma. The granulocyte harvesting efficiency was 25%, and the mean labeling efficiency was 87%. The grafts were harvested 3 hours after labeled granulocyte injection and 2 hours after reperfusion. Granulocyte adherence was estimated from radioactivity in the blood and in anastomotic and graft sections, the area of graft sections, and neutrophilic granulocyte and differential leukocyte counts.

The midsections of Goretex grafts retained more neutrophilic granulocytes than the midsections of vein grafts. In vein grafts the anastomotic regions retained more neutrophilic granulocytes than the midsections, but the reverse was the case for Goretex grafts. In the latter grafts, a major fraction of neutrophilic granulocytes was incorporated into thrombus. The deposition of neutrophilic granulocytes on vascular grafts was confirmed by semiquantitative data obtained by scintigraphy.

The use of ^{111}In-labeled granulocytes provides an approach to evaluating new cardiovascular prostheses and vascular grafts, just as ^{111}In-labeled platelets have been used to evaluate the effects of platelet inhibitors on vascular grafts.

▶ Graft behavior following implantation continues to be of interest to vascular surgeons. The wisdom of using woven, rather than knitted, grafts in younger patients should be kept in mind. Other factors in addition to graft patency, such as mechanical failure and degeneration of grafts, must be included in the attribution of graft failure.

Several investigators have engaged in the study of absorbable prostheses, in particular for transluminal implantation. The work by Greisler et al. is of importance to understand the healing process of this graft. It is too soon to conclude the validity of this approach. Aneurysmal formation is a real concern in absorbable prostheses.

The role of platelet-vessel wall interaction in the pathogenesis of intimal hyperplasia may be overplayed. Perhaps inflammatory reaction, especially white cells, plays an important role in endothelial cell coverage and anastomotic hyperplasia. The technique of ^{111}In-labeled granulocytes described by the Mayo group should shed some light on the pathogenesis of intimal hyperplasia.

Evaluation of Czechoslovakian Polyester Arterial Prostheses

Martin W. King, Robert Guidoin, Kingsley Gunasekera, Louisette Martin, Michel Marois, Pierre Blais, Jean-Michel Maarek, and Camille Gosselin

ASAIO 7:114–133, July–Sept. 1984 16–8

Polyester arterial prostheses have recently been developed in Czechoslovakia, and four different models of Czechoslovakian prostheses made of knitted polyester have now been analyzed in vitro and in a thoracoabdominal bypass model in dogs. Noncrimped, crimped, crimped and reinforced, and noncrimped and tapered designs were evaluated. The prostheses were compared with U.S. models of arterial prostheses. The Czechoslovakian models were implanted for up to 6 months.

The yarns of the Czechoslovakian models were thicker and heavier than those of U.S. prostheses. The generally high burst strengths of the Czechoslovakian models were equaled only by the De Bakey standard knitted prosthesis. An acceptable level of healing was generally found after implantation of the prostheses, with good encapsulation, fair dimensional stability, and adequate strength retention. The incidence of embolization was low; very few renal infarcts were found. The crimped models performed like standard weft-knit prostheses, but the noncrimped models lost tension distally after a month of implantation, leading to shrinkage and folding of the prosthetic wall. Higher rates of mural thrombi and distal embolization resulted.

The Czechoslovakian polyester arterial prostheses provide acceptable healing and adequate strength with a low rate of embolization. The crimped models merit further clinical evaluation, although western surgeons appear to prefer the more dimensionally stable warp-knit fabrics. Noncrimped models of the polyester prostheses have performed less satisfactorily.

▶ It is doubtful this article would influence the choice of prosthesis by U.S. surgeons. Nevertheless, it is good to know about the arterial prostheses manufactured by other countries.

17 Surgery of the Sympathetics

Radiofrequency Percutaneous Upper Thoracic Sympathectomy: Technique and Review of Indications
Harold A. Wilkinson (Univ. of Massachusetts, Worcester)
N. Engl. J. Med. 311:34–36, July 5, 1984 17–1

Fifteen upper thoracic sympathectomies, 4 bilateral, were carried out by percutaneous radiofrequency destruction of the appropriate sympathetic ganglia. Patient age range was 14 to 71 years. Follow-up averaged 22 months. The procedure was usually carried out in day surgery with local anesthesia. Generally six radiofrequency lesions were made on each side under fluoroscopic control with standard radiofrequency equipment. The tip temperature was first raised to 60 C for 1 minute to produce a reversible block, and the patient was tested for Horner's syndrome and for sympathetic denervation by finger plethysmography and skin temperature measurement. Lesions were produced with a tip temperature of 90 C for 3 minutes.

All but 1 of the 19 procedures produced good to excellent results. Three patients treated for palmar hyperhidrosis had excellent relief from abnormal sweating in 5 of 6 hands and partial relief in 1 hand. Nine of 10 patients treated for vascular occlusive disease or Raynaud's disease had good improvement in blood flow. Three of these patients had troublesome brachial hyperpathia and pain for 2 months. One patient had recurrent vascular symptoms 7 months after a partial sympathectomy and responded well to a repeat procedure. Both patients treated for causalgia had excellent results, but only 1 had satisfactory pain relief.

Percutaneous radiofrequency destruction of upper thoracic sympathetic ganglia can be done on an outpatient basis. It is effective, safe, and less costly than open operation. Good results have been obtained in patients with occlusive vascular disease, causalgia, and palmar hyperhidrosis.

▶ This technique, if proved to be effective by other investigators, offers an alternate method of sympathetic ablation. The attractiveness of the technique is that it is done without surgical exposure. It can be done on an outpatient basis.

Iatrogenic Causalgia: Classification, Clinical Findings, and Legal Ramifications
Steven H. Horowitz (New Hyde Park, N.J.)
Arch. Neurol. 41:821–824, August 1984 17–2

Since its original description by S. Weir Mitchell in American Civil War soldiers, the classification of major or true causalgia has been reserved, almost without exception, for cases resulting from wartime nerve injuries. Cases occurring in civilian life are relegated to the minor causalgia groups.

In this study of 11 patients, a prolonged excruciating pain having an intense burning quality resulted from an iatrogenically induced nerve injury. The pain initially occurred in the distribution of the affected nerve and later spread to contiguous cutaneous areas. The burning character of the pain, its focal nature, intensity, and endurance, and its occurrence immediately or shortly after an injury to a specific nerve, define the causalgia state.

The cases presented illustrate that a distinction between major and minor causalgias is not clinically realistic. Perhaps most convincing was the persistence of the burning pain for 1.5–7 years, far longer than in the vast majority of cases previously reported with major causalgia.

Unfortunately, causalgia is often either unknown or poorly understood by clinicians in civilian practice. The emphasis in the medical literature has been on cases occurring during wartime. Not one of the patients described herein was diagnosed as having causalgia at the time of injury. As early therapy is deemed crucial to any success in relieving causalgia, failure to appreciate promptly the significance of the burning pain may result in a long-standing pain syndrome with dire consequences.

Iatrogenic causalgia has been alluded to in the medical literature but not detailed. The frequency of its occurrence is unknown. Certain procedures must hold a greater risk for its development than others, but aside from excessive nerve traction, the risk factors are obscure. If it is determined that a definite risk of causalgia exists for a specific procedure, the patient should be apprised of that risk during preoperative informed-consent discussions. If no risk should exist for a procedure, such as intramuscular injections, then the production of causalgia constitutes malpractice. Eight of the patients in this study have sought legal redress for their symptoms. In 5 cases the legal issues of malpractice have been settled in favor of the plaintiffs; 3 are still pending.

▸ With increasing frequency of litigation, the readers need to know about causalgia, especially of iatrogenic origin. It is interesting to note that 2 of 11 patients developed causalgia following first rib resection for thoracic outlet syndrome. Missed diagnosis may be responsible for the recurrent problem following thoracic outlet decompression.

18 Dialysis and Vascular Access

Results From Use of 826 Vascular Access Devices in Cancer Patients
John H. Raaf (Cleveland Clinic Cancer Center
Cancer 55:1312–1321, Mar. 15, 1985 18–1

A review was made of experience with the use of 826 vascular access devices in 681 patients with neoplastic disease seen in the past 7 years. The devices included 103 polytetrafluoroethylene (PTFE) arteriovenous grafts, 358 Broviac 2.2-mm and 135 Hickman 3.2-mm right atrial catheters, 161 2.2-mm and 44 4.5-mm dual-lumen right atrial catheters, 12 venous infusion ports, and 13 large-bore, staggered-tip, dual-lumen catheters. The PTFE grafts were placed in the arm or leg for access to chemotherapy. Silastic right atrial catheters have been used in increasing numbers of patients with access problems because of the time needed to insert and revise PTFE grafts. The HemoCath is a large-bore right atrial catheter composed of Silastic. The Infuse-A-Port venous infusion port consists of a totally implanted plastic injection disk containing a chamber connected to a Silastic catheter.

All of the devices provided satisfactory venous access. However, 28% of the PTFE arteriovenous grafts eventually became occluded, as did only 0.7% of the Silastic right atrial catheters. Also, only 7% of the Silastic right atrial catheters were removed or lost because of complications. A tendency toward higher complication rates with use of the 4.5-mm dual-lumen catheter was observed. In some patients with a HemoCath, it proved difficult to draw adequate blood into the dialyzer. The venous infusion port seemed suitable for administering adjuvant chemotherapy to outpatients.

The Silastic right atrial catheter presently is preferred because of its simplicity of use and low long-term complication rate. The second channel of the 2.2-mm dual-lumen catheter can be used for parenteral nutrition or blood sampling, or to replace the first lumen should this become occluded. These devices can be used with relative safety even in immunosuppressed cancer patients. The catheter is left in place in most patients with chemotherapy-induced neutropenia and fever or bacteremia. Larger-bore dual-lumen catheters provide effective access for acute hemodialysis or plasmapheresis, as well as for routine venous access.

Prospective Study of End-to-Side vs. Side-to-Side Arteriovenous Fistulas for Hemodialysis
K. R. Wedgwood, P. A. Wiggins, and P. J. Guillou (St. James' Univ. Hosp., Leeds, England)
Br. J. Surg. 71:640–642, August 1984 18–2

Retrospective studies have yielded opposing results regarding the optimum configuration of arteriovenous (A-V) fistulas for hemodialysis. The authors conducted a randomized, prospective trial in 71 patients of the two most common types of A-V fistula, side to side (32 patients) and end of vein to side of artery (39), to define the optimum configuration for hemodialysis. Measurements include arterial diameter and flow, anastomotic length before anastomosis, and flow rates in the vessels proximal and distal to the anastomosis. Venous diameter was also measured.

Arterial diameter and arterial flow before anastomosis and anastomotic length were similar in both groups, as were arterial and venous flows after anastomosis. Retrograde flow was observed in the artery distal to the anastomosis in 25 end-to-side and 22 side-to-side fistulas. Caudal flow occurred in the vein distal to the anastomosis in 19 patients with side-to-side anastomoses. Nine months after operation, the patency rate in the end-to-side group (78.6%) was similar to that of the side-to-side group (79.2%). However, 7 of the 32 patients with side-to-side fistula developed hyperemia of the hand, and 3 required revision operations. No hyperemia was seen in the end-to-side group. Primary failure due to thrombosis occurred in 4 patients with end-to-side fistulas (10.3%), compared with 3 who had side-to-side fistulas (9.4%). Failed fistulas in the end-to-side group had significantly lower flow rates than successful fistulas, whereas in the side-to-side group flow rates in failed and successful fistulas were identical. Fistula flow rate showed a high degree of correlation ($r = 0.756$) and significance at 0.1% level with venous diameter; however, no significant difference was found between the two groups.

Seven of 19 patients with net caudal flow in the vein distal to the anastomosis developed hyperemia as a result of proximal venous thrombosis. Failed fistulas in the end-to-side group showed lower flow rates, suggesting that in the absence of proximal venous stenosis in end-to-side anastomosis, failure may be related to other variables like turbulence or coagulation factors. Peroperative measurements of fistula flow may have prognostic value in end-to-side but not side-to-side fistulas. Since there was no significant difference in venous diameter between the two groups, this cannot account for the incidence of venous hypertension in the side-to-side group.

End-to-side anastomosis is the configuration of choice for formation of A-V fistulas for hemodialysis.

Dialysis Access Fistulas: Treatment of Stenoses by Transluminal Angioplasty

Sidney Glanz, David Gordon, Khalid M. H. Butt, Joon Hong, Roland Adamson, and Salvatore J. A. Sclafani (Downstate Med. Center, Brooklyn, N.Y.)
Radiology 152:637–642, September 1984 18–3

Stenotic lesions are common in patients with internal and graft fistulas inserted for adequate access for dialysis. Experience with percutaneous transluminal angioplasty (PTA) for the treatment of stenosed dialysis access fistulas in upper extremities of 51 patients over 4 years is described. A total of 56 balloon dilatations were performed, including 44 for venous anastomotic lesions in patients with either internal or graft fistulas, 3 for arterial anastomotic lesions, and 9 for distant venous stenoses.

After the lesion was delineated by angiography, the stenosis was crossed with a straight wire or a 3-mm J-wire, and a 5-F catheter was introduced for a pressure pullback. An appropriate-sized catheter was then introduced. (There have been no problems with the use of 9- or 10-mm balloons). The patient was given 5,000 units of heparin prior to inflation of the balloon. Infiltration of lidocaine around the stenotic lesions alleviated the often painful dilatation. Postprocedure compression with Surgicel facilitated hemostasis. Most procedures were performed on an outpatient basis. Results were evaluated by postprocedure angiography, pressure pullback, and clinical response.

Thirty-nine of 56 dilatations (70%) were initially successful. Twenty-eight of 35 dilatations (80%) followed up for 3 months were clinically patent, 19 of 27 (70%) were patent at 6 months, 12 of 22 (55%) were patent at 1 year, 6 of 12 (50%) were patent at 2 years, and 3 of 9 (33%) were patent at 3 years. Venous anastomotic lesions showed an initial patency rate of 66% (29 of 44) and a 6-month patency rate of 61% (14 of 23); in cases of far proximal venous stenoses 80% (8 of 9) dilatations were initially successful and 80% (4 of 5) were still patent after 6 months.

Three complications (5%) were encountered: 1 case of thrombosed internal fistula, 1 of graft thrombosis and 1 of pseudoaneurysm at the dilatation site 1 year after the procedure. Two total occlusions were treated: 1 involved a short segment occlusion (less than 1 cm) at the venous anastomosis of the graft to the axillary vein which reoccluded 2 weeks later; the other involved a hypertrophied valve in the subclavian vein and remained patent 3 months after dilatation.

The study indicates that although long-term patency rates of PTA for fistulas are not high, balloon dilatation is a technically simple procedure that can be performed on an outpatient basis and repeated on recurrent lesions. However, selection of patients for angioplasty is important. No successful dilatations of lesions longer than 4 cm have been reported by these authors. Venous anastomotic lesions may be quite resistant to dilatation because of dense perivenous and endovenous fibrosis; however, polyethylene rather than polyvinyl chloride balloons have been used to generate the higher pressures needed to dilate fibrotic lesions. In addition, several resistant venous stenoses have been dilated by leaving the balloon inflated up to 5 minutes. The use of heparin prior to balloon inflation is useful with long balloon inflation times because it decreases the likelihood of graft thrombosis.

▶ Vascular access surgery is now an integral part of vascular surgical practice. These three articles provide some new thoughts on this technically demanding procedure. The ability of the percutaneous transluminal balloon catheter to dilate stenotic lesions is a welcome adjunct, especially in patients who have had multiple fistula reconstructions. Vascular access is now done with increasing frequency for cancer patients. The Sloan-Kettering experience should prove to be informative to those who are interested in these new vascular access devices.

19 Lymphedema

Lymphatic Hypoplasia Without Lymphedema

James McIvor and Girish Tyagi (London)
Clin. Radiol. 35:503–505, November 1984 19–1

The occurrence of lymphatic hypoplasia was determined in a prospective study of lymph vessel abnormalities in the lower limbs of 744 adult patients without lymphedema, begun in 1976 when lower extremity films were included in all pedal lymphographic studies. Hypoplastic lymph vessels (Fig 19–1) were found in the thighs of 2 patients with clinically normal limbs in the first year of the study, and in 5 others over the next 6 years. The prevalence rate was 0.94%: 1.1% for men, and 0.5% for women. Hypoplasia of lymph vessels was limited to the left lower limb in all instances.

This relatively high prevalence of lymphatic hypoplasia not associated

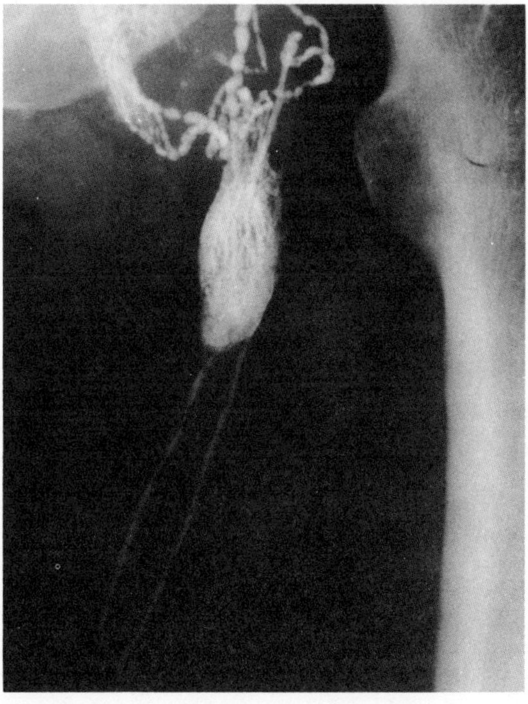

Fig 19–1.—Single lymphatic vessel in left thigh of patient, aged 76 years, with carcinoma of the prostate. The patient died 4 years later with no evidence of lymphedema. (Courtesy of McIvor, J., and Tyagi, G.: Clin. Radiol. 35:503–505, November 1984.)

with lymphedema suggests that lymphatic hypoplasia is only one factor in the development of clinical lymphedema. Other unidentified factors must contribute to the development of clinical lymphedema in subjects with lymphatic hypoplasia.

▶ This extensive prospective study of lymphedema by lymphangiography reveals two interesting findings. First, that hypoplastic lymphatics can occur without edema, and second, males predominate in lymphatic hypoplasia. The latter is in contrast to the usual finding of frequency of lymphedema in females. Indeed, there may actually be unidentified factors that cause lymphedema.

Role of CT in Diagnosis of Primary Lymphedema of the Lower Limb

N. S. Hadjis, D. H. Carr, Linda Banks, and J. J. Pflug (Royal Postgrad. Med. School, London)

AJR 144:361–364, February 1985 19–2

Secondary lymphedema after damage to and obstruction of the lymphatic pathways is a well-known cause of chronic leg swelling. Primary lymphedema also occurs; lymphangiography is time consuming and may produce complications such as cellulitis. Exacerbation of edema is also possible. The value of computed tomography (CT) was examined in 12

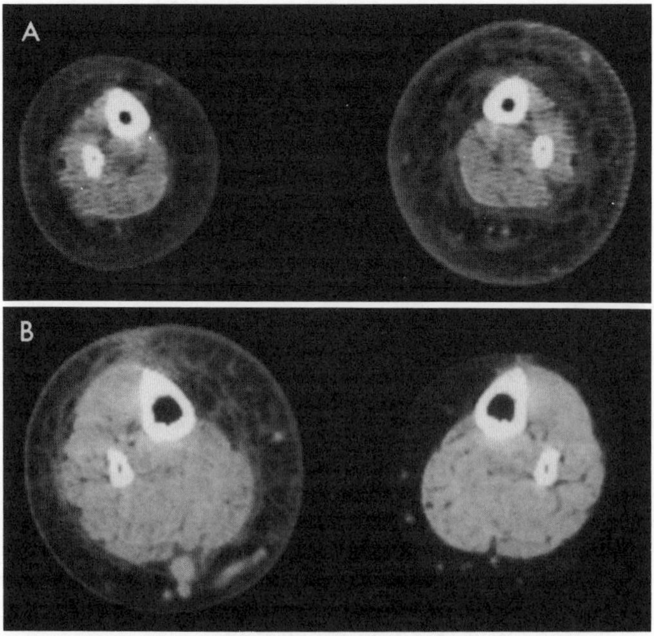

Fig 19–2.—Two patients with bilateral lymphedema. Characteristic honeycomb appearance of subcutaneous compartment; bilateral (**A**) and unilateral (**B**) distribution. Normal organization of subfascial compartment. (Courtesy of Hadjis, N.S., et al.: AJR 144:361–364, February 1985.)

patients (10 women) with primary lymphedema of the lower extremity, who had had symptoms for an average of 45 months. Ten patients were younger than age 35 years at onset of lymphedema. All patients were operated on after conservative measures had been tried. Computed tomography was also performed on 9 patients with swollen legs, 6 of whom had chronic venous disease and 3, bilateral lipedema.

Operation revealed thick, fibrous subcutaneous tissue or lakes of encapsulated fluid in all patients with lymphedema. Computed tomography showed an increase in thickness of the subcutaneous tissue compartment and, in all patients but 1, skin thickening. A honeycomb appearance of the subcutaneous tissue (Fig 19–2) was seen in 10 patients, apparently representing fat pockets surrounded by fluid, fibrous tissue, or both. These features did not enhance after intravenous contrast administration in 2 cases. The honeycomb appearance was not seen in patients with chronic venous disease. No specific CT pattern was apparent in the cases of lipedema. The CT attenuation numbers for the subcutaneous compartment were similar to those in patients with lymphedema.

Computed tomography may be helpful in the differential diagnosis of leg swelling and may preclude the need for venography or lymphangiography. A honeycomb appearance of the subcutaneous tissue was seen in primary lymphedema, but not in chronic venous disease or lipedema. The pattern was evident in most but not all cases of lymphedema.

▶ Lymphangiography is a difficult diagnostic procedure and is not readily available in many hospitals. In contrast, the CT scan is now a common testing procedure in many hospitals. The ability to detect lymphedema by CT should be of value in the workup of "swollen leg."

Subject Index

A

B

F

G

H

N

O

P

R

S

U

V

Index to Authors